The Clinical Orthopedic Assessment Guide

SECOND EDITION

Janice Loudon, PhD, PT, SCS, ATC
University of Kansas Medical Center

Marcie Swift, PT, PhD, FAAOMPT
University of Kansas Medical Center

Stephania Bell, MS, PT, OCS, CSCS
Injury Analyst/Senior Writer, ESPN

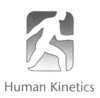

Human Kinetics

Library of Congress Cataloging-in-Publication Data

Loudon, Janice K. (Janice Kaye), 1959–
　The clinical orthopedic assessment guide / Janice Loudon, Marcie Swift, Stephania Bell. -- 2nd ed.
　　p. ; cm.
　Includes bibliographical references and index.
　ISBN-13: 978-0-7360-6709-6 (soft cover)
　ISBN-10: 0-7360-6709-4 (soft cover)
　1. Orthopedics--Diagnosis--Handbooks, manuals, etc. I. Swift, Marcie, 1973- II. Bell, Stephania, 1966- III. Title.
　[DNLM: 1. Musculoskeletal Diseases--diagnosis--Handbooks. 2. Joints--physiology--Handbooks. 3. Joints--physiopathology--Handbooks. 4. Orthopedics--Handbooks. 5. Physical Examination--Handbooks. WE 39 L886c 2008]
　RD734.L68 2008
　616.7'075--dc22

　　　　　　　　　　2007049478

ISBN-10: 0-7360-6709-4
ISBN-13: 978-0-7360-6709-6

Acquisitions Editor: Loarn D. Robertson, PhD; **Developmental Editor:** Maureen Eckstein; **Assistant Editors:** Christine Bryant Cohen and Anne Rumery; **Copyeditor:** Bob Replinger; **Proofreader:** Joanna Hatzopoulos Portman; **Indexer:** Betty Frizzell; **Permission Manager:** Dalene Reeder; **Graphic Designer:** Nancy Rasmus; **Graphic Artists:** Patrick Sandberg, Denise Lowery, and Yvonne Griffith; **Cover Designer:** Keith Blomberg; **Photographer (cover):** Neil Bernstein; **Photographer (interior):** Neil Bernstein; **Visual Production Assistant:** Jason Allen; **Art Manager:** Kelly Hendren; **Associate Art Manager:** Alan J. Wilborn; **Illustrator:** Tim Brummett; **Printer:** Versa Press

We thank the University of Kansas Medical Center in Kansas City, Kansas, for assistance in providing the location for the photo shoot for this book.

Printed in the United States of America　　　　10　9　8　7　6　5　4　3　2　1

Human Kinetics
Web site: www.HumanKinetics.com

United States: Human Kinetics
P.O. Box 5076
Champaign, IL 61825-5076
800-747-4457
e-mail: humank@hkusa.com

Canada: Human Kinetics
475 Devonshire Road Unit 100
Windsor, ON N8Y 2L5
800-465-7301 (in Canada only)
e-mail: info@hkcanada.com

Europe: Human Kinetics
107 Bradford Road, Stanningley
Leeds LS28 6AT, United Kingdom
+44 (0) 113 255 5665
e-mail: hk@hkeurope.com

Australia: Human Kinetics
57A Price Avenue
Lower Mitcham, South Australia 5062
08 8372 0999
e-mail: info@hkaustralia.com

New Zealand: Human Kinetics
Division of Sports Distributors NZ Ltd.
P.O. Box 300 226 Albany
North Shore City
Auckland
0064 9 448 1207
e-mail: info@humankinetics.co.nz

CONTENTS

This is the second edition to the text *The Clinical Orthopedic Assessment Guide*. This edition has the same goal as the first—to provide the orthopedic therapist with a handy and inexpensive reference to assist with patient assessment. The improved layout and the addition of photographs promote easier understanding of information. Each major chapter follows a common format and focuses on one anatomical section.

The new edition is divided into six parts and contains two new chapters—one dealing with the pelvis and the other with neurodynamics. Clinical syndromes are updated. Additionally, a suggested examination sequence for the history and tests and measures is provided for each peripheral and spinal joint. Many of the special tests included in each chapter are accompanied with the sensitivity and specificity values reported in the literature.

The new edition is now even more user friendly than before. The reader will appreciate the following:

- A compact size that makes it easier to transport.
- A special binding allows clinicians to lay the book open on a flat surface without damaging the text's spine.
- Significantly more photos, many of which are enhanced with arrows showing direction of movement or highlighting specific elements.
- Five special symbols have been added to the top of test and measurement pages so information can be located with a quick flip through the pages. Refer to the figure below for an example of each symbol:

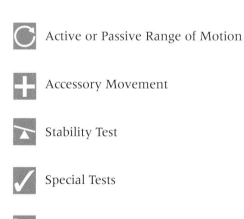

Active or Passive Range of Motion

Accessory Movement

Stability Test

Special Tests

Degrees of Freedom

This improved design will provide clear guidance in executing multiple assessments and empower you in your own practice. Our hope is that this second edition of *The Clinical Orthopedic Assessment Guide* becomes a very useful reference in your own medical library.

Introduction to Biomechanical Principles

The aim of part I is to familiarize the reader with terminology and the examination sequence used throughout the text. Chapter 1 provides operational definitions for basic principles related to joint function. These basic principles include osteokinematics, arthrokinematics, end feel, capsular patterns, and close- and loose-packed positions. Chapter 2 focuses on the subjective examination based on the teachings of Geoffrey Maitland. Topics discussed include patient profile, symptom description, behavior of symptoms, special questions, history, and previous history.

Classifications and Definitions

The basis for good orthopedic treatment is good orthopedic assessment. This chapter provides a review of terminology and serves as a layout for chapters 3 to 10 and 12 to 14. To develop an appropriate treatment plan, an orthopedic clinician must have a solid working knowledge of joint biomechanics. This chapter defines the bases of biomechanics including articulation, types of joints, degrees of freedom, active range of motion, passive accessory movement, end feel, capsular pattern, close- and loose-packed positions, stability, special tests, and arthrokinematics. Further detailed information on arthrokinematics can be found in the bibliography. Finally, this chapter includes a review of terminology related to neurology, surface palpation, muscle origin and insertion, muscle action and innervation, and clinical syndromes.

Joint Basics

Articulation   The segment on articulation in each chapter of this book is used to describe joint shape and define the actual contact area between the bones that make up the joint articulation.

Types of Joints   The literature offers many forms of joint classification. This text uses the joint classification presented in *Cunningham's Textbook of Anatomy*. The three classifications of joints are fibrous joints, cartilaginous joints, and synovial joints. The following section describes 12 types of joints within these three broad classes, beginning with the least mobile joints and progressing to the joints with the most motion.

Fibrous Joint (Synarthrosis)

Suture   A fibrous joint, found only in the skull, with minimal or no movement (figure 1.1).

Syndesmosis   Two bones connected by fibrous tissue that allows minimal movement; much denser than a suture. Example: membranous connection (interosseous) between the tibia and fibula (figure 1.2).

Gomphosis   Fibrous joint analogous to a peg fitting into a socket, resulting in minimal movement. Example: tooth in socket.

Cartilaginous Joint (Amphiarthrosis)

Synchondrosis   Cartilaginous connection between two bones that eventually ossifies with maturity; virtually immobile. Example: epiphyseal plate (figure 1.3).

Symphysis   Joint consisting of two bones connected by hyaline cartilage and fibrocartilage; slightly movable. Example: pubic symphysis (figure 1.4).

Synovial Joint (Diarthrosis)

Plane   Gliding joint with opposing surfaces relatively flat. Example: superior tibiofibular joint (figure 1.5).

Sellar (saddle)   Two bones each with reciprocal concavoconvex articular surfaces that fit together like a puzzle; biaxial; produces flexion and extension, abduction and adduction. Example: carpometacarpal of thumb (figure 1.6).

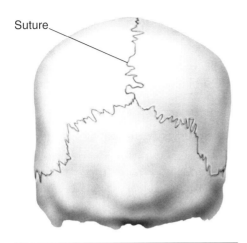

Suture

Figure 1.1 A suture in the skull.

Reprinted from R. Behnke, *Kinetic Anatomy*, 2nd ed. (Champaign, IL: Human Kinetics), 12.

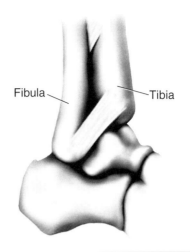

Fibula — Tibia

Figure 1.2 Syndesmosis between the tibia and fibula.

Reprinted from R. Behnke, *Kinetic Anatomy*, 2nd ed. (Champaign, IL: Human Kinetics), 12.

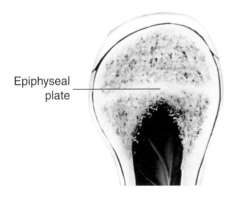

Epiphyseal plate

Figure 1.3 Synchondrosis of the epiphyseal plate.

Reprinted from R. Behnke, *Kinetic Anatomy*, 2nd ed. (Champaign, IL: Human Kinetics), 5.

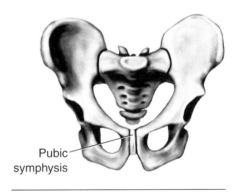

Pubic symphysis

Figure 1.4 Pubic symphysis.

Reprinted from R. Behnke, *Kinetic Anatomy*, 2nd ed. (Champaign, IL: Human Kinetics), 137.

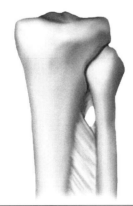

Figure 1.5 Plane joint: superior tibiofibular joint.

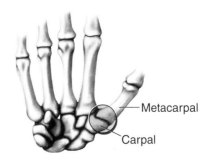

Metacarpal

Carpal

Figure 1.6 Sellar joint of the carpo-metacarpal of the thumb.

Reprinted from R. Behnke, *Kinetic Anatomy*, 2nd ed. (Champaign, IL: Human Kinetics), 10.

Ginglymus (hinge) Two bones that articulate and permit motion in only one plane; uniaxial; flexion and extension. Example: ulnohumeral joint (figure 1.7).

Trochoid (pivot) One articulating surface, cylindrical in shape, that rotates within a ring formed by bone or ligament; allows supination, pronation, and rotation. Example: atlantoaxial joint (figure 1.8).

Spheroid An articulation in which one bone is convex (ball shaped) and rotates about a concave surface (socket) of a second bone; triaxial; all joint movements. Example: glenohumeral joint (figure 1.9).

Condyloid Ball-and-socket type, but ligamentous constraints prevent rotation about a vertical axis. Example: metacarpophalangeal joints of digits 2 through 5 (figure 1.10).

Ellipsoid Modified ball and socket in which one articulating surface is ellipsoidal instead of spheroidal; biaxial; flexion and extension, abduction and adduction. Example: radiocarpal joint (figure 1.11).

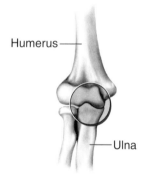

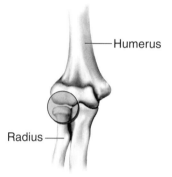

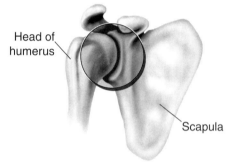

Figure 1.7 Ginglymus joint: ulnohumeral joint.

Reprinted from R. Behnke, *Kinetic Anatomy*, 2nd ed. (Champaign, IL: Human Kinetics), 10.

Figure 1.8 Trochoid joint: atlantoaxial joint.

Reprinted from R. Behnke, *Kinetic Anatomy*, 2nd ed. (Champaign, IL: Human Kinetics), 10.

Figure 1.9 Spheroid joint: glenohumeral joint.

Reprinted from R. Behnke, *Kinetic Anatomy*, 2nd ed. (Champaign, IL: Human Kinetics), 10.

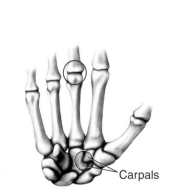

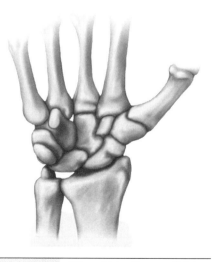

Figure 1.10 Condyloid (MCP) joint.

Figure 1.11 Ellipsoid (radiocarpal) joint.

Degrees of Freedom

Degrees of freedom refer to the number of movements that occur at a specific joint. For example, the knee has six degrees of freedom: rotational and linear motion occurring in three planes (coronal, sagittal, and transverse). An axis of motion of a joint is the axis about which it rotates.

Rotation

Flexion and extension   Occurs in a sagittal plane about a coronal axis (figure 1.12*a*).

Internal and external rotation   Occurs in a transverse plane about a longitudinal axis (figure 1.12*b*).

Adduction and abduction   Occurs in a coronal plane about a sagittal axis (figure 1.12*c*).

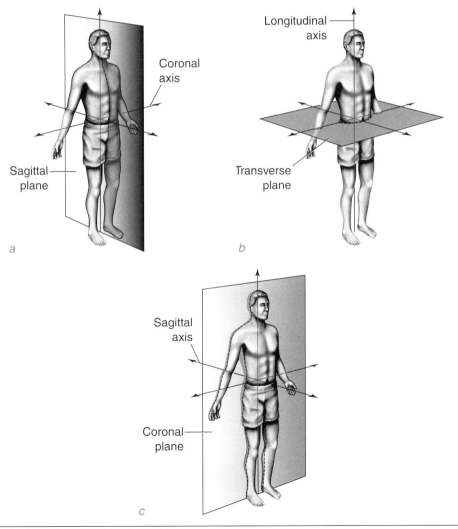

Figure 1.12   Rotation movement patterns.

Reprinted from R. Behnke, *Kinetic Anatomy*, 2nd ed. (Champaign, IL: Human Kinetics), 27.

Concave–Convex Rule (Kaltenborn)

When a concave surface moves on a convex surface, roll and slide occur in the same direction. For example, in non-weight-bearing knee extension, the tibia rolls and slides anteriorly on the fixed femur. When a convex surface moves on a concave surface, roll and slide are in the opposite direction. For example, in weight-bearing knee extension, the femur rolls anteriorly and slides posteriorly on a fixed tibia. This is the primary principle by which joint mobilization treatment is determined (figures 1.11 and 1.12). Clinicians primarily will use the glide component during mobilization as shown in figure 1.12.

Translation

Anterior and posterior   Occurs about a sagittal axis; linear movement volar and dorsal.

Lateral and medial   Occurs about a coronal axis; linear movement side to side.

Superior and inferior   Occurs about a longitudinal axis; linear movement cranial and caudal.

For purposes of this text, the degrees of freedom are described for rotational motion only. Translation is described as a glide and is included in the material on accessory movement.

Active Range of Motion

Active range of motion is the normal amount of motion that occurs in a joint in one of the three cardinal planes. Active range of motion is measured in degrees and depends on the type of joint.

Passive Accessory Movement

Accessory movement is the movement that occurs between the articulating surfaces. Accessory movement needs to take place to maintain minimal torquing or shearing between joint surfaces. For example, the accessory movement that accompanies shoulder abduction is humeral spin on the glenoid and humeral inferior glide.

Roll   One portion of the joint surface rolls on another.

- Surfaces are incongruent.

- New points on one surface contact new points at similar intervals on opposing surface.

- Rolling is always in the same direction as angular movement. Example: The distal femur rolls posteriorly during knee flexion.

Treatment Direction

The direction of treatment for accessory motion is generally dictated by the concave–convex rule (figure 1.13). The operator moves the convex bone in the opposite direction as the restriction. The concave bone glides in the same direction as the restriction. For a tibiofemoral joint that lacks full extension, the clinician would apply an anterior glide to the tibia (figure 1.14).

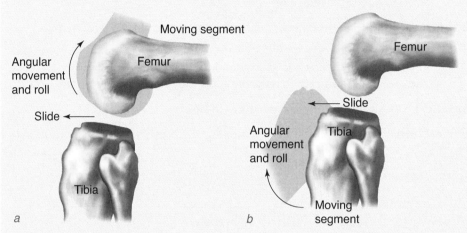

Figure 1.13 Joint mobilization: (*a*) movement of the femur on the tibia and (*b*) movement of the tibia on the femur.

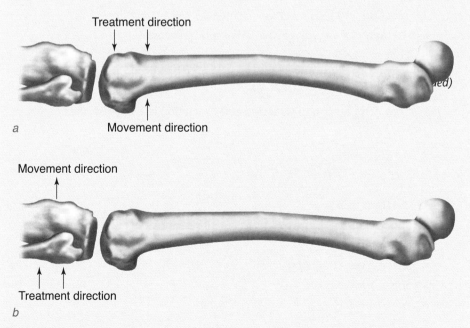

Figure 1.14 Gliding movement of bone depends on concave–convex surface.

Slide   One bone slides across another.

- Surfaces are congruent.
- Same point on moving joint surface contacts various points on opposing surface.
- Sliding occurs in the opposite direction of angular movement if the moving joint surface is convex, and sliding occurs in the same direction as angular movement if the moving surface is concave (most joint surfaces move with a combination of roll and slide). Example: The proximal tibia slides anteriorly during knee extension.

Spin   One bone rotates perpendicularly to joint plane of stationary bone.

- Rotation occurs about a stationary mechanical axis.
- Rotation usually occurs in conjunction with rolling and sliding. Example: The proximal radius spins posteriorly on the radial notch with pronation.

Traction   Separation of two articulating surfaces.

Distraction   Separation of two articulating surfaces perpendicular to axis of motion.

Compression   Approximation of two articulating surfaces.

Contraindications to Joint Mobilization

1. Hypermobility and instability
2. Joint effusion
3. Infection and inflammation (acute)
4. Rheumatoid arthritis (active inflammatory stage)
5. Cancer (active metastasis)
6. Disturbed bowel or bladder function and perineal anesthesia: indicative of cauda equina compression
7. Cord compression: pins-and-needles sensation in bilateral hands or feet

Precautions to Joint Mobilization

1. Osteoporosis
2. Spondylolisthesis
3. Pregnancy
4. Positive vertebral artery test
5. Spinal fractures
6. Spinal surgery
7. Spinal stenosis
8. Neurological changes: pain associated with disturbances of reflexes, muscle power, or sensation

End Feel: Physiological Limit of a Joint

Normal

Soft   Give of end point due to soft-tissue approximation. Example: elbow flexion.

Firm (capsular)   Hard or firm type of movement with some give. Example: external rotation of shoulder.

Hard (bony)   Hard unyielding sensation. Example: elbow extension.

Abnormal

Spasm   Sudden dramatic arrest of movement accompanied by pain. Example: inflamed joint.

Springy   Similar to firm end feel but in range where one would not expect to find end feel. Example: torn meniscus of knee.

Empty   The end feel in which the patient is in considerable pain with movement and will not allow the clinician to continue passive range. No mechanical resistance is encountered. Examples: subacute bursitis, neoplasm.

Firm (capsular)   A firm end feel in which the end feel is normally soft or hard. Example: synovitis or soft-tissue edema.

Hard   Abrupt halt in range at an abnormal range. Examples: fracture, arthropathy.

Pain-Resistance Sequence (Cyriax)

1. Pain before resistance indicates an acute lesion. During performance of passive range of motion, pain occurs before the clinician meets resistance.
2. Pain with resistance indicates a subacute lesion. Pain occurs at the same time as resistance.
3. Pain after resistance indicates chronic lesion. The clinician notes resistance before the patient notes pain.

Capsular Pattern

The capsule, constructed of fibrous connective tissue, helps maintain the integrity of synovial joints. A capsular pattern is a proportional limitation of movement in a joint that usually indicates injury or inflammation of the capsule. Tightness is noted within the joint capsule and ligaments. Each synovial joint has a characteristic capsular pattern. A noncapsular pattern, on the other hand, is a limitation in a joint that is not characteristic of the capsular pattern. Possible causes include internal derangement and bursitis.

Close-Packed Position

Close-packed position usually refers to the extreme end of range of motion. The joint surfaces are maximally congruent, the ligaments and capsules are taut, and the joint possesses its greatest stability.

Loose-Packed Position

In this text, loose packed denotes maximal loose-packed position. In loose-packed position the articular surfaces are relatively free to move in relation to one another.

In this position the largest amount of joint play occurs. Ligaments and capsules are lax and dynamically safe.

Stability

Each joint has soft-tissue structures that help maintain the stability of that joint. These structures include the capsule, ligaments, and menisci. The subsection on stability defines the major stabilizing structures of each joint.

Special Tests

The subsection on special tests presents common special tests for each joint. Special tests are performed to diagnose tissues that may be pathological or injured.

Arthrokinematics

The subsection on arthrokinematics summarizes the accessory and conjunct motion that accompanies each plane of motion for that joint. This information can help the clinician decide what mobilization technique is indicated to improve joint mobility.

Neurology

The neurology subsections present dermatomal, myotomal, and peripheral nerve information for each joint.

Surface Palpation

The subsection on surface palpation is designed to give the clinician a quick guide to common palpatory areas for each joint.

Muscle Origin and Insertion

The subsection on muscle origin and insertion lists the origin point and insertion point for muscles surrounding each joint.

Muscle Action and Innervation

The subsection on muscle action and innervation lists muscle action about each joint and the nerve innervation for each muscle.

Clinical Syndromes

Tables at the end of chapters 3 to 10 and 12 to 14 identify common musculoskeletal syndromes. These tables are intended to help the clinician differentiate the tissue at fault. The tables include names and descriptions of disorders, location and behavior of symptoms, history, objective exam and diagnostics, and intervention. Also included in the joint chapters is a recommended sequence for the subjective and objective exam. The subjective exam sequence lists special questions and common aggravating and easing symptoms. The objective exam is organized by test position.

CHAPTER 2

Examination Sequence for History and Tests and Measures

Although most of this text is directed at specific tests and measures, a detailed history performed at the outset of evaluation is a critical part of treatment. Geoffrey Maitland, an Australian physical therapist who has contributed volumes to the world of orthopedic physical therapy, highlighted the importance of thorough interrogation of the patient at the outset of treatment (Maitland 1991). A complete history should help the practitioner formulate a hypothesis regarding a patient's problem that can then be proved or altered accordingly as objective testing and treatment proceed.

The information obtained during the history should guide the clinician's selection of tests and measures and interventions, as well as the vigor with which they are carried out. The history enables the clinician to make an accurate assessment of the patient's problem. Additionally, a detailed history offers the clinician an opportunity to establish solid rapport with the patient. The patient learns that his or her information is valuable to the clinician, who in turn generally encourages the patient to participate in resolving the problem.

Maitland emphasized good communication between clinician and patient when obtaining information. Therefore, you, as the clinician, should know not only which questions to ask but also why you are asking those questions. In other words, predetermine what is to be gained by proceeding with a certain line of questioning. This forethought allows you to determine whether the patient is providing the appropriate information and, if not, the strategies that you can use to obtain the necessary information. For instance, if you ask the patient where her symptoms are located and she responds, "In my leg," you have not obtained information that will be particularly helpful in identifying the structure likely to be at fault. You can, however, follow up by asking for clarification: "Could you outline with your hands exactly where in your leg the symptoms are?" The patient, in outlining the specific area of symptoms, may then point you to a specific dermatome versus a peripheral nerve pattern. This information offers a small but important step in assisting you in differential diagnosis, and consequently, appropriate treatment.

The following guidelines summarize the types of questions that Maitland recommended be asked of all patients (Maitland 1986). Each chapter offers additional specific questions to ask patients that will guide clinical decision making about the appropriate tests and measures to perform for the various peripheral and spinal joint clinical syndromes.

Patient Profile

The patient profile refers to the patient's personal information such as age, occupation, current daily activity level (as compared with normal, if different), recreation or hobbies, and psychosocial factors such as dependents, litigation, or worker's compensation. Noting the specifics of occupation and activities gives the therapist an appreciation for what positions or movements the person must undergo on a daily basis. For instance, if a patient states that his occupation is office worker, the clinician knows only part of the story. Does he sit at a computer, talk on the phone, read, write? If the job entails multiple activities, how long does he engage in each one? Office work might mean different things to different people, and the details of what the term really means may affect the clinician's choice of treatment and development of appropriate goals.

Symptom Description—Location and Type

The second step is to identify the precise location of symptoms. Ask the patient to outline with his or her hands (with one finger if possible) exactly where the symptoms manifest themselves. Follow by retracing the symptom outline on the patient's body to verify the location. Then ask the patient to describe in his or her own words how the symptoms feel. Continue to use the patient's words when referring to the symptoms. This approach not only encourages you to think in more accurate terms but also conveys to the patient that you were listening to his or her original description. If the patient does not volunteer any of the following information when describing his or her symptoms, then be sure to determine whether the symptoms are deep or superficial, constant or intermittent, sharp or dull, variable or nonvariable, and whether numbness or tingling is present. All these factors can provide insight into the nature of the patient's condition and the structure or structures that are at fault. Precise description of symptom location and type often provides an early clue for the clinician about the structure or structures responsible for the patient's complaints. As a final step, be sure to verify that the patient has no complaints in the joints above or below the symptom areas all along the kinetic chain. For any upper-extremity complaint, check the wrist and hand, the elbow, the shoulder, and the neck. For any lower-extremity complaint, be sure to clear the foot and ankle, the knee, the hip, and the lumbar spine.

Behavior of Symptoms

Now establish how the symptoms behave. If more than one area of symptoms is present, is there a relationship between the areas? For instance, if a patient complains of back pain and leg pain, does she describe a scenario in which the back pain worsens and then the leg pain worsens, or do the two behave independently of one another? Also, to help you assess the severity and irritability of the patient's condition, determine what activities, movements, or positions aggravate the patient's symptoms. Ask the patient what frequency or what duration of an aggravating activity is required to reproduce symptoms, to what extent they are reproduced, and then how long after cessation of the aggravating activity the symptoms disappear. Additionally, determine factors that ease the symptoms such as movements, positions, medications, and so on. Determine the behavior of the patient's symptoms over a 24-hour period. Do the patient's symptoms wake her from sleep? If so, how long until she is able to return to sleep? Symptoms that wake a patient from sleep suggest a more severe condition. How are the symptoms first thing in the morning? How do the symptoms behave throughout the day? Again, answers to these questions may provide clues about the nature and severity of the patient's problem.

Special Questions

Besides interviewing the patient regarding his or her specific complaint, ask several questions to help rule out any contraindications to treatment or identifying factors that warrant caution in physical evaluation and treatment of the patient. We recommend asking the following questions of all patients presenting with any complaint of lumbar pain or extremity pain of unknown etiology.

1. How is your general health? (The answer to this question informs you of other ongoing medical processes and provides insight about the patient's impression of his or her own health.)
2. Have you experienced any recent unexplained weight loss or weight gain? (This may point to possible systemic disease or tumor.)
3. Are you taking any medications currently? (Again, the patient's response gives information about general health and potential exercise precautions.)

4. Do you have any history of long-term steroid or anticoagulant use? (Either of these situations might present a precaution to joint mobilization because of increased risk of tissue damage or bleeding.)

5. Have you had any special tests such as X ray, CT, or MRI for this problem? If yes, are you aware of the results? (This may provide you with information if the results are not present in the patient's chart. Alternatively, the results may be available, but the patient may be unaware of what they are.)

6. Have you had any trouble initiating urination or controlling bowels? Are you experiencing any numbness in the saddle area? (A positive response may be suggestive of possible cauda equina compression.)

7. Does coughing or sneezing affect your symptoms? (Increased intra-abdominal pressure typically aggravates disc symptoms.)

8. Have you experienced any numbness or tingling in both hands or both feet at the same time? Have you experienced any loss of coordination with gait? (This circumstance may suggest possible cord compression.)

History of the Current Episode

You must carefully interrogate the patient regarding the history of the current problem. A thorough history may provide you with many clues about the nature of the problem as well as its progression. This information will help you be more efficient when determining a treatment plan and setting goals. Ask the patient when and how this episode began (did it come on suddenly or was it gradual?). Also ask the patient to identify which symptoms appeared first and then how they progressed. Note any treatment to date for this episode as well as its effects. Finally, ask the patient to assess the evolution of the problem; in other words, ask whether it is getting better, getting worse, or staying the same.

Previous History

Note as well whether the patient has experienced any prior episodes of this nature and how they compare, in terms of both intensity and duration, to the current event. Determine whether the location of the symptoms has varied across episodes. Ask whether there has been previous treatment for this problem, what it was, and what the effects were, if any. Did the patient improve after the last episode and to what extent (100%, 50%, and so forth)? If the patient reports less than 100% improvement, ask him or her to explain further so that you can better determine the prognosis for this occurrence. Identify any other significant medical history, including surgeries or hospitalizations, at this time.

Head and Spine

Part II contains five chapters related to the head and spine. The temporomandibular joint, cervical spine, thoracic spine, lumbar spine, and pelvis each has its own chapter. The focus of part II is to provide detailed information to the clinician about the spine along with an objective sequence. Each chapter begins with a description of the basics of each joint including joint articulation, type of joint, degrees of freedom and active range of motion, passive accessory movement, capsular pattern, close-packed and loose-packed positions, and arthrokinematics. The remainder of each chapter describes stability of the joint, special tests, neurological assessment, surface palpation, muscle origins and insertions, and actions and innervations. Finally, a clinical syndrome table is included that serves to help the clinician with musculoskeletal differential diagnoses.

Temporomandibular Joint

This chapter addresses the temporomandibular joint, or TMJ. This complex joint is closely related to the upper cervical spine. Therefore, when examining a patient with this type of dysfunction, the clinician must rule out the cervical spine as a source of the patient's symptoms or as an associated factor. This chapter covers osteology, arthrokinematics, range of motion, muscle origin and insertion, muscle action, neurology, and special tests for the TMJ. Clinical syndromes are presented in a table at the end of the chapter.

Joint Basics

Articulation   The temporal bone along the surfaces of the articular eminence, glenoid fossa, and posterior glenoid spine articulate with the disc, which in turn articulates with the mandibular condyle (figure 3.1).

Type of Joint   The condyle of the mandible and inferior surface of the disc form a ginglymus joint; the superior surface of the disc and the articular eminence constitute a cartilaginous joint.

Degrees of Freedom

The axis of rotation through the lower joint is generally a line passing through both poles of the condyle (remember that anatomical variances may occur, even from one side to another in the same individual, that may affect this axis). Translation and gliding occur along the inferior surface of the temporal bone and the superior surface of the articulating disc.

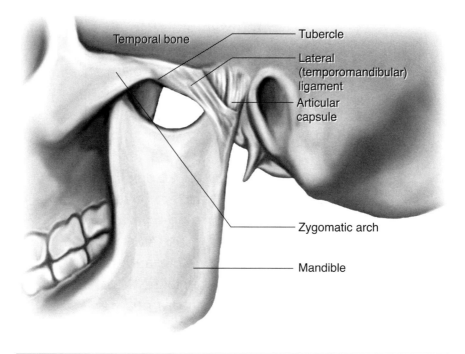

Figure 3.1   Temporomandibular joint.

Active Range of Motion

Mouth opening (mandibular depression): 40–55 mm (two or three flexed proximal interphalangeal joints). To calculate mouth opening correctly, add degree of overbite, or vertical overlap of maxillary teeth to mandibular teeth (measure in millimeters).

Mouth closing (mandibular elevation): Complete approximation of teeth.

Lateral deviation: approximately one-fourth opening range (generally 8–10 mm); symmetrical.

Protrusion (mandible moves anteriorly): 3–6 mm. To calculate protrusion correctly, add degree of overjet, or anterior-posterior distance between overlapping maxillary and mandibular teeth (measure in millimeters).

Retrusion (mandible moves posteriorly): 3 mm.

During active range of motion (AROM) assessment, look for any deviation as well as limitation in range:

1. A C-curve during opening may indicate joint hypomobility on the side of deviation.
2. An S-curve during opening may suggest a muscle imbalance or capsulitis.

Distraction (Unilateral)

Assessment: To assess or increase joint mobility.

Patient position: Sitting or supine with the jaw relaxed.

Clinician position: Place gloved thumb (opposite side being worked on) on the patient's back molars with the fingers outside the mouth and encircled about the jaw. Also support the patient's head with the other hand if the patient is sitting.

Method: Caudal direction; may be used for pain, mobility, disc reduction (if the patient tolerates).

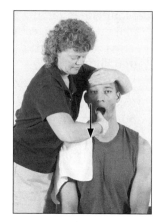

Distraction With Anterior Glide (Unilateral)

Assessment: To assess or increase joint mobility.

Patient position: As previous.

Clinician position: As previous.

Method: As previous, but after distracting, add anterior translation force; may be used for similar purposes.

Lateral Glide (Unilateral)

Assessment: To assess or increase joint mobility.

Patient position: As previous.

Clinician position: As previous.

Method: Apply lateral force against the molars with the thumb; simultaneously apply medial force against the body of the mandible with the fingers (with supination-type motion); may be used for similar purposes, especially medial disc displacement.

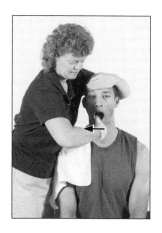

End Feel

Mouth opening: firm (tissue stretch secondary to tension on capsule, ligaments)

Mouth closing: bone on bone (teeth approximate)

Protrusion: firm (tissue stretch of posterior portion of disc)

Retrusion: firm (tissue stretch of temporomandibular ligament)

Lateral deviation: firm

Capsular Pattern

Limitation in mouth opening.

Close-Packed Position

Both extremes of range of motion.

1. Maximum opening: anterior joint close-packed limited by soft tissue and capsule
2. Maximum closing: posterior joint close-packed limited by teeth

Loose-Packed Position

Midrange at freeway space. Soft tissue of TMJ is the most relaxed, the mandible is slightly depressed, and the tongue rests against the hard palate (roughly 2–4 mm space between maxillary and mandibular teeth). The clinician may palpate by placing a finger (pad forward) in each external auditory canal with the patient's mouth open and feeling for the point at which the mandibular condyle makes contact with the finger when the patient closes his or her mouth (figure 3.2, *a* and *b*).

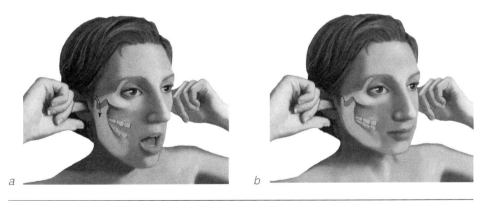

a   *b*

Figure 3.2 (*a*) To palpate the TMJ, place the index finger in the auditory canal; (*b*) feel for the point at which the mandibular condyle makes contact with the finger on closing.

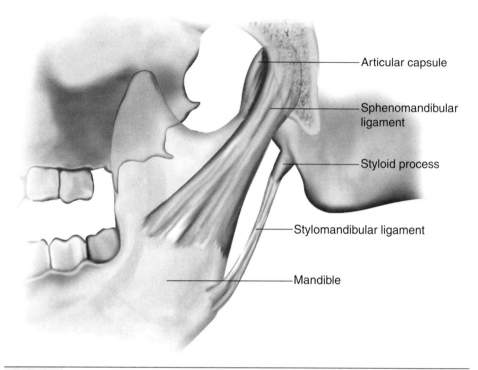

Articular capsule

Sphenomandibular ligament

Styloid process

Stylomandibular ligament

Mandible

Figure 3.3 TMJ ligaments.

Stability

Capsular Ligament Attaches at mandibular fossa, articular tubercle, and mandibular condyle; helps provide stability for disc atop mandible.

Temporomandibular Ligament Thickening of joint capsule that provides lateral reinforcement; attaches at zygomatic arch articular eminence and neck of mandible; restrains motion of lower jaw and prevents impingement of tissues behind mandibular condyle.

Sphenomandibular Ligament From the spine of the sphenoid to the middle ramus of the mandible; provides suspension for the mandible and prevents excessive anterior translation.

Stylomandibular Ligament A thickening of deep cerebral fascia running from the styloid process of the temporal bone to the posterior ramus of the mandible and inserting between the medial pterygoid and the masseter muscles; may assist in limiting protrusion.

The sphenomandibular and stylomandibular ligaments together are thought to keep the mandibular condyle, articular disc, and temporal bone opposed.

Disc Biconcave shape provides increased congruency of joint in various positions; the thin center and wider anterior-posterior dimensions allow increased adaptability of the disc to its bony articular surfaces, thereby creating greater congruency.

Chvostek's Test

Assessment: Pathology of cranial nerve VII.

Patient position: Sitting or supine with jaw relaxed and mouth closed.

Clinician position: Standing beside the patient.

Method: Tap parotid gland over the masseter muscle.

Positive response: Twitching of facial muscles.

Reciprocal Clicking

Assessment: Anterior displacement of disc.

Patient position: Sitting or supine.

Clinician position: Standing beside the patient and palpating lateral poles of condyles.

Method: The patient begins with mouth closed and then performs full opening followed by full closing.

Positive response: The patient feels a click during opening and again during closing (may be at different positions); the opening click is generally the louder of the two.

Arthrokinematics

Mandibular Depression The convex condyles rotate anteriorly on a concave articular eminence during the first 10–25 mm of mandibular opening. After 10–25 mm, the condyle–disc complex translates anteriorly in conjunction with continued rotation to permit full mouth opening.

Mandibular Elevation During mouth closing, the reverse actions take place. The condyle–disc complex translates posteriorly followed by posterior rotation of the condyle on the disc.

Protrusion Both mandibular condyles along with the discs translate anteriorly to produce this motion.

Retrusion Both mandibular condyles along with the discs translate posteriorly to produce this motion.

Lateral Deviation The condyle on the ipsilateral side spins, while the condyle on the contralateral side translates anteriorly.

Distraction Distraction occurs ipsilaterally at the condyle during biting unilaterally against resistance (such as food) placed between the upper and lower third molars.

Compression Compression occurs contralaterally at the condyle during biting unilaterally against resistance (such as food) placed between the upper and lower third molars. Compression may also occur secondary to muscular contraction during functional activities.

Lateral glide is an accessory motion that may accompany any or all of the arthrokinematics described to provide more available movement at the joint.

Neurology

Because the neurology of the TMJ region is rather complex, it is easy to confuse pain of TMJ origin with other types of facial pain. Clinicians should have a general idea of the motor and sensory nerves that supply the general region.

Motor Most of the muscles around the TMJ are supplied by the mandibular branch of the fifth cranial nerve (temporalis, medial and lateral pterygoid, and masseter) and by the seventh cranial nerve (digastric, stylohyoid).

Sensory The auriculotemporal and masseteric branches of the mandibular nerve supply the majority of sensory innervation to the TMJ.

Structures innervated by the afferents of cervical vertebrae 1 through 3 can all refer pain to the head, TMJ, and face. Additionally, the ganglia of cranial nerve V is located at about C3, thus presenting the possibility for cervical pathology to result in pain referrals along the sensory distribution of the trigeminal nerve.

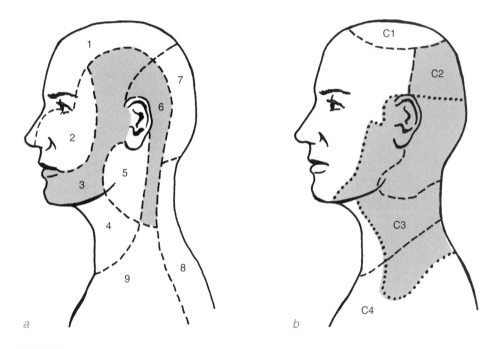

(a) Sensory nerve distribution of head, neck, and face: (1) ophthalmic nerve, (2) maxillary nerve, (3) mandibular nerve, (4) transverse cutaneous nerve of neck (C2–C3), (5) greater auricular nerve (C2-C3), (6) lesser auricular nerve (C2), (7) greater occipital nerve (C2–C3), (8) cervical dorsal rami (C3–C5), and (9) suprascapular nerve (C5–C6); (b) dermatome pattern of the head, neck, and face. C3 is shown in dotted lines because of overlap.

Adapted from *Orthopedic Physical Assessment*, 2nd ed., D.J. Magee, pg. 57. Copyright 1992, with permission from W.B. Saunders.

Surface Palpation

TMJ (by external auditory canal)

Mandibular condyles

Pterygoid, temporalis, and masseter muscles

Mandible

Teeth

Hyoid bone (anterior to C2–C3)

Thyroid cartilage (anterior to C4–C5)

Mastoid process

Cervical spine (for details see "Cervical Spine," chapter 4)

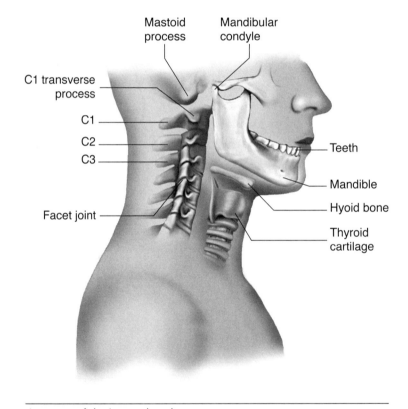

Anatomy of the jaw and neck.

Muscle Origin and Insertion

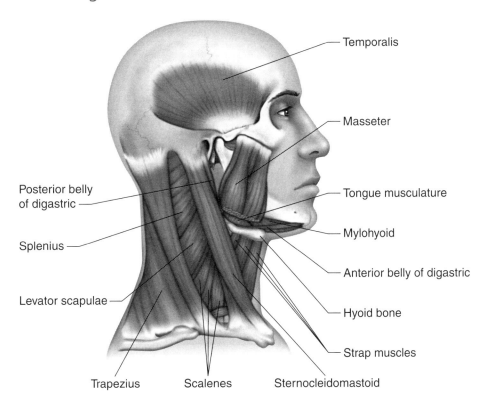

Temporalis

Masseter

Tongue musculature

Mylohyoid

Anterior belly of digastric

Hyoid bone

Strap muscles

Posterior belly of digastric

Splenius

Levator scapulae

Trapezius

Scalenes

Sternocleidomastoid

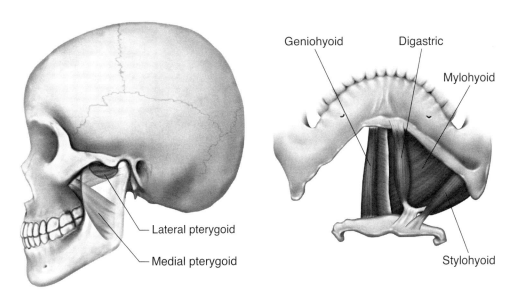

Lateral pterygoid

Medial pterygoid

Geniohyoid

Digastric

Mylohyoid

Stylohyoid

Muscles of the jaw and neck.

Muscle	Origin and insertion
Lateral pterygoid	Pterygoid process and base of skull to mandibular neck and articular disc
Mylohyoid	Mylohyoid line of body of mandible to hyoid bone
Geniohyoid	Inferior mental spine of mandible to hyoid bone
Digastric	Mastoid process of temporal bone to posterior chin (body of mandible) with slip of fascia connecting tendon to hyoid bone
Masseter	Zygomatic arch to ramus and angle of mandible
Temporalis	Lateral skull to coronoid process and anterior ramus of mandible
Medial pterygoid	Pterygoid process to angle of mandible
Stylohyoid	Styloid process of temporal bone to hyoid bone

Based on J. Hamill and K. Knutzen, 1995, *Biomechanical basis of human movement* (Baltimore, MD: Lippincott, Williams, and Wilkins).

Muscle Action and Innervation

Action	Muscle involved	Nerve supply
Mandibular depression (mouth opening)	Lateral pterygoid Mylohyoid* Geniohyoid* Digastric*	Mandibular (CN V) Inferior alveolar (CN V) Hypoglossal (CN XII) Inferior alveolar (CN V) Facial (CN VII)
Mandibular elevation (mouth closing)	Masseter Temporalis Medial pterygoid	Mandibular (CN V) Mandibular (CN V) Mandibular (CN V)
Mandibular protrusion	Lateral pterygoid Medial pterygoid Masseter* Mylohyoid* Geniohyoid* Digastric* Stylohyoid* Temporalis (anterior fibers)*	Mandibular (CN V) Mandibular (CN V) Mandibular (CN V) Inferior alveolar (CN V) Hypoglossal (CN XII) Inferior alveolar (CN V) Facial (CN VII) Facial (CN VII) Mandibular (CN V)
Mandibular retrusion	Temporalis (posterior fibers) Masseter* Digastric* Stylohyoid* Mylohyoid* Geniohyoid*	Mandibular (CN V) Mandibular (CN V) Inferior alveolar (CN V) Facial (CN VII) Facial (CN VII) Inferior alveolar (CN V) Hypoglossal (CN XII)
Mandibular deviation (lateral)	Lateral pterygoid (ipsilateral) Medial pterygoid (contra-lateral) Temporalis* Masseter*	Mandibular (CN V) Mandibular (CN V) Mandibular (CN V) Mandibular (CN V)

Act only when assistance is required. CN = cranial nerve.

Adapted from *Orthopedic Physical Assessment,* 2nd ed., D.J. Magee, pg. 83. Copyright 1992, with permission from W.B. Saunders.

Clinical Syndromes

Description	Location and behavior of symptoms	History or onset	Tests and measures, diagnostics
SYNOVITIS			
Inflammation of synovium; may be accompanied by joint effusion.	Pain in periauricular area; increased or decreased with functional activities; better with rest.	Gradual or acute trauma.	May be unable to close fully or open secondary to pain; pain with TMJ palpation while closing; (+) forced biting; (+) retrusive overpressure.
CAPSULITIS			
Inflammation of joint capsule.	Pain in periauricular area; increased or decreased with functional activities; better with rest.	Gradual or acute trauma.	May be unable to open fully secondary to pain; pain with TMJ palpation with mouth closed and with mouth opened 30 mm; (+) forced biting; (+) retrusive overpressure.
FIBROSIS			
Fibrosis of joint capsule.	Stiffness possibly accompanied by pain.	Follows history of prolonged capsulitis, prolonged immobilization or mandibular restriction, trauma, repetitive microtrauma, or arthritis.	Decreased mandibular mobility and deflection from midline suggesting decrease in translation.
HYPERMOBILITY			
Excessive joint mobility.	Feeling of jaw going out of place may describe joint noises.	May report history of "catching" when mouth opened, making closing difficult.	Large indentation palpable posterior to condyle when mouth opened, deviation of mandible to contralateral side at end opening; depression > 40 mm.

» continued

» continued

Description	Location and behavior of symptoms	History or onset	Tests and measures, diagnostics
DISLOCATION			
Joint locked in open position.	Inability to close mouth.	May report history of "catching" or feeling of jaw going out of place; may or may not have pain.	Mouth opened and deviated to contralateral side.
DISC DISPLACEMENT WITH REDUCTION			
Disc rests in dislocated position, is reduced with mouth opening, and returns to position with closing.	Reports joint noises during mouth opening and closing; may describe a click with opening and again with closing.	Trauma or gradual onset.	Clicking with mouth opening or closing over lateral poles; lifting angle of mandible anterior or superior, while patient opens and closes; check for noise and/or pain worsening.
DISC DISPLACEMENT WITHOUT REDUCTION (ACUTE)			
Displacement of disc anteriorly that does not reduce with mandibular motion.	Inability to open mouth fully; difficulty with functional activities such as yawning and chewing.	Previous history of joint noise and intermittent locking.	Mandibular depression and protrusion limited with deviation toward the involved side; lateral deviation limited toward the opposite side.
DISC DISPLACEMENT WITHOUT REDUCTION (CHRONIC)			
Displacement of disc anteriorly that does not reduce with mandibular motion.	Not functionally limited but complains of joint noise with motion (crepitus).	Previous history of joint noise and intermittent locking.	As previous, but slight or no limitations in range; palpable crepitus.
OSTEOARTHRITIS			
Degenerative joint disease.	Same as for inflammatory (capsulitis, synovitis); with joint noise.	Gradual following prolonged inflammatory condition or after acute trauma.	Same as for inflammatory (capsulitis, synovitis), but palpable crepitus; (+) X-ray for structural changes.

Description	Location and behavior of symptoms	History or onset	Tests and measures, diagnostics
OSTEOARTHROSIS			
Degenerative joint disease (progression).	Primary complaint is joint noise; pain often decreases.	End result of osteoarthritis.	Close to functional depression and protrusion with slight deviation toward involved side at end ranges; close to functional lateral deviation to opposite side; (+) X-ray for structural changes.
FIBROUS ANKYLOSIS			
Fibrous adhesions in joint.	Multidirectional limitation in movement.	Usually result of major trauma or surgery.	Multidirectional limitation in movement, generally a result of decreased translation.

(+) positive response

Adapted from C. Wadsworth, 1988, *Manual examination and treatment of the spine and extremities* (Baltimore, MD: Lippincott, Williams, and Wilkins).

Cervical Spine

This chapter addresses the cervical spine (figure 4.1, *a* and *b*). The cervical spine may be responsible for symptoms in the neck, shoulder, arm, head, or face or may be a secondary factor contributing to shoulder, arm, head, or face pain. Therefore, clinicians must have an appreciation of the many possible presentations of cervical spine dysfunction.

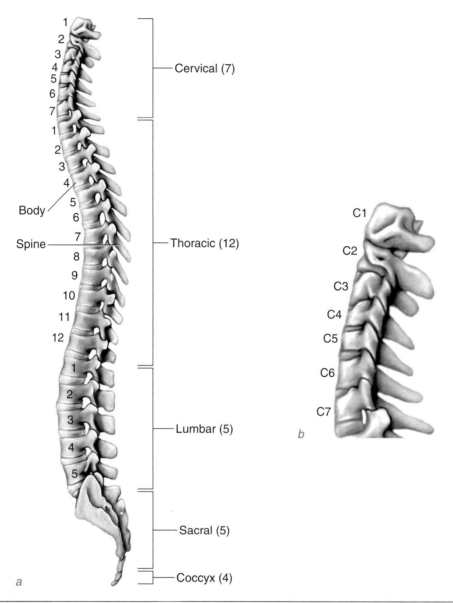

Cervical (7)

Thoracic (12)

Lumbar (5)

Sacral (5)

Coccyx (4)

Body

Spine

C1
C2
C3
C4
C5
C6
C7

a

b

Figure 4.1 Spinal column: (*a*) cervical vertebrae; (*b*) cervical vertebrae (lateral view).

Reprinted, by permission, from R. Behnke, *Kinetic anatomy*, 2nd ed. (Champaign, IL: Human Kinetics), 120.

Joint Basics

Articulation   Two unique articulations are present within the cervical spine: the occipitoatlantal (OA) joint between the skull and C1 and the atlantoaxial (AA) joint between C1 and C2. At the OA, the two convex occipital condyles articulate with the two concave superior facets of the atlas. The AA joint is actually made up of three joints: the median AA (atlanto–odontoid articulation) and two lateral joints. The median AA is the articulation of the dens and the atlas, and the lateral joints are the articulations between the convex inferior facets of the atlas and the concave superior facets of the axis. Vertebrae C3–C7 are intervertebral joints much like the remaining joints in the spine. The articulations occur between the intervertebral body and the intervertebral disc, as well as between the right and left superior facets of one vertebra with the right and left inferior facets of the body above. Cervical vertebrae are unique in that on the anterior aspect bilaterally they possess an additional articulation. The uncovertebral joints, or joints of von Luschka, are not present at birth but develop around the age of 10 as a result of upright weight bearing. The right and left superior uncovertebral joints of one cervical vertebra articulate with the right and left inferior uncovertebral joints of the cervical body above (figure 4.2).

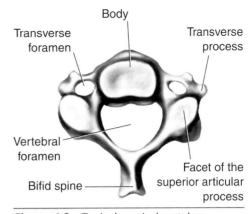

Figure 4.2 Typical cervical vertebra.

Reprinted, by permission, from R. Behnke, *Kinetic anatomy*, 2nd ed. (Champaign, IL: Human Kinetics), 123.

Type of Joint   The OA joint is a plane synovial joint. At the AA joint, the median AA is a synovial trochoid joint, whereas the lateral joints are plane synovial joints. For the remaining spinal segments, a cartilaginous joint exists between the vertebral body and the disc, whereas the articulation of the superior articular process (facet) and the inferior articular process (facet) constitutes a plane diarthrodial joint.

Degrees of Freedom

- Flexion and extension in a sagittal plane about a coronal axis
- Side bending in a frontal plane about a sagittal axis
- Rotation in a transverse plane about an axis in the frontal and sagittal planes

The motions described may occur at any one motion segment, but because vertebral motion segments function as part of an articular system, motion between any two vertebrae is generally limited to a small amount of translation (or glide) and rotation. Furthermore, because each intervertebral joint functions as part of an articular system, the axis of motion of any given joint changes in response to motion at segments above and below.

Active Range of Motion

The facets of the AA joint lie parallel to the transverse plane, thus permitting rotation around a vertical axis. The superior facets of C3–C7 facets are oriented upward, posteriorly, and medially, whereas the inferior facets are oriented downward, anteriorly, and laterally. The facet orientation within the cervical spine allows the following degrees of movement for gross cervical motion: 80–90° flexion, 70° extension, 20–45° side bending, 70–90° rotation. Further, each joint within the cervical spine contributes to varying degrees of flexion, extension, side bending, and rotation.

OA: approximately 17° of flexion, 12° of extension, 3–5° of side bending, 3–5° of rotation (2–3° with initial motion, 2–3° more at end of physiological rotation range)

AA: 47° rotation, 10° flexion and extension, little to no side bending

C3–C7: 45° rotation, 40° flexion, 24° extension, 50° side bending (fairly evenly distributed among these segments)

Upper Cervical Spine Flexion

Patient position: Sitting.

Clinician position: Standing in front of the patient.

Method: The clinician asks the patient to tuck in the chin and then observes the quality and quantity of movement (*a*).

Alternative method: Can apply overpressure (*b*).

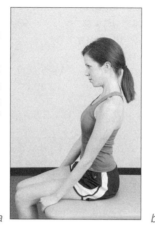 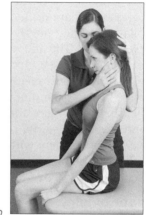

a   *b*

Cervical Spine Flexion

Patient position: Sitting.

Clinician position: Standing on the side of the patient for AROM. After the patient has achieved the available range of motion, the clinician places one hand over the patient's CT junction and the other hand on the patient's occiput.

Method: Gently apply overpressure into flexion oscillating into the end range.

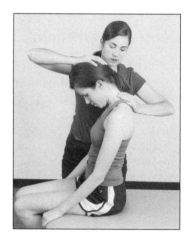

Upper Cervical Spine Extension

Patient position: Sitting (*a*).

Clinician position: Standing in front of the patient.

Method: The clinician asks the patient to poke the chin forward and then observes quality and quantity of movement (*b*).

Alternative method: Can apply overpressure.

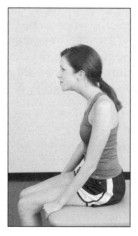 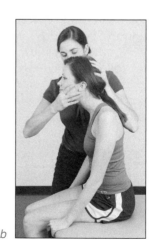

a   *b*

Cervical Spine Extension

Patient position: Sitting.

Clinician position: Standing on the side of the patient for AROM. After the patient has achieved the available range of motion, the clinician places one hand over the patient's CT junction and the web space of the other hand on the patient's chin.

Method: Gently apply overpressure into extension oscillating into the end range.

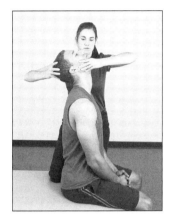

Cervical Spine Rotation

Patient position: Sitting.

Clinician position: Standing in front of the patient for AROM. After the patient has achieved the available range of motion, the clinician stands to the left side of the patient and places the left hand on the patient's right lateral head with the forearm stabilizing the patient's anterior shoulder. The clinician places the left hand on the patient's left lateral head with the forearm stabilizing the patient's posterior shoulder.

Method: Gently apply overpressure into rotation oscillating into the end range.

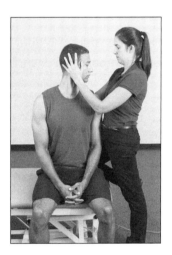

Upper Cervical Spine Side Bending

Patient position: Sitting.

Clinician position: Standing in front of the patient.

Method: The clinician places the ulnar border of the left hand along C2. The clinician asks the patient to drop the ear to the shoulder and then observes quality and quantity of movement.

Alternative method: Can apply overpressure.

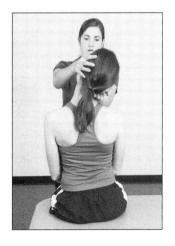

Cervical Spine Side Bending

Patient position: Sitting.

Clinician position: Standing in front of the patient for AROM. After the patient has achieved the available range of motion, the clinician places the left hand on the lateral side of the patient's head and the right hand on the patient's shoulder.

Method: Gently apply overpressure into side bending oscillating into the end range.

Alternative method: Localize overpressure to individual levels.

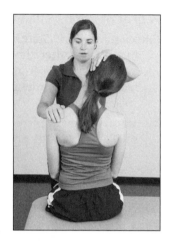

Quadrant

Patient position: Sitting.

Clinician position: Standing in front of the patient.

Method: The clinician asks the patient to look up to the ceiling (cervical spine extension). The clinician then asks the patient to follow his or her finger into the right corner of the room, combining movements of cervical spine extension, side bending, and rotation (see *a*). The clinician can then can apply overpressure if appropriate (*b*).

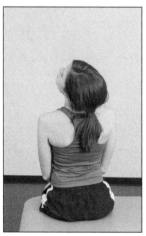
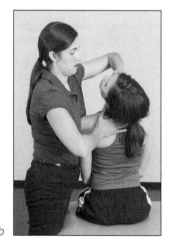

a　　　　　　*b*

Central PAIVM

Assessment: To assess or increase central P-A mobility.

Patient position: Lying on abdomen with hands cupping forehead. A pillow is placed under lower legs for comfort.

Clinician position: Standing at the head of the table with the tips of the thumbs (back to back) on the spinous process to be examined. The clinician's fingers straddle the side of the patient's neck and gather up soft tissue. Shoulders should be relaxed and elbows slightly flexed.

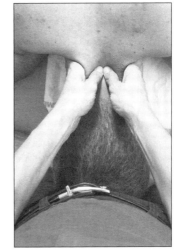

Method: The clinician applies a posterior-to-anterior force on each spinous process being examined. Perform a total of three passes. Apply first pressures gently; increase amplitude and depth of the movement if no pain response occurs. Assess quality of movement through the range and end feel; compare with levels above and below.

Positive response: Movements that reproduce the comparable sign (pain versus resistance versus spasm).

Unilateral PAIVM

Assessment: To assess or increase unilateral P-A mobility.

Patient position: Lying on abdomen with hands cupping forehead. A pillow is placed under lower legs for comfort.

Clinician position: Standing at the head of the table on the side in which the technique is to be performed. The clinician places thumb tips (back to back) on articular process to be mobilized. The fingers straddle the neck and take up soft tissue. Shoulders should be relaxed and elbows slightly flexed.

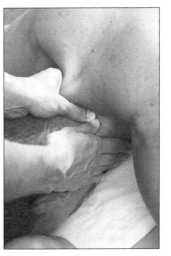

Method: The clinician applies a posterior-to-anterior force on each articular process being examined. Perform a total of three passes. Apply first pressures gently; increase amplitude and depth of the movement if no pain response occurs. Assess quality of movement through the range and end feel; compare with levels above and below.

Positive response: Movements that reproduce the comparable sign (pain versus resistance versus spasm).

Manual Traction

Assessment: To unload spinal segments.

Patient position: Supine, head resting on pillow. Adjust the head plate of the table to allow the patient's neck to lie in a neutral position.

Clinician position: Standing at the head of the table. The right hand supports the occiput with the palm (the index finger should lie over the superior nuchal line,

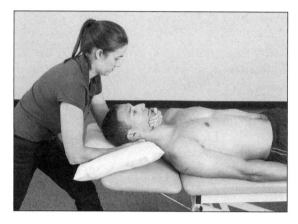

and the thumb should be behind the patient's right ear). The clinician holds the patient's chin with the left hand, and the left forearm lies along the left side of the patient's face. The clinician stands in a walk-stance position, has elbows flexed, and crouches over the patient's head to hold the crown of the patient's head against the front of the clinician's left shoulder.

Method: The clinician applies a gentle longitudinal pull through the forearms combined with a slight backward movement of the body.

Alternative method: Cervical self-traction.

Fold a towel lengthwise twice. Take the end of a durable 5 ft (1.5 m) rope and securely tie the two ends of the towel together so that they do not come undone. Position the folded towel so that it barely touches the floor and tie the other end of the rope around a secure doorknob. The patient lies on his or her back on the floor and places the back of the head in the towel sling. The patient should be comfortably resting in the sling, approximately 1 to 2 in. (2.5 to 5 cm) from the floor. Instruct the patient to scoot his or her body away from the door to achieve a slight pull in the neck. The patient's head should be slightly flexed.

End Feel

Flexion: firm

Extension: firm

Side bending: firm

Rotation: firm

Capsular Pattern

Side bending and rotation limited equally, then extension.

Close-Packed Position

Extension (facets).

Loose-Packed Position

Slightly extended.

Stability

Transverse Atlantal Ligament (Atlantal Cruciform Ligament)   The transverse atlantal ligament traverses the ring of the atlas, dividing it into a larger posterior section that houses the spinal cord and a smaller anterior space for the dens (see figure 4.3). Longitudinal fibers extend superiorly to attach to the occiput; inferior fibers descend to the posterior portion of the axis; the transverse portion maintains the dens and the atlas in close approximation. The primary function of this ligament is to prevent anterior displacement of C1 on C2.

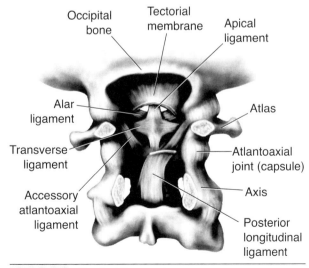

Figure 4.3   Cervical ligaments.

Reprinted, by permission, from R. Behnke, *Kinetic anatomy*, 2nd ed. (Champaign, IL: Human Kinetics), 125.

Alar Ligaments   Alar ligaments travel from either side of the dens to the medial aspect of the occiput; they are taut in flexion but relaxed in extension. The left ligament checks rotation of the head and neck to the right; the right lower portion and the left upper portion limit side bending of the head and neck to the right. This ligament also functions to prevent distraction of C1 on C2.

Posterior AA   The posterior AA is a continuation of the ligamentum flavum in the upper cervical; it runs from posterior arch of atlas to arch of axis.

Anterior AA   The anterior AA is a continuation of the anterior longitudinal ligament in the upper cervical; it runs from anterior-inferior atlas to anterior axis.

Tectorial Membrane   The tectorial membrane is the continuation of the posterior longitudinal ligament above the axis; it is a thin membrane between the occiput and C2.

Ligamentum Nuchae   This ligament runs posteriorly from C1 and connects all cervical spinous processes.

Muscle Length Test: Upper Trapezius

Patient position: Supine, with the head and upper thoracic spine off the edge of the table to T2.

Clinician position: Standing behind the patient and slightly to the left. The left hand holds the patient's head at the occiput, with the head supported by the abdomen. The right hand is on the superior aspect of the right shoulder, and the fingers are pointing toward the feet.

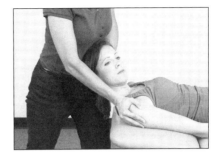

Method: Using the left hand, the clinician places the patient's neck into upper cervical flexion and then adds full ventral flexion. Add left lateral flexion and right rotation. Slowly apply pressure through right shoulder, feeling for resistance. Compare to the other side.

Muscle Length Test: Levator Scapula

Patient position: Supine, with the head and upper thoracic spine off the edge of the table to T2.

Clinician position: Standing behind the patient and slightly to the left. The left hand holds the patient's head at the occiput, with the head supported by the abdomen. The right hand is on the superior angle of the spine of the scapula.

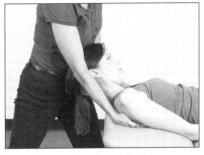

Method: Using the left hand, the clinician places the patient's neck into upper cervical flexion and then adds full ventral flexion. Add left lateral flexion and left rotation. Slowly apply pressure through the scapula feeling for resistance. Compare to the other side.

Muscle Length Test: Suboccipitals

Patient position: Supine, with the head and neck in a position of comfort, with or without a pillow.

Clinician position: Standing at the head of the table in a walk-stance position. The clinician places the left hand on the table and holds C2 at the articular pillars with the thumb and index finger. The right hand is at the base of the occipital bone. The clinician's right shoulder rests lightly on the patient's forehead.

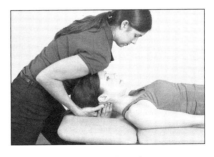

Method: Slowly apply an arclike motion with the right arm and hand, feeling for the resistance.

Vertebral Artery

Patient position: Sitting with the head in (*a*) cervical spine extension, (*b*) cervical spine rotation, (*c*) cervical spine extension in rotation (rotates first, then extends).

Clinician position: The clinician is standing to the side of the patient with the hands supporting both sides of the patient's head.

Method: Sustain each position for at least 20 seconds. Observe the patient's eyes for nystagmus.

Wait at least 10 seconds between tests or until dizziness settles. Limited cervical mobility may limit your ability to test the VBA. Use caution with irritable patients.

Alternative method: Supine (see figure *d*, *e*, and *f*).

Indications: Subjective complaints of dizziness, facial paresthesias, diplopia, blurring of vision, nausea, vomiting, nystagmus, or unsteadiness. Patients who present with an upper-quarter dysfunction with a coexisting cervical spine dysfunction on whom you plan to perform end-range techniques or grade V techniques.

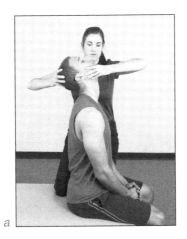
a

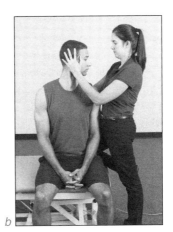
b

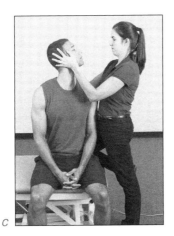
c

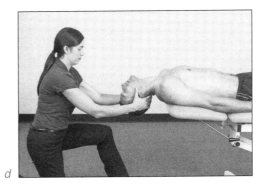
d

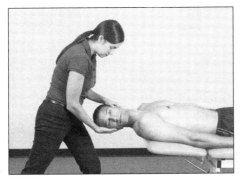
e

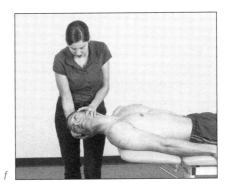
f

Transverse Ligament Stability Test

Assessment: Integrity of transverse ligament.

Patient position: Supine, head resting in neutral position on the bed (with or without pillow), and eyes open.

Clinician position: Standing at the head of the bed in a walk-stance position. The left hand is under the patient's occiput, producing craniovertebral flexion, and the left shoulder is gently stabilizing the

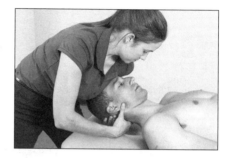

patient's forehead. The radial border of the index finger of the right hand is placed against the spinous process of C2.

Method: The clinician uses the radial border of the index finger of the right hand to push posteriorly to anteriorly against the spinous process of C2. Hold until no further motion is detected or until positive signs or symptoms are produced. Assess response.

Alternative method: Sitting (Sharp-Purser test).

Normal response: No movement present.

Positive response: If the ligament is lax, the clinician will find a lag time and a palpable clunk as dens abuts against the atlas. The patient may report easing of symptoms.

Alar Ligament Stability Test

Patient position: Supine, head resting in neutral position on the bed or pillow, and eyes open.

Clinician position: Standing at the head of the bed in a walk-stance position. The right hand fixates C2 spinous process using lumbrical grip, and the left hand grasps the occiput over the crown of the head.

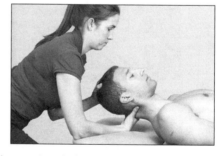

Method: Using the left hand, side bend the patient's head to the left. Assess response. Using the left hand, side bend the patient's head to the right. Assess response. Repeat in craniovertebral flexion and extension.

Normal response: Very little movement present—end feel should be firm. If the ligament is lax some sidebend (SB) will occur.

Positive response: The test is positive if excessive occipital motion is found in all three positions.

Arthrokinematics

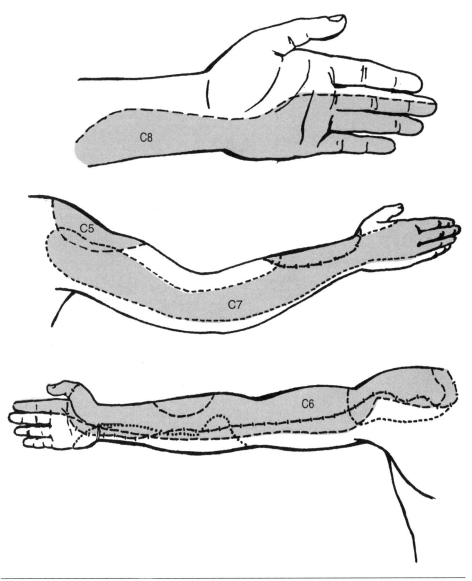

Dermatomes of C4 through T1.

Upper Cervical

Flexion   The occiput glides posteriorly on the atlas; the atlas then glides forward and tilts anteriorly.

Extension   The occiput glides anteriorly on the atlas; the atlas glides backward and then tilts posteriorly.

Side Bending   Occipital condyles glide opposite the direction of side bending; the atlas then slides ipsilaterally and rotates contralaterally secondary to tension in the alar ligament.

Rotation   The occiput rotates only 2–3° on the atlas; the occiput and atlas then rotate together to the same side; tension on the alar ligament causes the occiput to side bend contralaterally near end range.

Mid and Lower Cervical   The cervical facets (C2–C7) are oriented at a 45° angle to the transverse plane.

Flexion   The disc is compressed anteriorly; facets glide cranially.

Extension   The disc is compressed posteriorly; facets glide caudally.

Side Bending   The disc is compressed on the side of the concavity; facets on the side of the concavity glide caudally, while those contralateral to concavity glide cranially.

Rotation   The disc undergoes torsion; facets glide in the same direction as vertebral body rotation.

Neurology

Nerve root	Reflex	Motor	Sensory
C1		Rectus capitis anterior and lateral	
C2		Rectus capitis posterior	Side of head
C3		Scalenes, erector spinae	Anterior and lateral neck
C4		Levator scapulae, trapezius	Lateral neck to shoulder
C5	Biceps	Deltoid	Lateral shoulder
C6	Brachioradialis	Biceps, extensor carpi, radialis longus and brevis	Posterior and radial aspect of thumb
C7	Triceps	Triceps, flexor carpi radialis	Long finger
C8	Abductor digiti minimi	Flexor digitorum profundus, extensor pollicis longus	Ulnar aspect of little finger
T1		Hand intrinsics	Medial forearm and arm

Cranial Nerve Examination

Nerve tested	Test	Positive
1 Olfactory	Soap smell	Complete loss of sense of smell or distorted sense
2 Optic	Confrontation	Hemi or quadranopsia
3 Oculomotor (EW)	Consensual reflex	Absent, sluggish, oscillating
3, 4, 6 Oculomotor, trochlear, abducens	H test, convergence	Paresis or paralysis
5 Trigeminal	Facial sensation Jaw jerk	Absence or lack of sensation Hyperreflexia or clonus
7 Facial	Smile, frown	UMNL, LMNL
8 Vestibular	Tilt, Hallpike-Dix	Dizziness, nystagmus
8 Cochlear	Finger rustle bone conduction	Loss of hearing or asymmetrical hearing Heard in deaf ear = conduction deafness Heard in good ear = sensorineural deafness
9 Glossopharyngeal	Not tested	NA
10 Vagus	Uvula test	Deviation toward strong side
11 Accessory	Trapezius or SCM strength	Weakness
12 Hypoglossal	Tongue protrusion	Deviation toward weak side

Surface Palpation

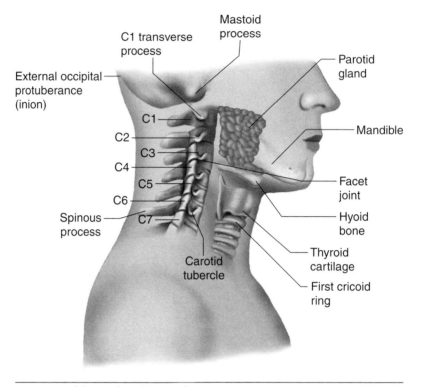

Anatomy of the neck and cervical spine.

Posterior
External occipital protuberance
Inion
Cervical spinous processes
Cervical faccts
Mastoid process

Lateral
Cervical transverse processes
Temporomandibular joint
Mandible
Parotid

Anterior
Hyoid
Thyroid
First cricoid ring
First rib
Supraclavicular fossa

Muscle Origin and Insertion

Muscle	Origin and insertion
Rectus capitis anterior	Occiput to anterior portion of lateral mass of C1
Rectus capitis lateralis	Occiput to transverse process of C1
Longus capitis	Inferior occiput to transverse processes of C3–C6
Obliquus capitis superior	Transverse process of C1–T4 to lateral portion of inferior nuchal line
Sternocleidomastoid	Clavicle and sternum to mastoid process
Splenius capitis nuchal	Spinous processes C2–T4 to lateral portion of superior line and mastoid process
Semispinalis capitis	Transverse processes C7–T6 and articular processes of C4–C6 to superior and inferior nuchal lines
Longissimus capitis	Transverse processes T1–T5 and articular processes of C4–C7 to mastoid process
Spinalis capitis	Medial portion of semispinalis capitis
Trapezius	Occiput, ligamentum nuchae, and spinous processes of C7–T12 to lateral one-third of the clavicle, scapular spine, and acromion
Rectus capitis posterior major	Spinous process of C2 to inferior nuchal line
Rectus capitis posterior minor	Posterior arch of C1 to inferior nuchal line
Obliquus capitis inferior	Spinous process of C2 to transverse process of C1
Longus colli	Anterior vertebral bodies T3–midcervical to transverse processes of vertebrae above or anterior bodies of vertebrae above up to anterior arch atlas
Scalenus anterior	Transverse processes of C3–C6 to upper surface of first rib (near sternum)
Scalenus medius	Transverse processes of C2–C7 to first rib
Scalenus posterior	Transverse processes of C5–C6 to second rib
Splenius cervicis	Spinous processes of C2–T4 to transverse processes of C1–C3
Semispinalis cervicis	Transverse processes of T1–T6 to spinous processes C2–C5
Longissimus cervicis	Transverse processes of T1–T5 to transverse processes of C2–C6
Levator scapulae	Superior angle of scapula to transverse processes of C2–C4
Iliocostalis cervicis	Upper six ribs to transverse processes of C4–C6
Rotatores	Transverse processes to spinous processes from sacrum to C2; span of each fascicle only one or two segments
Multifidus	Transverse processes to spinous processes from sacrum to C2; span of each fascicle only two to four segments
Intertransversarii	Transverse processes to spinous processes from sacrum C2; span of each fascicle only one or two segments

Adapted from J. Hamill and K. Knudzen, 1995, *Biomechanical basis of human movement* (Baltimore, MD: Lippincott, Williams, and Wilkins), 499, 509, 510.

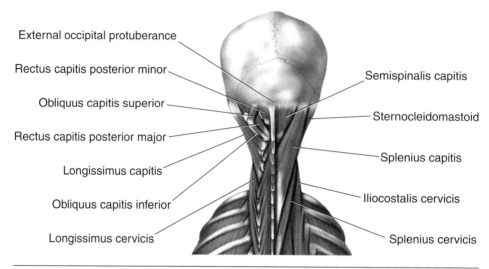

External occipital protuberance

Rectus capitis posterior minor

Obliquus capitis superior

Rectus capitis posterior major

Longissimus capitis

Obliquus capitis inferior

Longissimus cervicis

Semispinalis capitis

Sternocleidomastoid

Splenius capitis

Iliocostalis cervicis

Splenius cervicis

Major muscles of the neck.

Reprinted, by permission, from R. Behnke, *Kinetic anatomy*, 2nd ed. (Champaign, IL: Human Kinetics), 134.

Muscle Action and Innervation

Action	Muscle involved	Nerve supply
Upper cervical flexion	Rectus capitis anterior	C1–C2
	Rectus capitis lateralis	C1–C2
	Longus capitis	C1–C3
	Hyoid muscles	Inferior alveolar nerve
		Facial nerve
		Hypoglossal nerve
		Ansa cervicalis
	Obliquus capitis superior	C1
	Sternocleidomastoid (if head neutral or flexed)	Accessory C2
Upper cervical extension	Splenius capitis	C4–C6
	Semispinalis capitis	C1–C8
	Longissimus capitis	C6–C8
	Spinalis capitis	C6–C8
	Trapezius	Accessory C3–C4
	Rectus capitis posterior minor	C1
	Rectus capitis posterior major	C1
	Obliquus capitis superior	C1
	Obliquus capitis inferior	C1
	Sternocleidomastoid (if head slightly extended)	Accessory C2
Upper cervical rotation (muscles contract unilaterally)	Trapezius (face moves to opposite side)	Accessory C3, C4
	Splenius capitis (face moves to same side)	C4–C6
	Longissimus capitis (face moves to same side)	C6–C8
	Semispinalis capitis (face moves to same side)	C1–C8
	Obliquus capitis inferior (face moves to same side)	C1
	Sternocleidomastoid (face moves to opposite side)	Accessory C2
Upper cervical side bending (muscles contract unilaterally)	Trapezius	Accessory C3, C4
	Splenius capitis	C4–C6
	Longissimus capitis	C6–C8
	Semispinalis capitis	C1–C8
	Obliquus capitis inferior	C1
	Rectus capitis lateralis	C1–C2
	Longus capitis	C1–C3
	Sternocleidomastoid	Accessory C2
Neck flexion	Longus colli	C2–C6
	Scalenus anterior	C4–C6
	Scalenus medius	C3–C8
	Scalenus posterior	C6–C8

» continued

» continued

Action	Muscle involved	Nerve supply
Neck extension	Splenius cervicis	C6–C8
	Semispinalis cervicis	C1–C8
	Longissimus cervicis	C6–C8
	Levator scapulae	C3–C4
		Dorsal scapular
	Iliocostalis cervicis	C6–C8
	Spinalis cervicis	C6–C8
	Multifidus	C1–C8
	Interspinalis cervicis	C1–C8
	Trapezius	Accessory C3–C4
	Rectus capitis posterior major	C1
	Rotatores brevis	C1–C8
	Rotatores longi	C1–C8
Side bending of neck	Levator scapulae	C3–C4
		Dorsal scapular
	Splenius cervicis	C6–C8
	Iliocostalis cervicis	C6–C8
	Longissimus cervicis	C6–C8
	Semispinalis cervicis	C1–C8
	Multifidus	C1–C8
	Intertransversarii	C1–C8
	Scaleni	C3–C8
	Sternocleidomastoid	Accessory C2
	Obliquus capitis inferior	C1
	Rotatores brevis	C1–C8
	Rotatores longi	C1–C8
	Longus colli	C2–C6
Neck rotation (muscles contract unilaterally)	Levator scapulae (face moves to same side)	C3–C4 Dorsal scapular
	Splenius cervicis (face moves to same side)	C6–C8
	Iliocostalis cervicis (face moves to same side)	C6–C8
	Longissimus cervicis (face moves to same side)	C6–C8
	Semispinalis cervicis (face moves to same side)	C1–C8
	Multifidus (face moves to opposite side)	C1–C8
	Intertransversarii (face moves to same side)	C1–C8
	Scaleni (face moves to opposite side)	C3–C8
	Sternocleidomastoid (face moves to opposite side)	Accessory C2
	Obliquus capitis inferior (face moves to same side)	C1
	Rotatores brevis (face moves to same side)	C1–C8
	Rotatores longi (face moves to same side)	C1–C8

Adapted from D.J. Magee, 1992, *Orthopedic physical assessment*, 2nd ed. (Philadelphia, PA: W.B. Saunders), 44.

HISTORY

Location of Symptoms

Disc dysfunction: ache and stiffness to neck; a deep ache located along medial border of scapula (Cloward signs)

Spondylosis: bilateral or unilateral cervical ache that may radiate to supraspinous fossa; may complain of sharp pain

Acute nerve root: pain usually worse distally in dermatomal pattern

Chronic nerve root: pain in dermatome distribution (patchy), distal not dominant; intermittent symptoms

Aggravating factors: turning bilaterally, looking up, looking down, sustained flexion (sitting, reading)

Special Questions

Vertebral artery compromise: dizziness, ringing in ears

TESTS AND MEASURES

Standing

Observation

General appearance, affect, visual cues of symptoms

Willingness to move, undressing

Body structure, level of fitness

Posture—sitting and standing (presence of shift, dowager's hump, decreased CS lordosis, increased TS kyphosis)

Changes of body contour (atrophy, swelling, spasm)

Skin (scars and so on)

Functional tests

Sitting, looking up, looking down, turning head to look over shoulder

Implicate and clear shoulder when indicated

Shoulder flexion

Shoulder abduction

Horizontal adduction—hand across chest (HAC)

Hand behind back (HBB)

Static resisted tests for IR, ER, ABD, biceps

Sitting

Active Cervical Movements with overpressure

F = flexion (0–45°)

E = extension (0–45°)

L SB = left side bending (0–45°)

R SB = right side bending (0–45°)

L ROT = left rotation (0–60°)

R ROT = right rotation (0–60°)

Quadrant

When indicated

Correct deformity

Overpressures

Repeated movements

Sustained movements

Vertebral artery testing

Begin neurological examination: C4 myotome

MMT: cervical flexion, extension, side bending, rotation

Supine

Neurodynamic testing (ULNT1, ULNT 2A, ULNT 2B, ULNT3) (See chapter 19)

When indicated

Implicate and clear elbow, wrist, and hand

Neurological exam: C6–T1 myotomes, C5–T1 reflexes, C1–T2 dermatomes

Stability tests

Vertebral artery testing

MMT: deep cervical flexors

Prone

Palpation

Skin (temperature, sweating, skin rolling)

Soft-tissue muscle (upper traps, levator, middle trap), tone, presence of trigger points

Bony alignment (occiput, inion, superior nuchal line, mastoid process, spinous process, facet joints)

PAIVMs

-Central PAIVM

-Unilateral PAIVM

-Manual traction

Clinical Syndromes

With the spine, offering complete guidelines for differential diagnosis is not feasible. The clinician must always keep in mind that any pathology in the upper extremity or lower extremity could be of spinal origin or could have some relationship to spinal dysfunction.

The Clinical Syndromes table on page 59 lists common musculoskeletal disorders of the cervical spine. The clinical responses listed for each disorder represent possible responses rather than absolute responses. Use this table as a guideline to form a hypothesis of the nature of the problem. The patient may exhibit only partial components of a disorder or may be affected by a combination of disorders. This listing does not include all possible disorders. For example, several pathological disorders must be considered. Abbreviated treatment suggestions are included.

Clinical Syndromes

Description	Location and behavior of symptoms	History	Tests and measures, diagnostics	Intervention
FRACTURES				
Fracture of atlas (C1).	Upper cervical: Atlas	Hyperextension force (posterior arch fracture) or axial compression force (burst fracture or Jefferson fracture). These fractures are caused by diving into shallow water headfirst and MVAs.	Plain radiographs (AP open mouth) and CT.	Cervical orthosis, halo traction, screw fixation through the odontoid, or late fusion.
Fracture of the axis (C2).	Upper cervical: axis	Hyperextension force (traumatic spondylolisthesis or hangman's fracture). Typical mechanism of injury is MVA.	Plain radiographs and CT.	Cervical orthosis, halo traction or fusion.
Fracture of the axis (dens).	Upper cervical: axis.	Excessive rotation force.	Plain radiographs (AP open mouth) and CT.	Cervical orthosis, halo traction, screw fixation through the odontoid, or late fusion.
Fractures of C3–C7.	Mid to lower cervical spine	Hyperflexion forces (wedge fracture), axial compression (burst fracture), avulsion force during hyperextension or compressive force during hyperflexion (teardrop fracture).	Plain radiographs (AP, AP open mouth, and lateral views). MRI and CT may be used to determine the degree of spinal canal compromise.	Cervical orthosis, surgery to achieve stabilization (interspinous wiring, bilateral plating, anterior plating and bone grafts). Rehabilitation: restoration of mobility, strength and function.

» continued

» continued

Description	Location and behavior of symptoms	History	Tests and measures, diagnostics	Intervention
WHIPLASH				
Cervical sprains or injuries (hyperflexion or hyper-extension sprains) to the ligaments of the spine; like having many tiny sprained ankles in the neck Pathology: facet joints, discs, muscle, ligaments, cervical vertebrae, brain, meninges, arteries, nervous system	Suboccipital, neck, shoulders, scapulae, back; unilateral or bilateral; frontal HA; retro-orbital pain; facial or throat pain; patches of numbness; subjective laryngeal disturbances; numbness or paresthesia in either UE—patchy or dermatomal.	Acceleration–deceleration injury.	Acute: 24 hours to 1 week; pain is the dominant complaint; cautious or apprehensive active movements of the neck (may need to test in NWB), shoulders or arms may be tolerated. Patient may complain of dizziness with active movements—should be kept to a minimum; palpation deferred, VA testing usually deferred; difficult to perform neuro (check reflexes, Babinski and clonus). Subacute: 1 to 6 weeks; active movement to end range—limited by stiffness and spasm; complete neuro exam; increased complaints of thoracic and lumbar pain (possibly because of inflammation of nervous system); identify hypermobility or hypomobility with PAIVMs or cervical stability tests. Chronic: longer than 6 weeks; symptoms may become intermittent; limited active movements, weak muscles (postural stabilizers); palpation findings, neurodynamic tests performed. Diagnostics: plain radiographs (lateral) reveal a change in the normal lordotic curve. Lateral extension flexion and extension films will reveal joint stability. CT, myelography, and EMG are of no value unless neuro signs are evident.	Acute: Cervical orthoses (soft), modalities, ROM exercises (NWB may be tolerated better), soft tissue massage, rest, ice. Subacute or chronic: mobilize stiff segments as tolerated, muscle stretching, soft-tissue techniques, exercise for strengthening. Medical management: pain medications.

Description	Location and behavior of symptoms	History	Tests and measures, diagnostics	Intervention
CERVICOGENIC HEADACHES (HA)				
Arising from dysfunction of the cervical spine. Differential diagnosis: tension HA, migraine HA, cluster HA.	Dull ache, intermittent shooting pain, moderate to severe intensity. Unilateral—can be bilateral. Frontal, retro-orbital, temporal, occipital, associated with neck pain and stiffness. Associated symptoms: dizziness, nausea, light-headedness, visual disturbances, tinnitus, inability to concentrate, ear pain or fullness. Aggravation: neck movements or sustained head positions. May not know the pattern; stress or tension. Ease: lying down, change in posture, ice, analgesics.	Predisposing factors: poor posture, weak cervical flexors, facet joint arthropathy, cervical joint trauma, joint hypomobility and hypermobility. Episodic or chronic. Trauma (MVA); DJD of UCS joints.	ROM: reduced CS ROM. Neuro: no neuro signs. Soft tissue: tightness in levator scapula, upper trap, suboccipitals, SCM. Palpation: positive signs with PAIVMs. Muscle strength: weak cervical flexors.	Manual therapy: distraction, lower CS and thoracic mobilization or manipulation. Soft-tissue mobilization or muscle stretching. Postural education. Muscle strengthening. Body mechanics or ergonomics. Medical management: occipital nerve block with or without cortisone, biofeedback, NSAIDS, muscle relaxants.

» continued

» continued

Description	Location and behavior of symptoms	History	Tests and measures, diagnostics	Intervention
DISCOGENIC ACUTE DISC AND DEGENERATIVE DISC				
Discogenic acute disc: 20–35 years of age. Degenerative disc: 30–55 years of age.	Cloward sign. Ache or stiffness to neck. +/– distal symptoms if nerve root is involved. Aggravation: extension, rotation toward painful side; ADs can be limited, sitting, driving, and prolonged flexion, and speed of movement.	Not usually associated with incident but may be related to sustained posture. Slow onset or wake with pain. May have history of MVA.	Posture: may have deformity. ROM: CS F limited but not worse movement; ipsilateral CS E, ipsilateral CS ROT, and ipsilateral CS SB limited and painful. Neuro findings: +/–. Palpation: central PAs more comparable than unilateral PAs. Diagnostics: plain radiographs reveal little of diagnostic value. Plain radiographs may reveal previous degenerative changes. Myelography, CT-myelography, and MRI are used to assist in determining treatment or necessity for surgery.	Traction. Modalities. Manual therapy techniques (centrals and unilateral PAIVMs). Ergonomics. Body mechanics. Medical management: pain medication, surgery (rare).
SPONDYLOSIS				
Term used to describe DJD and DDD of the spine. Joint hypomobility and joint hypermobility can contribute to the development of DJD or DDD.	Bilateral or unilateral cervical ache that may radiate to SSF. May complain of sharp pain. Asymptomatic in many cases. Aggravation: sustained flexion, quick movements, EOR movements.	Long history of neck pain. May have history of MVA.	Posture. ROM: may have limited motion with pain (occasionally excessive). Palpation: central and unilateral PAs comparable. Diagnostics: plain radiographs (lateral) reveal decreased height of the disk space, Schmorl's nodes in the vertebral endplates, osteophytes at the uncovertebral joints.	Manual therapy techniques (central and unilaterals PAIVMs). Traction. Muscle stretching. Posture. Ergonomics. Medical management: pain management.

Thoracic Spine

The thoracic spine is a unique region because of the rib articulations present with each thoracic vertebra (figure 5.1*a-b*). The ribs connect the thoracic spine to the sternum, and the cage that is formed houses multiple vital organs including the lungs and heart. Because of the many visceral structures in proximity to the thoracic region, the clinician must recognize visceral pain referral patterns to assist with differential diagnoses. Likewise, many musculoskeletal complaints of thoracic origin may mimic visceral symptoms, so the clinician must be able to perform a complete assessment of this region.

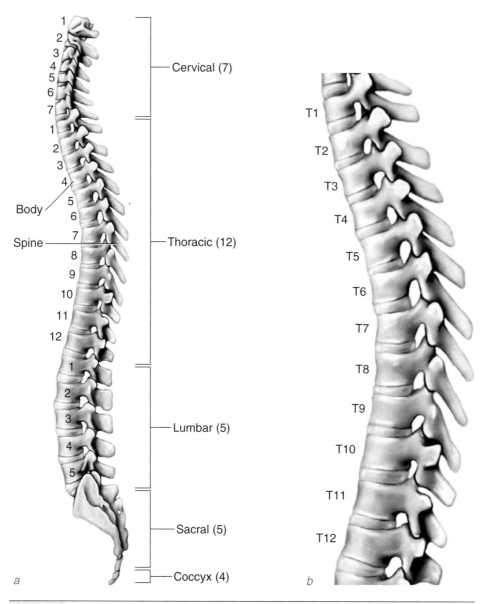

Figure 5.1 Spinal column: (*a*) thoracic vertebrae; (*b*) thoracic vertebrae (lateral view).

Reprinted, by permission, from R. Behnke, *Kinetic anatomy*, 2nd ed. (Champaign, IL: Human Kinetics), 120.

Joint Basics

Articulation   There are two primary types of articulations along the thoracic spine itself: one between the vertebral body and the intervertebral disc and another between the right and left superior articular processes (facets) and the right and left inferior articular processes (facets) of the body above (figure 5.2). Other joints in the thoracic region (considering ribs, costal cartilage, manubrium, and sternum) include the following.

Costotransverse   Convex costal tubercle of rib articulates with concave costal facet on transverse processes of T1–T10; costotransverse joints are not present at T11–T12 because ribs 11 and 12 do not articulate with transverse processes.

Costovertebral   Convex head of rib articulates with two concave demifacets on adjacent thoracic vertebrae; ribs 2–10 fit in this angle created by two demifacets and have some contact with the intervertebral disc; ribs 1, 11, and 12 articulate with one vertebra only.

Costochondral   Ribs 1–7 (true ribs) articulate with costal cartilage.

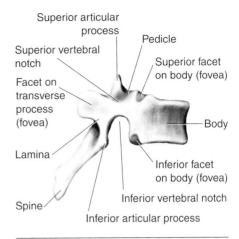

Figure 5.2   Thoracic vertebral segment.

Reprinted, by permission, from R. Behnke, *Kinetic anatomy*, 2nd ed. (Champaign, IL: Human Kinetics), 123.

Chondrosternal   The cartilage articulating with ribs 1–7 in turn articulates with the manubriosternum.

Interchondral   The costal cartilage of ribs 8–10 (false ribs) articulates with the cartilage above them (that of ribs 1–7), thereby attaching them to the sternum with a fused costal cartilage.

Manubriosternal   The manubrium articulates with the sternum.

Xiphisternal   The body of the sternum articulates with the xiphoid process.

Type of Joint   A thoracic spinal segment constitutes a symphysis between the vertebral body and the disc and a plane diarthrodial joint between the superior articular process (facet) of one vertebra and the inferior articular process (facet) of the vertebra above.

> **Costotransverse:** plane synovial
> **Costovertebral:** plane synovial
> **Costochondral:** synchondrosis
> **Chondrosternal:** synovial
> **Interchondral:** synovial
> **Manubriosternal:** synchondrosis
> **Xiphisternal:** synchondrosis

Degrees of Freedom

- Flexion and extension in a sagittal plane about a coronal axis.
- Side bending in a frontal plane about a sagittal axis.
- Rotation in a transverse plane about an axis in the frontal and sagittal planes.

The motions described may occur at any one motion segment; however, because vertebral motion segments function as part of an articular system, motion between any two vertebrae is generally limited to a small amount of translation (or glide) and rotation. Furthermore, because each intervertebral joint functions as part of an articular system, the axis of motion of any given joint changes in response to motion at segments above and below.

Active Range of Motion

The active range of motion includes gross thoracic motion; individual spinal segmental motion cannot be measured except by X ray.

Flexion: 20–45°

Extension: 25–45°

Side bending: 20–40°

Rotation: 35–50°

Costovertebral (Rib Cage) Expansion: 3 to 7.5 cm   Costovertebral expansion is measured by placing a tape measure around the individual's chest at the level of the fourth intercostal space. The measurement process begins by having the patient exhale as much as possible, at which point the initial measurement is made. The patient then inhales maximally, and a second measurement is made. The difference between the two is then noted.

Rib Motion   Rib motion is not quantifiable numerically. The clinician should assess it by placing his or her hands over the patient's upper chest and feeling for anteroposterior rib motion.

- Inspiration: Ribs 1 through 6 elevate and increase anteroposterior diameter (pump-handle motion); ribs 7 through 10 elevate and move laterally to increase lateral dimension (bucket-handle motion).
- Expiration: The reverse of inspiration.

Flexion

Assessment: Segmental forward bending in the thoracic spine.

Patient position: Sitting at the end of the table with the hands behind the neck and the elbows together.

Clinician position: Standing to the side of the patient for AROM. After the patient has achieved the available range of motion (without deviations), the clinician places one hand over the patient's hands (at the cervicothoracic junction) and one hand on the patient's elbows.

Method: The clinician gently applies overpressure into flexion (bowing-like manner) oscillating into the end range.

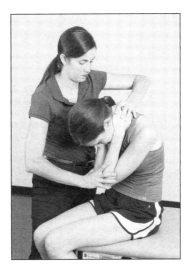

Extension

Assessment: Segmental backward bending in the thoracic spine.

Patient position: Sitting at the end of the table with the hands behind the neck and the elbows together.

Clinician position: Standing to the side of the patient for AROM. After the patient has achieved the available range of motion (without deviations), the clinician places the heel of one hand over the patient's midthoracic spine (fingers pointing downward along posterior thoracic chest wall) and grasps the patient's forearms with the other hand.

Method: The clinician gently applies overpressure into extension oscillating into the end range.

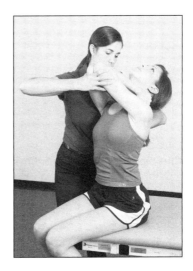

Side Bending

Assessment: Segmental side bending in the thoracic spine.

Patient position: Sitting at the end of the table with the hands crossed over the chest (hands on opposite shoulders) or behind the neck and the elbows together.

Clinician position: Standing in front of the patient for AROM. After the patient has achieved the available range of motion (without deviations), the clinician stands to the left side of the patient and places the left hand on the patient's right shoulder by crossing the arm and forearm over the patient's chest. The clinician places the web space of the right hand with palm side up below the patient's axilla.

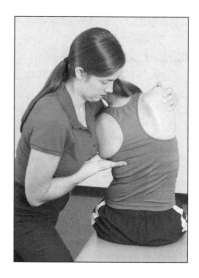

Method: The clinician gently applies overpressure into side bending oscillating into the end range.

Rotation

Assessment: Segmental rotation in thoracic spine.

Patient position: Sitting at the end of the table with the hands crossed over the chest (hands on opposite shoulders).

Clinician position: Standing in front of and to the side of the patient being tested for AROM. After the patient has achieved the available range of motion (without deviations), the clinician, with his or her thighs, blocks the patient's thighs from rotating farther and places both hands on the patient's shoulders.

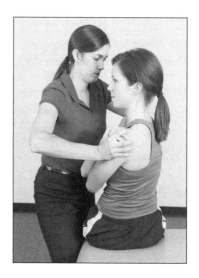

Method: The clinician gently applies overpressure into rotation oscillating into the end range.

Central PAIVM

Assessment: To assess or increase central PA mobility.

Patient position: Lying on the abdomen with the arms by the body or hanging off the edge of the table. Place a pillow under the lower legs for comfort.

Clinician position:

Grade I, II (see figure *a*): The clinician stands on the side of the patient in which the technique is to be performed with thumbs placed longitudinally along the vertebral column so that they point toward each other. The fingers can spread over the posterior chest wall above and below the thumbs. The shoulders are directly over the patient, and the elbows are slightly flexed.

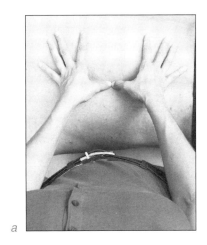

a

Grade III, IV (see figure *b*): The clinician stands on the side of the patient in which the technique is to be performed and places the left or right hand on the patient's back so that the ulnar border of hand (between pisiform and hook of hamate) is in contact with the spinous process of the vertebrae to be mobilized. The shoulders are directly over the patient. The right wrist is fully extended with the forearm midway between supination and pronation. The right hand is reinforced with the left hand. The elbows are allowed to flex slightly.

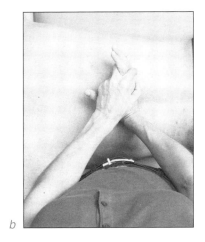

b

Method: The clinician applies a posterior-to-anterior force on the spinous process being examined. Perform three passes. Apply first pressures gently; increase amplitude and depth of the movement if no pain response occurs. Assess quality of movement through the range and end feel; compare with levels above and below.

Positive response: Movements that reproduce the comparable sign (pain versus resistance versus spasm).

Alternative method: T1–T2 (see figure *c*)—also see description for cervical spine central posteroanterior pressure.

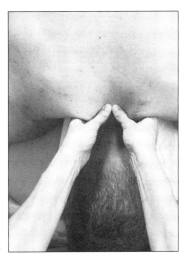

c

Unilateral PAIVM

Assessment: To assess or increase unilateral PA mobility.

Patient position: Lying prone with the arms by the side and the head and legs supported.

Clinician position: The clinician stands on the side of the patient in which the technique is to be performed. Place thumb pads on the back (pointing toward each other) over the transverse process or costotransverse joint. Spread the fingers around the thumbs to provide stability. Position the shoulders above the hands and transmit pressure from the trunk through the arms to the thumbs (the thumb flexors should not be primary movers).

Method (see figure *a*): The clinician applies a posterior-to-anterior force on the articular process being examined. Perform three passes. Apply first pressures gently; increase amplitude and depth of the movement if no pain response occurs. Assess quality of movement through the range and end feel; compare with levels above, below, and to opposite side.

Alternative method: T1–T3—see figure *b* and see description for cervical spine PAs.

Positive response: Movements that reproduce the comparable sign (pain versus resistance versus spasm).

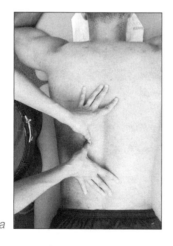
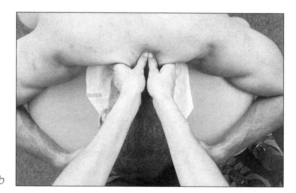

a *b*

Traction

Assessment: To apply vertical distraction and gapping.

Patient position: Sitting with the hands clasped behind the head and the elbows forward for upper thoracic or the arms crossed across the body for lower thoracic.

Clinician position: Standing behind the patient with the knees slightly flexed; arms placed between patient's arms and forearms, grasping onto the forearms for upper thoracic and around patient's arms (above shoulders and grasping forearms) for lower thoracic.

Mobilizing force: Straighten the knees and lean slightly back to provide traction force.

Transverse Pressure

Assessment: To assess or increase rotation.

Patient position: The patient lies prone with the arms by the side and the head and legs supported.

Clinician position: Standing on the left side of the patient in a walk-stance position. The table height is near groin level. The clinician takes up a small amount of soft tissue with the distal phalanx of the right thumb against the side of the spinous process being examined using forearm pronation (see figure *a*). The rest of the fingers of the left hand are comfortably resting on the patient's posterior chest wall. The left thumb is placed on the thumbnail of the right thumb, forming a right angle. The rest of the fingers of the left hand are in a comfortable cuplike grip.

Method: The clinician applies a lateral force on the spinous process being examined. Movement is produced from the clinician's trunk and arms. The thumb remains in contact with the spinous process so that the movement is localized to the segment (see figure *b*). Apply first pressures gently; increase amplitude and depth of the movement if no pain response occurs. Assess quality of movement through the range and end feel; compare with levels above and below.

Positive response: Movements that reproduce the comparable sign (pain versus resistance versus spasm).

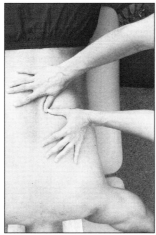
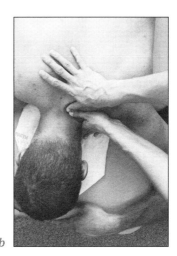

a   *b*

First Rib Mobility

Assessment: Mobility of the first rib.

Patient position: Supine with or without a pillow under the head; arms at the side of the body.

Clinician position: Standing at the head of the bed, the clinician's right hand is placed at the posterior superior aspect of the first rib, under the posterior portion of the upper trapezius.

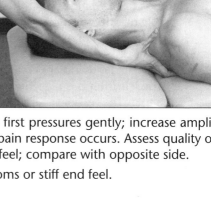

Method: The clinician places an inferior and anterior force to the first rib. Apply first pressures gently; increase amplitude and depth of the movement if no pain response occurs. Assess quality of movement through the range and end feel; compare with opposite side.

Positive response: Reproduction of symptoms or stiff end feel.

Rib Spring

Assessment: Rib mobility.

Patient position: Lying supine with the arms by the side and head supported.

Clinician position: Standing on the side of the patient in which the technique is to be performed. Place the thumb pads (pointing toward each other) over the rib being examined. Spread the fingers around the thumbs to provide stability. Position the shoulders above the hands and transmit pressure from the trunk through the arms to the thumbs (thumb flexors should not be primary movers).

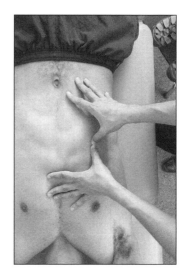

Method: The clinician applies an anterior-to-posterior force on the rib being examined. Perform three passes. Apply first pressures gently; increase amplitude and depth of the movement if no pain response occurs. Assess quality of movement through the range and end feel; compare with levels above and below.

Positive response: Movements that reproduce the comparable sign (pain versus resistance versus spasm).

Rib Screw

Patient position: Lying prone with the arms by the side or hanging over the edge of the table.

Clinician position (see figure *a*): Standing on the side of the patient adjacent to the level being examined (chin directly over the segment being examined). The clinician places the pisiform of the right semicupped hand over the proximal rib (rib 4) and the pisiform of the left semicupped hand on the distal rib (rib 5). The hands and forearms should be parallel to each other and relatively perpendicular to the spine. The wrists are slightly radially deviated.

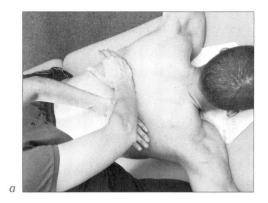

a

Method: The clinician takes up the soft-tissue slack by applying a PA force with a rotatory force such that the hands and forearms change orientation from the start position to face somewhat cephalad and caudad. The right hand moves caudally, and the left hand moves cephalad (see figure *b*). The clinician can repeat the technique in the opposite direction by reversing hands and moving his or her body in the direction of the passes. Perform three passes. Apply first pressures gently; increase amplitude and depth of the movement if no pain response occurs. Assess quality of movement through the range and end feel; compare with levels above and below.

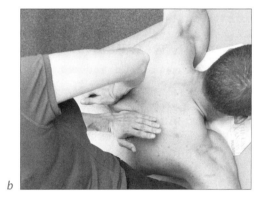

b

Positive response: Movements that reproduce the comparable sign (pain versus resistance versus spasm).

End Feel

Flexion: firm (tension in posterior longitudinal ligament, ligamentum flavum, interspinous ligaments, and facet joint capsules)

Extension: bone on bone; firm because of contact of spinous processes and facets; disc size; tension in anterior longitudinal ligament, joint capsule, and abdominal muscles

Side bending: bone on bone (limited by facets and rib cage)

Rotation: bone on bone (limited structurally by rib cage)

Capsular Pattern

Side bending and rotation limited equally; then extension.

Close-Packed Position

Extension (facets).

Loose-Packed Position

Midway between flexion and extension.

Stability

The ligamentum flavum and the anterior longitudinal ligament are thicker in the thoracic region, thereby enhancing stability there. Facet joint capsule laxity is decreased in the thoracic spine. Decreased flexibility and increased stability is generally present in the thoracic region secondary to structural features such as the presence of ribs, elongated spinous processes, tighter facet capsules, thicker ligamentum flavum, and increased vertebral body dimensions.

Dynamic Stability Test for Posterior Translation in the Thoracic Spine

Assessment: This test stresses the anatomical structures (ligament, capsule, disc, muscle, and so on) that resist posterior translation of a segmental spinal unit.

Patient position: Sitting at end of the table with the hands crossed over the chest (hands on opposite shoulders).

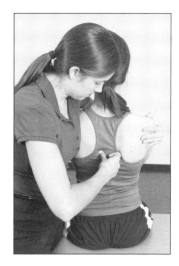

Clinician position: Standing to the left side of the patient. The clinician stabilizes the thorax with the left hand on the patient's right shoulder or scapula by crossing the arm and forearm over the patient's chest. The clinician stabilizes the transverse processes of the inferior vertebra by placing the right hand with the flat posterior surface of the middle phalanx of the second digit on the right transverse process and the pad of the thumb on the left transverse process, forming a "V" with the web space.

Method: Gently resist elevation of the patient's crossed arms (isometric contraction).

Normal response: If the segmental musculature and ligamentous system are able to control the excessive posterior translation, no posterior translation will be felt and the segment is dynamically stable.

Positive response: Reproduction of symptoms and an increase in the quantity of motion observed or palpated by the tester.

Passive Neck Flexion

Assessment: Dural tension.

Patient: Supine; no pillow if tolerable.

Test position: Passively flex the patient's head until encountering resistance or symptoms.

Clinician position: Standing to the patient's side, supporting the head.

Positive response: Resistance encountered before end of range, reproduction of patient's symptoms; note that mild pulling or a stretching sensation in the lower cervical or midthoracic is a normal response.

Thoracic Outlet Tests

Assessment: Compression of the neurovascular bundle at the thoracic outlet; often characterized by compression of any or all of the following: subclavian artery, subclavian vein, brachial plexus.

Positive response: Various tests are performed to target different structures; however, the tests alone should not be used to diagnose but rather to support clinical presentation. During all tests the patient is observed for the following signs: reproduction of symptoms, decreased radial pulse, trophic changes, pallor, cyanosis.

Thoracic Outlet (Inlet) Syndrome Tests: Three-Minute Elevated Arm Test

Assessment: Possible neurovascular compression in the area of the thoracic outlet and inlet.

Patient position: Sitting or standing.

Clinician position: Next to the patient and monitoring symptoms.

Method: The patient abducts both shoulders to 90° and flexes the elbows to 90°. The patient is to maintain this position for three full minutes while opening and closing fists slowly.

Positive response: Inability to complete the task or onset of symptoms.

Thoracic Outlet Test: Hyperabduction Maneuver

Patient position: Sitting.

Clinician position: Maintain upper extremity in abduction and palpate radial pulse.

Test position: The patient's arm is raised overhead in abduction.

Thoracic Outlet (Inlet) Syndrome Tests: Roos Test

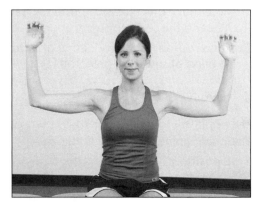

Patient position: Sitting or standing, the patient abducts the arms to 90°, laterally rotates the shoulder, and flexes the elbow to 90° so that the elbows are slightly behind the frontal plane.

Clinician position: Standing in front of the patient.

Method: Instruct the patient to open and close the hands slowly for three minutes.

Positive response: Inability to hold the test position for three minutes or complaints of ischemic pain, heaviness or profound weakness of the arm, or numbness and tingling of the hand.

Arthrokinematics

Flexion   The disc is compressed anteriorly; facets glide cranially.

Extension   The disc is compressed posteriorly; facets glide caudally.

Side Bending   The disc is compressed on the side of the concavity; facets on the side of the concavity glide caudally while those contralateral to concavity glide cranially.

Rotation   The disc undergoes torsion; facets glide relative to one another; direction depends on relative position of spine (i.e., neutral, flexed, extended).

Neurology

There are 12 thoracic nerves on each side of the body. The first 11 lie between the ribs, and the 12th lies below rib 12. These 12 nerves, or intercostal nerves, supply primarily the thoracic and abdominal walls, although the first two thoracic nerves also provide some innervation to the upper limb. Note that the sympathetic ganglia in the thoracic region lie in close proximity to the heads of the ribs.

Surface Palpation

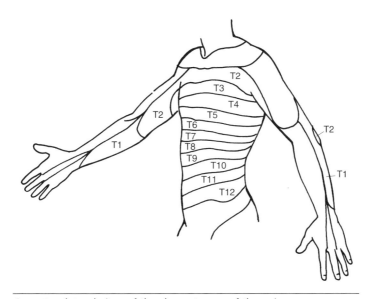

An anterolateral view of the dermatomes of the spine.

Adapted from *Peripheral Nerve Injuries,* 2nd ed., W. Haymaker and B. Woodall, eds., pg. 27. Copyright 1953, with permission from W.B. Saunders.

Anterior chest

Sternum

Manubrium

Body

Xiphoid

Clavicle

Abdominal quadrants

Ribs (anterior and lateral)

Sternocostal cartilages

Costochondral cartilages

Posterior chest

Ribs (posterior and lateral)

Scapulae

Spine (spinous processes, facets, muscles, ligaments)

Muscle Origin and Insertion

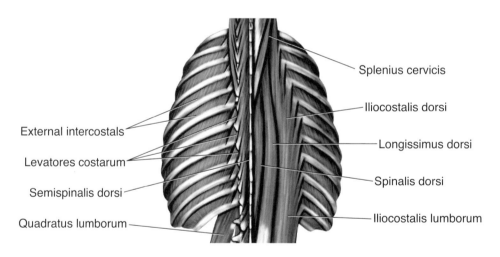

Major muscles of the midback.

Reprinted from R. Behnke, *Kinetic anatomy,* 2nd ed. (Champaign, IL: Human Kinetics), 134.

Muscle	Origin and insertion
External abdominal oblique	Lower 6 ribs to anterior iliac crest, pubis, and linea alba
Internal abdominal oblique	Iliopsoas fascia, anterior iliac crest, and lumbar fascia to lower 3 ribs, xiphoid process, linea alba, and symphysis pubis
Spinalis thoracis	Common tendon of erector spinae and lower thoracic spinous processes to upper thoracic spinous processes
Iliocostalis thoracis	Upper borders of lower 6 ribs to lower borders of upper 6 ribs
Longissimus thoracis	Common tendon of erector spinae to lower 9 or 10 ribs and adjacent transverse processes
Semispinalis thoracis	Transverse processes of thoracic vertebrae to spinous processes of upper thoracic and lower cervical vertebrae
Multifidus	Transverse processes to spinous process from sacrum to C2; each fascicle spanning only 2 to 4 segments
Rotatores	Transverse processes to spinous processes from sacrum to C2; each fascicle spanning only 1 or 2 segments
Interspinalis	Shorter group of rotatores to spinous processes of contiguous vertebrae
Intertransversii	Shorter group of rotatores to transverse processes of contiguous vertebrae
Transversus abdominis	Lower 6 ribs, lumbar fascia, iliac crest, and inguinal ligament to xiphoid process, linea alba, symphysis pubis
Scalenus anterior	Transverse process of C3–C6 to upper surface of first rib (near sternum)
Scalenus medius	Transverse processes of C2–C7 to first rib
Scalenus posterior	Transverse processes of C5–C6 to second rib
Serratus posterior superior	Lower ligamentum nuchae, spinous process of C7–T3 to ribs 2 to 5
Iliocostalis cervicis	Upper 6 ribs to transverse processes of C4–C6
Levatores costarum	Transverse processes of C7–T11 to upper edge of rib below
Pectoralis major	Medial two-thirds of clavicle, sternum, upper 6 ribs to lateral intertubercular groove

» continued

Muscle	Origin and insertion
Pectoralis minor	Ribs 3–5 to coracoid process of scapula
Serratus anterior	Anterolateral ribs 1–8 to costal surface of medial border of scapula
Sternocleidomastoid	Clavicle and sternum to mastoid process
Serratus posterior inferior	Lower 2 thoracic and upper 2 lumbar spinous processes to lower 4 ribs
Iliocostalis lumborum	Iliac crest and sacrum to lower 6 or 7 ribs
Quadratus lumborum	Medial iliac crest and last rib to lumbar transverse processes
Intercostals	Rib to rib all levels
Diaphragm	Inner surfaces of sternum and lower ribs and upper lumbar bodies to central tendon that divides thoracic and abdominal cavities
Latissimus dorsi	Lower 6 thoracic and all lumbar and sacral spinous processes and iliac crest to medial lip of intertubercular groove

Adapted from J. Hamill and K. Knudzen, 1995, *Biomechanical basis of human movement* (Baltimore, MD: Lippincott, Williams, and Wilkins), 498, 506, 509.

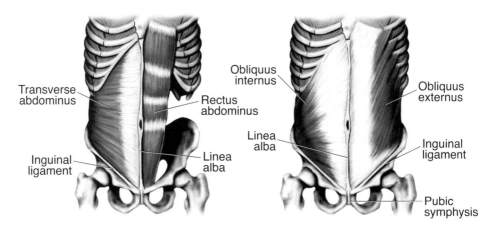

Musculature of the anterolateral abdominal wall.

Reprinted from R. Behnke, *Kinetic anatomy,* 2nd ed. (champaign, IL: Human Kinetics), 132.

Muscle Action and Innervation

Action	Muscle involved	Nerve supply
Thoracic flexion	Rectus abdominis	T6–T12
	External abdominal oblique (bilateral)	T7–T12
	Internal abdominal oblique (bilateral)	T7–T12, L1
Thoracic extension	Spinalis thoracis	T1–T12
	Iliocostalis thoracis (bilateral)	T1–T12
	Longissimus thoracis (bilateral)	T1–T12
	Semispinalis thoracis (bilateral)	T1–T12
	Multifidus (bilateral)	T1–T12
	Rotatores (bilateral)	T1–T12
	Interspinalis	T1–T12
Thoracic rotation and side bending	Iliocostalis thoracis (same side)	T1–T12
	Longissimus thoracis (same side)	T1–T12
	Intertransversii (same side)	T1–T12
	Internal abdominal oblique (same side)	T7–T12, L1
	Semispinalis thoracis (opposite side)	T1–T12
	Multifidus (opposite side)	T1–T12
	Rotatores (opposite side)	T1–T12
	External abdominal oblique (opposite side)	T7–T12
	Transversus abdominis (opposite side)	T7–T12, L1
Rib elevation	Scalenus anterior (1st rib)	C4–C6
	Scalenus medius (1st rib)	C3–C8
	Scalenus posterior (2nd rib)	C6–C8
	Serratus posterior superior (ribs 2–5)	Intercostal 2–5
	Iliocostalis cervicis (ribs 1–6)	C6–C8
	Levatores costarum (all ribs)	T1–T12
	Pectoralis major (arm fixed)	Lateral pectoral (C6–C7)
	Serratus anterior (lower ribs if scapula fixed)	Medial pectoral (C7–C8, T1)
	Pectoralis minor (ribs 2–5 if scapula fixed)	Long thoracic (C5–C7)
	Sternocleidomastoid (if head fixed)	Lateral pectoral (C6–C7)
		Medial pectoral (C7–C8, T1)
		Accessory (C3–C3)
Rib depression	Serratus posterior inferior (lower 4 ribs)	T9–T12
	Iliocostalis lumborum (lower 6 ribs)	L1–L3
	Longissimus thoracis	T1–T12
	Rectus abdominis	T6–T12
	External abdominal oblique (lower 5–6 ribs)	T7–T12
	Internal abdominal oblique (lower 5–6 ribs)	T7–T12, L1
	Transversus abdominis	T7–T12, L1
	Quadratus lumborum (12th rib)	T12, L1–L4
	Transversus thoracis	T1–T12

» continued

Action	Muscle involved	Nerve supply
Rib approximation	Iliocostalis thoracis	T1–T12
	Intercostals (internal and external)	Intercostal 1–11
	Diaphragm	Phrenic
	External intercostals	Intercostal 1–11
	Transverse thoracis (sternocostals)	Intercostal 1–11
	Diaphragm	Phrenic
	Sternocleidomastoid	Accessory (C2–C3)
	Scalenus anterior	C4–C6
	Scalenus medius	C3–C8
	Scalenus posterior	C6–C8
	Pectoralis major	Lateral pectoral (C6–C7)
		Medial pectoral (C7–C8, T1)
	Pectoralis minor	Lateral pectoral (C6–C7)
		Medial pectoral (C7–C8, T1)
	Serratus anterior	Long thoracic (C5–C7)
	Latissimus dorsi	Thoracodorsal (C6–C8)
	Serratus posterior superior	Intercostal 2–5
	Iliocostalis thoracis	T1–T12
Expiration	Internal intercostals	Intercostal 1–11
	Rectus abdominis	T6–T12
	External abdominal oblique	T7–T12
	Internal abdominal oblique	T7–T12, L1
	Iliocostalis lumborum	L1–L3
	Longissimus	T1–L3
	Serratus posterior inferior	T9–T12
	Quadratus lumborum	T12, L1–L4

Reprinted from *Orthopedic Physical Assessment,* 2nd ed., D.J. Magee, pg. 235. Copyright 1992, with permission from W.B. Saunders.

EXAMINATION SEQUENCE

HISTORY

Location of Symptoms

Nerve root: pain that runs posterior to anterior along the line of the rib; sudden shooting pain

Costotransverse joint: horizontal band of pain (posterior to anterior); does not match the rib line; ache

Disc dysfunction: deep central ache with pain piercing through chest; deep ache, sharp or dull, may result in secondary nerve root symptoms

Spondylosis: deep central ache

Postural dysfunction: generalized diffuse dull ache

Lower cervical dysfunction: upper trapezius or supraspinous fossa ache

Spinal facet or costotransverse joint: unilateral posterior pain

Local anterior structures or disc dysfunction: unilateral anterior pain

Manubriosternal joint or thoracic disc: central anterior pain

Other: visceral referral, T-4 pain pattern, sympathetic symptoms

Aggravating Factors

Twisting, sustained flexion, extension (standing up straight), coughing, sneezing, deep breath, sustained overhead arm positions, supine on firm surface, carrying, pushing or pulling

Ease Factors

Resting propped up on pillows, side lying, improving sitting posture (sitting up straight), supporting weight of arms on arm of chair or pillow, lumbar roll, rib belt

24 Hours

Can have pain at night because of need for frequent position changes; red flag—unremitting, prolonged night pain

Special Questions

Prolonged oral steroid use with possible osteoporotic complications

TESTS AND MEASURES

Standing

Observation

Dressing

Body type and structure

Posture (increased TS kyphosis, TS position relative to pelvis and scapulae, lateral deviation, anterior view—anterior ribs and rotation of vertebrae as seen in the rib and sternum)

Changes in body contour (atrophy, swelling, spasm)

Breathing pattern

Willingness to move

Implicate or Clear: Shoulder as Indicated

Functional Tests

Deep breaths

Quick breaths

Any movement to reproduce symptoms

Sitting

Implicate or Clear: Cervical Spine

Active Thorax Movement with Overpressure

F = flexion (0–80°or 4 in. [10 cm])

E = extension (0–25°)

R SB = right side bending (0–35°)

L SB = left side bending (0–35°)

R Rot = right rotation (0–45°)

L Rot = left rotation (0–45°)

Breathing—Palpate Upper, Middle, and Lower Ribs

Stability Test: Posterior Translation in Thoracic Spine

When Indicated

Correct deformity

Overpressure

Repeated movements

Sustained movements

Neurological examination (sensation)

Supine

Peripheral Joint Tests

SIJ

First Rib Mobility

Anterior Chest Palpation

Manubrium

Sternum

Sternomanubrial junction

Sternochondral junctions

Costochondral junctions

Costocartilage

Passive accessory movements of ribs anteriorly, R2–9

Neurological Examination

Sensation

Beevor's sign

MMT

Transverse abdominis

Rectus abdominis

Internal and external oblique

Quadratus lumborum

Side Lying

Scapulothoracic Mobility

Palpation

Skin—temperature, skin rolling, scratch test

Soft tissue

Bony alignment (vertebrae, spinous process [SP], transverse process [TP], costotransverse joint [CTJ])—assess for positional faults and determine whether positional fault or anatomical anomaly exists

-C7

-T2: same level as superior angle of scapula

-T3: same level as spine of scapula

-T7: same level as inferior angle of scapula

-Spinous processes of T1–3: level with the corresponding transverse processes

-Spinous processes of T4–6: half level below its corresponding TP

-Spinous processes of T7–9: one full level below corresponding TP

-Spinous process of T10–12: gradually return to the level of the corresponding TP

Cervical spine palpation as indicated

PAIVMs

-Central PAIVM

-Unilateral PAIVM (TP, CTJ)

-Transverse glide

-Rib screw

MMT

Thoracic extension

Back extension

Clinical Syndromes

With the spine, offering complete guidelines for differential diagnosis is not feasible. The practitioner must always keep in mind that any pathology in the upper extremity or lower extremity could be of spinal origin or could have some relationship to spinal dysfunction.

The Clinical Syndromes table on page 86 lists common musculoskeletal disorders of the thoracic spine. The clinical responses listed for each disorder represent possible responses rather than absolute responses. Use this table as a guideline to form a hypothesis of the nature of the problem. The patient may exhibit only partial components of a disorder or may be affected by a combination of disorders. This listing does not include all possible disorders. For example, several pathological disorders must be considered. Abbreviated treatment suggestions are included.

Clinical Syndromes

Description	Location and behavior of symptoms	History	Tests and measures, diagnostics	Intervention
UPPER RIB CONDITIONS				
Usually relates to elevation of the ribs or thoracic outlet syndrome.	Upper-extremity symptoms of numbness and tingling, pain, or vascular symptoms.	The patient is typically an open-mouth breather because of allergies, deviated septum, and forward head.	Stiff elevated first or second ribs. Diagnostics: X rays may reveal the presence of a cervical rib.	Intervention aimed at treating the dysfunction and not the diagnosis will result in success with most of these patients. Surgical management: resection of cervical rib.
FLATTENED UPPER THORACIC SPINE				
May be related to increased tension in the nervous system of the thoracic region.	Has been associated with intractable head, neck, shoulder girdle, arm, and rib joint pain.	Long history of mid-back pain.	The C7–T1 segments can be quite stiff with variable mobility in the flattened section of the thoracic spine. Diagnostics: X rays: lateral view shows flattened or lordotic thoracic curve.	This condition is somewhat resistant to treatment; changing the contour of the flattened curve is difficult. As the therapist selects treatment, it is important to think of positions and movements to unload the joints from the close-packed extension.
CHRONIC GENERALIZED UPPER THORACIC STIFFNESS				
The patient is typically a middle-aged woman.	Generalized tightness and pain at the CT junction.	Work history of prolonged positions (typing, computer work, surgeon).	The upper thoracic region is stiff, hardened, and forward-curved. The upper rib joints are typically fixed. Limited upper-extremity movement and muscle imbalances are present.	Cervicothoracic junction mobilization, thoracolumbar mobilization and exercises.

Description	Location and behavior of symptoms	History	Tests and measures, diagnostics	Intervention
UPPER OR MIDTHORACIC SPONDYLOSIS				
With stiffness T4 syndrome	T4 syndrome, an uncommon variation, can include unilateral or bilateral glove paresthesia of the upper limbs, generalized headache, and joint abnormalities in segments ranging from T2 to T6.	History of microtrauma or macrotrauma to upper to midthoracic spine.	Stiffness or stiffness combined with hypermobility of adjacent segments characterizes this condition.	Central PAs. Indirect treatment for rotation of the spine to influence the sympathetic nervous system.
With hypermobility	The hypermobile patient will complain of interscapular pain. Pain that worsens with prolonged positioning (patients feel as if they need to change positions frequently), pain with upper-limb movement or lifting, and a history of trauma (vomiting, childbirth).	History of trauma (MVA or falls) or microtrauma (gymnast or ballet dancer).	Hypermobility and stiffness occur frequently in adjacent segments.	Spinal stabilization training, strengthening, mobilization of hypomobile adjacent segments.
COSTAL JOINT DERANGEMENT				
	Breathing is often painful in some portion of the inhalation or exhalation phase.	Acute onset caused by trunk twisting or reaching.	Pain with unilateral palpation over CTJ or with trunk rotation, limited rib excursion during breathing, stiffness with rib mobility testing.	Joint mobilization. Retrain breathing patterns. If acute, limit trunk movement with tape. If chronic, exercise to encourage mobility.

» continued

» continued

Description	Location and behavior of symptoms	History	Tests and measures, diagnostics	Intervention
ACUTE LUMBAR PAIN OF THORACIC ORIGIN				
Maigne (in *Greive's Common Vertebral Joint Problems*) suggests these lower thoracic and upper lumbar facet changes can represent 60% of acute and chronic back-ache and coexist with primary lumbar dysfunc-tion in another 20% of the cases. Positive signs from these levels carry less weight if careful exam of the lumbar spine shows frank lumbar or L-S signs. (These thoracic levels also refer to the anterior and lateral abdominal walls.)	T9 to L2 facet lesions can refer pain unilaterally to the low back and upper buttock region.		Posture: long trunk in com-parison to body height, at times a low thoracic kyphosis and an ectomorphic body type. Positive palpation responses at the thoracic spine or reproduction of symptoms at the lumbar pain with AROM.	Mobilization to the TL junction: transverse glides and unilateral PAs. Exercises to improve mobil-ity of TL junction and strength of trunk stabiliz-ers and prime movers.
THORACIC DISC LESIONS				
UMN or LMN signs can be present, but bowel or blad-der disturbance is not common. Disc lesions are more common at the T7, T8, and T9 levels.	Pain may shoot directly through the chest wall or around the chest wall. Any movement, even breathing, can exacer-bate pain. Pain can increase with cough or sneeze.	If the patient is young, history usu-ally includes a forceful injury. The onset can be insidious in older patients (because of degenerative changes).	Reproduction of symptoms with palpation responses or AROM. Trunk rotation or deep or sudden breath repro-duce symptoms. Positive Beevor's sign on abdomi-nal reflex test-ing.	Grade I mobilization—central PAs, transverse, distraction. Postural and positional instruction. Tape to avoid prevocational positions.

Description	Location and behavior of symptoms	History	Tests and measures, diagnostics	Intervention
SCAPULOCOSTAL SYNDROME				
	Noise or crepitus when the scapula is moved on the rib cage.	Has been hypothesized to be due to soft tissue fasciculi in the interscapular region or scapulothoracic soft tissue. The etiology is unknown.	Posture—increased thoracic kyphosis, forward shoulders, abducted scapulae with weak or lengthened interscapular musculature.	Soft-tissue treatment and treat related muscle imbalances, trunk mobility.
TIETZE'S SYNDROME				
Inflammation of the costosternal junction, usually unilateral on the second rib.	Anterior chest pain, local and superficial, is worse with breathing and with trunk twisting.	It has been suggested that a rib or vertebral lesion posteriorly could precipitate this condition or a history of repetitive or acute overloading of the rib cage.	Pain, tenderness, and swelling over the costosternal junction—second rib most common. Posterior rib lesion is possible. Abnormal breathing pattern because of pain.	Treat posterior rib lesion, train in proper breathing technique.
CHRONIC ANTERIOR CHEST WALL PAIN				
	Continuous but varying in intensity, without radiation to the neck or upper limb. Pain is more severe in the sternal region and no sympathetic or cardiac symptoms are present. Chest wall pain does not respond to glycerin.	Possible chronic condition occurs in patients over 45 and post-cardiac artery occlusion. Patient able to differentiate pain with cardiac pain.	Pain in chest wall, more in sternal region, not r adiating to the jaw, neck or arms. Absence of cardiac symptoms (vasomotor changes, blood counts, pain does not respond to nitroglycerin). Diagnostics: EKG, chest wall pain relieved with corticosteroid injection.	Treatment of somatic changes because of visceral referral and viscerosomatic relationship.

» continued

Description	Location and behavior of symptoms	History	Tests and measures, diagnostics	Intervention
ANKYLOSING SPONDYLITIS				
	Pain usually starts in pelvis and migrates up the spine. After fusion occurs, the pain decreases.	More common in young men, gradual onset of progressive stiffness. Peripheral joint involvement more prevalent in females.	The ability to side bend the spine is markedly restricted, limited chest excursion. Diagnostics: X ray: reveal early sacroiliitis, positive bone scan.	Exercises to maintain thoracic mobility and promote active lifestyle.
OSTEOPOROSIS				
	Compression fractures more likely in T-L junction with resultant wedging and increased kyphosis.	Elderly females or those with chronic use of corticosteroids.	Can be symptomless. Usually increased kyphosis with overall loss of height in advanced cases. Diagnostics: X ray (bone loss only when greater than 35%), bone density scan.	Exercises to restore postural muscle imbalances, weight-bearing exercise, strength training.
SCHEUERMANN'S DISEASE				
	Symptoms usually worsen as the day goes on (symptoms are more time dependent than position dependent).	Schmorl's nodes develop (vertebral endplate fractures—vertebral osteochondrosis) in the thoracic or the lumbar vertebrae. Also known as juvenile arthritic kyphoscoliosis or vertebral osteochondrosis.	Usually a marked thoracic kyphosis because of pathology of the vertebral bodies and the disc, not because of poor posture. The deformity will progress until skeletal maturity is reached. When the T-L junction is involved, the T-L and midlumbar segments become quite stiff and appear flat, whereas the more mobile lumbosacral junction becomes painful.	Exercises to improve mobility of TL junction, instruction in back care and body mechanics.

Lumbar Spine

This chapter addresses the lumbar spine (figure 6.1, *a-b*). Low back pain is one of the most common complaints of patients who present to physical therapy. Therefore, the clinician must be able to perform a thorough assessment of the area and differentiate the origin of various spinal pathologies. The clinician should also be suspicious of lumbar involvement whenever a patient complains of lower-extremity pain, tingling, or weakness of unknown etiology. The spine is often overlooked in these cases, but when it is correctly identified as the problem source, it may be very responsive to physical therapy interventions.

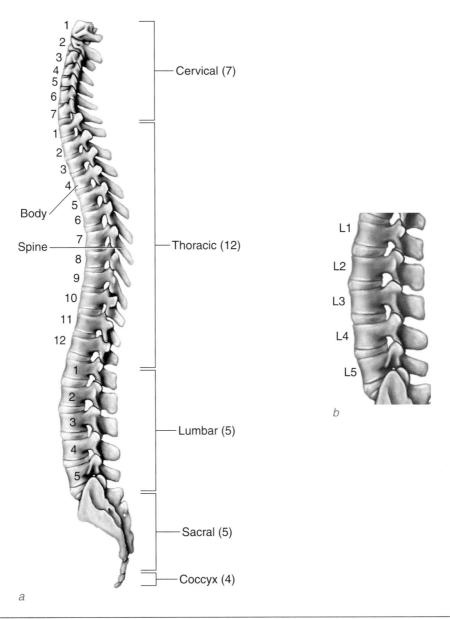

Figure 6.1 (*a*) Lumbar vertebrae; (*b*) lumbar vertebrae (lateral view).

Reprinted, by permission, from R. Behnke, *Kinetic anatomy*, 2nd ed. (Champaign, IL: Human Kinetics), 120.

Joint Basics

Articulation   Two primary types of articulations are present along the lumbar spine: one between the vertebral body and the intervertebral disc and the other between the right and left superior facets and the right and left inferior facets of the body above. The lumbar region contains five pairs of facets. The facets from L1 to L4 are oriented primarily in the sagittal plane, with the concave superior facets facing medially and posteriorly and the convex inferior facets directed anteriorly and laterally. The facets at L5 shift their orientation primarily to the frontal plane, and they are more widely spaced than those of the lumbar vertebrae above.

Type of Joint   A lumbar spinal segment constitutes a cartilaginous joint between the vertebral body and the disc and a plane diarthrodial joint between the superior articular process (facet) of one vertebra and the inferior articular process (facet) of the vertebra above.

Degrees of Freedom

- Flexion and extension in a sagittal plane about a coronal axis
- Side bending in a frontal plane about a sagittal axis
- Rotation in a transverse plane about an axis in the frontal and sagittal planes

These motions may occur at any one motion segment, but because vertebral motion segments function as part of an articular system, motion between any two vertebrae is generally limited to a small amount of translation (or glide) and rotation. Furthermore, because each intervertebral joint functions as part of an articular system, the axis of motion of any given joint changes in response to motion at segments above and below.

Active Range of Motion

Individual spinal segmental motion cannot be measured except by X ray. The L1–L4 facet orientation is such that rotation and side bending are more limited and flexion and extension are more available. Of the latter two, flexion is typically more limited in the lumbar region. The exception is at the L5–S1 articulation, which has little to no rotation but constitutes most of the flexion in the lumbar region.

Flexion: 40–60°

Extension: 20–35°

Rotation: 3–18°

Side Bending: 15–20°

Flexion

Assessment: Segmental forward bending in the lumbar spine.

Patient position: Standing with the arms at the side and the knees straight.

Clinician position: Standing behind the patient for AROM. After the patient has achieved the available range of motion (without deviations), the clinician stands in a squat-stance position on the side of the patient and places the palmar side of one hand and forearm across the patient's shoulders and upper thoracic spine and the other hand and forearm across the patient's pelvis and SI.

Method: Gently apply overpressure into flexion (in a bowing manner) oscillating into the end range.

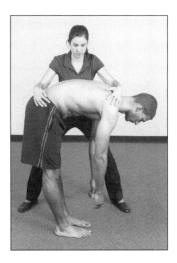

Extension

Assessment: Segmental backward bending in the lumbar spine.

Patient position: Standing with the arms at the side and the knees straight.

Clinician position: Standing behind the patient for AROM. After the patient has achieved the available range of motion (without deviations), the clinician stands to the side of the patient in a squat-stance position with the lead foot perpendicular to the patient's heels. The clinician then places one hand over the patient's anterior shoulders (to support the patient for the overpressure that will be given) and the other hand (the middle phalanx of the second metacarpal) on lumbosacral area.

Method: Gently apply overpressure into extension oscillating into the end range.

Alternative method: Patient's arms crossed over the chest.

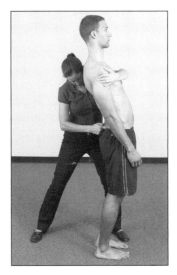

Rotation

Assessment: Segmental rotation in the lumbar spine.

Patient position: Prone.

Clinician position: Standing at the patient's side with one hand at the patient's opposite iliac crest and the other hand palpating the interspinous space at the desired level. The clinician palpates motion of the spinous process above relative to the spinous process below.

Side Bending

Assessment: Segmental side bending in the lumbar spine.

Patient position: Standing with the arms at the sides and the knees straight.

Clinician position: Standing behind the patient for AROM (the clinician should have the patient perform both left and right side bending AROM before applying overpressure, observing any deviations and correcting if appropriate). After the patient has achieved the available range of motion (without deviations), the clinician blocks the patient's left foot by placing his or her left foot on the outside of the patient's left foot. The clinician places his or her hands on the patient's shoulders.

Method: Gently apply overpressure into right side bending (in the direction of the patient's iliac crest) oscillating into the end range.

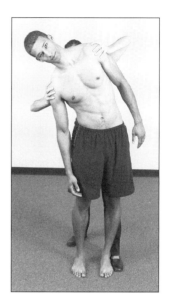

Combined Movements: Extension and Rotation (Quadrant)

Patient position: Standing.

Clinician position: Standing behind the patient.

Method: The clinician instructs the patient to keep the knees straight, bend backward, and maintain balance (lumbar extension). Then the clinician instructs the patient to drop the shoulder (see figure *a*), combining movements of lumbar extension, side bending, and rotation. The clinician then applies overpressure if appropriate (see figure *b*).

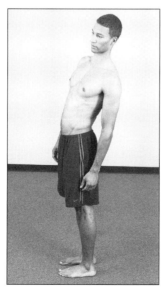
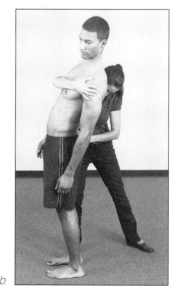

a   *b*

Central PAIVM

Assessment: To assess or increase central PA mobility.

Patient position: Lying on abdomen with the arms by the body or hanging off the edge of the table. Place a pillow under the lower legs for comfort.

Clinician position:

Grade I, II: The clinician stands at left or right side of the patient with the thumbs placed longitudinally along the vertebral column so that they point toward each other. The fingers can spread over the posterior chest wall above and below the thumbs. The shoulders are directly over the patient, and the elbows are slightly flexed (see figure *a*).

Grade III, IV: The clinician stands at the left or right side of the patient and places the right (or left) hand on the patient's back so that the ulnar border of the hand (between pisiform and hook of hamate) is in contact with the spinous process of the vertebrae to be mobilized. The shoulders are directly over the patient. The right wrist is fully extended with the forearm midway between supination and pronation. The right hand is reinforced with the left hand. The elbows are allowed to flex slightly (see figure *b*).

Method: The clinician applies a posterior-to-anterior force on each spinous process being examined. Perform three passes. Apply first pressures gently; increase amplitude and depth of the movement if no pain response occurs. Assess quality of movement through the range and end feel; compare with levels above and below.

Positive response: Movements that reproduce the comparable sign (pain versus resistance versus spasm).

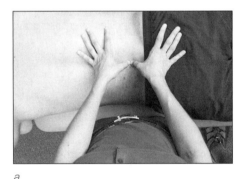

a

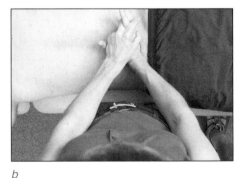

b

Unilateral PAIVM

Assessment: To assess or increase unilateral PA mobility.

Patient position: Lying prone with the arms by the sides and the head and legs supported.

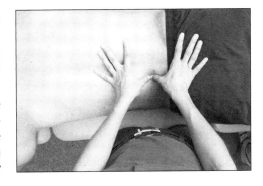

Clinician position: Standing on the side of the patient in which the technique is to be performed. Place the thumb pads on the back (pointing toward each other), immediately adjacent to the spinous process. Spread the fingers around the thumbs to provide stability. Position the shoulders above the hands and transmit pressure from the trunk through the arms to the thumbs (thumb flexors should not be primary movers).

Method: The clinician applies a posterior-to-anterior force on each articular process being examined. Perform three passes. Apply first pressures gently; increase amplitude and depth of the movement if no pain response occurs. Assess the quality of movement through the range and end feel; compare with levels above, below, and to the opposite side.

Positive response: Movements that reproduce the comparable sign (pain versus resistance versus spasm).

Rotation

Patient position:

Grade I, II: Lying on left side (painless side) with pillows supporting the head, in a position of comfort.

Grade III, IV (general): Lying on left side (painless side). The clinician positions the patient's left leg in a slightly flexed position at the hip in relation to the trunk with the knee in extension and the medial tibial condyle resting just beyond the table. The patient's right leg is positioned so that the hip and knee are flexed and the ankle is hooked in the popliteal fossa of the left leg.

Clinician position:

Grade I, II: The clinician stands behind the patient and places both hands on the patient's pelvis (see figure *a*).

Grade III, IV (general): The clinician flexes the patient's trunk and rotates the patient's thorax to the right by lifting the patient's left arm toward the ceiling so that the chest faces upward. The clinician kneels on the table with the right knee behind the patient and the left hand on the head of the humerus with the fingers spreading forward over the pectoral muscles and the right hand over the patient's pelvis (see figure *b*).

Method:

Grade I, II: Apply small oscillatory movements with both hands; apply no counter pressure to prevent thoracic movement.

Grade III, IV: Apply oscillatory movements with the right hand through the pelvis.

Alternative method: Localized to a specific level.

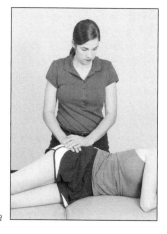
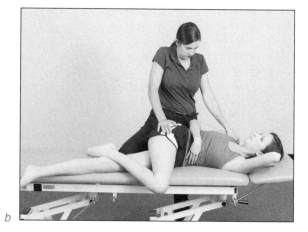

a *b*

Transverse Pressure

Assessment: To assess or increase rotation.

Patient position: Prone.

Clinician position: At patient's side to be mobilized. The thumb pads are adjacent to the spinous process on the same side.

Method: Apply transverse pressure (perpendicular to spinous processes) away from the clinician's body (see thoracic spine description for transverse pressure on page 71).

Traction

Assessment: To unload spinal segments.

Patient position: Lying on side of comfort (right) with the hips and knees flexed to allow the lumbar spine to relax midway between flexion and extension. May need to use a towel roll under the lumbar spine to prevent it from sagging into lateral flexion.

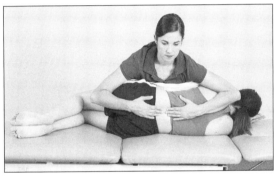

a

Clinician position: Standing in front of patient resting her or his lower ribs against the side of the patient. The clinician places the left forearm, pointing caudad, along the spine. The clinician's right forearm grasps around the pelvis under the ischial tuberosity. Place the pad of the index or middle fingers at the desired level's interspinous space (see figure *a*).

Method: Use body weight to apply longitudinal force inferiorly. Assess the results of a lighter pull before increasing. Monitor the patient's symptoms.

Alternative method: Manual lumbar traction—hook lying (see figure *b*).

The patient lies on his or her back with a pillow under the head and the knees bent. The clinician can kneel on the end of the table or stand at the end of the table. The clinician places a mobilization

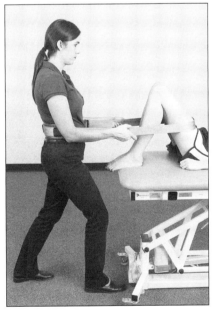

b

belt (also effective using a sheet) around his or her own waist and the patient's thighs. The clinician gently pulls back away from the patient.

End Feel

Flexion: firm (tension in posterior longitudinal ligament, ligamentum flavum, interspinous ligaments, and facet joint capsules)

Extension: bone on bone, firm (contact of spinous processes, facets, disc size, tension in anterior longitudinal ligament, joint capsule, and abdominal muscles)

Side bending: firm (facet approximation, rib cage, joint capsule tension)

Rotation: firm (impact of articular processes, intertransverse ligaments)

Capsular Pattern

Side bending and rotation limited equally (may be to same or opposite sides, depending on segmental level); then extension.

Close-Packed Position

Extension (facets).

Loose-Packed Position

Midway between flexion and extension.

Stability

Together, the following ligaments in the lumbar spine contribute to overall stability:

1. The anterior longitudinal ligament attaches anteriorly from the vertebral body above to the vertebral body below.
2. The posterior longitudinal ligament attaches posteriorly from bony rim to bony rim with some attachments to the disc as well.
3. The ligamentum flavum lamina to lamina with attachments to facet capsule.
4. The interspinous runs between spinous processes.
5. The supraspinous runs superiorly along spinous processes.
6. The iliolumbar ligament runs from transverse processes of L4 and L5 to iliac crests; it is composed of five bands—anterior, posterior, superior, inferior, and vertical. This broad, strong ligament helps stabilize the fifth lumbar vertebra on the sacrum (prevent anterior displacement). This ligament is present only in adults and is thought to develop from the lower fibers of the quadratus lumborum as a result of age-related changes and stress associated with upright posture and ambulation.
7. The thoracolumbar fascia surrounds the muscles of the lumbar spine; it is composed of three layers—anterior, middle, and posterior. The anterior layer, or passive layer, is a thin layer thought to be derived from the fascia of the quadratus lumborum. The middle layer lies posterior to the quadratus lumborum. The posterior, or active, layer is a fascial layer that fuses with the transversus abdominis, thereby providing an indirect attachment for this muscle to the lumbar vertebrae by the spinous processes. Tension in the fascia is thus transmitted to the spinous processes of L1–L4 and may assist the spinal extensor musculature in resisting an applied load.

The annulus, facet joint capsules, facet structural configurations, and increased disc and vertebral body size in the lumbar region all contribute to stability.

Lumbar Anterior Stability Test

Rationale: This test is performed to confirm the subjective information of possible hypermobility or instability. This test is used primarily to stress the integrity of the supraspinous ligament.

Patient position: The patient is positioned in side lying; the knees and hips are passively drawn up into flexion by palpating intersegmental motion.

Clinician position and procedure: The clinician stands in front of the patient, flexing the patient's knees with the caudal hand and palpating intersegmental motion with the cranial hand. After achieving neutral range of the desired segment, the clinician allows the patient's knees to rest on his or her thighs (see figure *a*).

The upper spinous process is fixed using the index and middle finger of the cranial hand and further stabilized by placing the other hand over it. The inferior interspinous space is palpated with the ring finger, leaving the small finger over the inferior spinous process. This set allows the clinician to sense the mobility and end feel of the segment through the interspinous space and inferior spinous process (see figure *b*).

Method: To stress the segment, the clinician pushes with his or her thighs, through the patient's knees, along the line of the femur. The position is held for about 15 seconds or until an end feel is achieved or until the patient reports reproduction of cord symptoms. At least three segments (segment above and below the desired level) should be assessed to compare the results. Note that some movement is expected because the segment is being stressed in its neutral range (middle range of its flexion and extension).

Responses: Positive responses may include pain, muscle spasms, increased mobility, lack of firm end feel, and crepitation, in a severe case. The determination of a positive instability is based on the judgment of the clinician, increase in motion compared with the other segment, and signs or symptoms associated with the stress test.

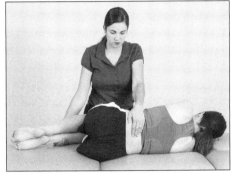

a

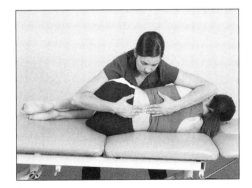

b

Babinski

Assessment: Upper motor neuron lesion.

Patient position: Supine and relaxed.

Clinician position: Standing alongside the patient toward the feet.

Method: Use the thumb or handle of a reflex hammer; apply a swift stroke along the plantar surface of the foot, moving from the heel along the lateral surface and then crossing the ball of the foot.

Positive response: Great toe extension, possibly with splaying of other toes into abduction.

Shift Assessment

Assessment: Possible disc or root involvement; the patient tends to shift away from the painful side as a protective mechanism. Standing; may be further assessed in supine position.

Clinician position: Standing behind the patient.

Method: View position of the shoulders in relation to the pelvis.

Positive response: If the shoulders are shifted to one side of the pelvis, then shift is present; shift is named by the side that the shoulders are leaning toward.

Shift Correction

Assessment: Provides information about whether the patient will tolerate attempts at correcting shift.

Patient position: Standing; may also be done in supine or prone position, depending on patient comfort.

Clinician position: Standing alongside the patient.

Method: Stance—place one hand at the patient's shoulders on the side that the patient is shifted toward; place the other hand on the patient's pelvis on the opposite side. Gently attempt to bring the shoulders and pelvis in line with one another. Supine or prone, place the hands at the patient's hips. Gently lift the patient's hips and slide in an attempt to bring the hips in line with the shoulders.

Positive response: If the patient can tolerate the position, then shift-correcting activities can and should be encouraged. If the patient cannot tolerate the position (either markedly increased back pain or reproduction or increase of peripheral symptoms), then shift-correcting activities should not be promoted at this time.

Arthrokinematics

Flexion   The disc is compressed anteriorly; facets glide cranially.

Extension   The disc is compressed posteriorly; facets glide caudally.

Side Bending   The disc is compressed on the side of the concavity; facets on the side of the concavity glide caudally, whereas those contralateral to concavity glide cranially.

Rotation   The disc undergoes torsion; facets glide relative to one another; direction depends on the relative position of the spine (neutral, flexed, extended).

Neurology

Nerve root	Reflex	Motor	Sensory
L1			Inguinal region
L2		Hip flexors	Proximal anterior thigh
L3		Quadriceps	Middle anteromedial and thigh
L4	Patellar tendon	Tibialis anterior	Anteromedial thigh and knee
L5	Medial hamstring	Extensor hallucis longus, extensor digitorum	Lateral thigh, leg, dorsum of foot
S1	Achilles	Peroneals and hamstrings	Lateral foot
S2		Toe flexors	Sole of foot

Surface Palpation

Posterior
Lumbar spinous process
Lumbar facets, transverse processes
Sacral spine
Iliac crest
Posterior superior iliac spine
Coccyx
Ischial tuberosity
Sciatic nerve
Piriformis
Supraspinous ligament
Paraspinal muscles
Inferior lateral angles
Sacral sulcus

Anterior
Abdominal quadrants
Inguinal region
Iliac crest
Anterior superior iliac spine
Symphysis pubis
Greater trochanter

Muscle Origin and Insertion

Muscle	Origin and insertion
Psoas major	Anterolateral aspect of lumbar vertebral bodies and transverse processes to below lesser trochanter
Rectus abdominis	Pubis to sternum and lower costal cartilages
External abdominal oblique	Lower six ribs to anterior iliac crest, pubis, and linea alba
Internal abdominal oblique	Iliopsoas fascia, anterior iliac crest, and lumbar fascia to lower three ribs, xiphoid process, linea alba, and symphysis pubis
Transversus abdominis	Lower six ribs, lumbar fascia, iliac crest, and inguinal ligament to xiphoid process, linea alba, symphysis pubis
Latissimus dorsi	Lower six thoracic and all lumbar and sacral spinous processes and iliac crest to medial lip of intertubercular groove
Erector spinae	Posterior surface of sacrum, iliac crest, and spinous processes of lumbar and last two thoracic vertebrae to all vertebrae and skull via three divisions
Transversospinalis	Rotator muscles from sacrum to C2; run transverse process to spinous process varying from one or two segments to two through four segments
Interspinales	Transverse processes to spinous processes from sacrum to C2; each fascicle spanning only one or two segments
Quadratus lumborum	Medial iliac crest and last rib to lumbar transverse processes
Intertransversarii	Transverse processes to spinous processes from sacrum to C2; each fascicle spanning only one or two segments

Based on J. Hamill and K. Knudzen, 1995, *Biomechanical basis of human movement* (Baltimore, MD: Lippincott, Williams, and Wilkins).

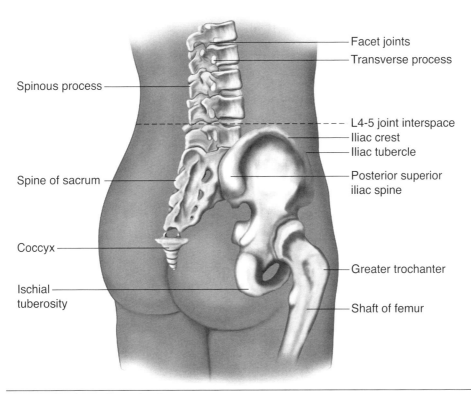

Facet joints
Transverse process
Spinous process
L4-5 joint interspace
Iliac crest
Iliac tubercle
Spine of sacrum
Posterior superior
iliac spine
Coccyx
Greater trochanter
Ischial
tuberosity
Shaft of femur

Posterior lumbar spine palpation.

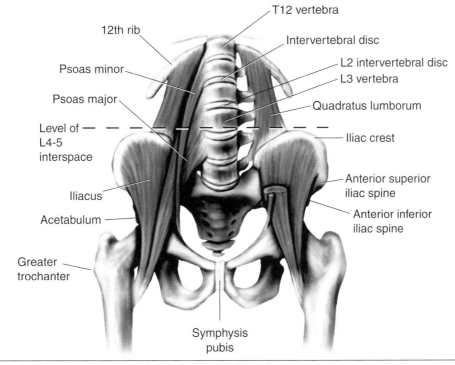

T12 vertebra
12th rib
Intervertebral disc
Psoas minor
L2 intervertebral disc
L3 vertebra
Psoas major
Quadratus lumborum
Level of
L4-5
interspace
Iliac crest
Iliacus
Anterior superior
iliac spine
Acetabulum
Anterior inferior
iliac spine
Greater
trochanter
Symphysis
pubis

Anterior view of the bony landmarks of the lumbar spine.

Reprinted, by permission, from R. Behnke, *Kinetic anatomy*, 2nd ed. (Champaign, IL: Human Kinetics), 178.

Muscle Action and Innervation

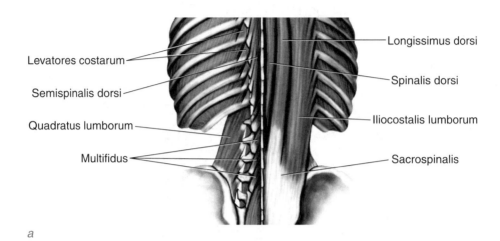

Levatores costarum

Semispinalis dorsi

Quadratus lumborum

Multifidus

Longissimus dorsi

Spinalis dorsi

Iliocostalis lumborum

Sacrospinalis

a

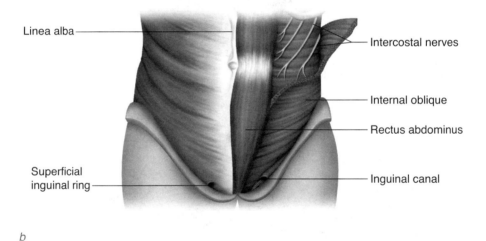

Linea alba

Superficial
inguinal ring

Intercostal nerves

Internal oblique

Rectus abdominus

Inguinal canal

b

(a) Major muscles of the back; (b) musculature of the anterolateral abdominal wall.

Reprinted, by permission, from R. Behnke, *Kinetic anatomy*, 2nd ed. (Champaign, IL: Human Kinetics), 134, 132.

Action	Muscle involved	Nerve supply
Forward bending	Psoas major	L1–L3
	Rectus abdominis	T6–T12
	External abdominal oblique	T7–T12
	Internal abdominal oblique	T7–T12, L1
	Transversus abdominis	T7–T12, L1
Backward bending	Latissimus dorsi	Thoracodorsal (C6–C8)
	Erector spinae	L1–L3
	Transversospinalis	L1–L5
	Interspinalis	L1–L5
	Quadratus lumborum	T12, L1–L4
Side bending	Latissimus dorsi	C6–C8
	Erector spinae	L1–L3
	Transversospinalis	L1–L5
	Interspinales	L1–L5
	Quadratus lumborum	T12, L1–L4
	Psoas major	L1–L3
	External abdominal oblique	T7–T12

Adapted from *Orthopedic Physical Assessment*, 2nd ed., D.J. Magee, Copyright 1992, with permission from W. B. Saunders.

EXAMINATION SEQUENCE

HISTORY

Aggravating Factors

Sitting, sitting to standing, standing, walking, lying, squatting, bending, half bending, maneuvers to unload spine, coughing

24 Hours

Always ask about pain and stiffness in the morning.

History

Mechanism of injury, progression of injury, previous episodes of injury

TESTS AND MEASURES

Standing

Observation

General appearance, affect, visual cues of symptoms

Willingness to move, gait, undressing

Body structure, level of fitness

Posture (shift correction if appropriate)

Changes of body contour (atrophy, swelling, spasm)

Skin (scars and so forth)

Functional Tests

AROM: Lumbar Spine

F = Flexion (0–80° or 4 in. [10 cm])

E = Extension (0–25°)

L SB = Left side bending (0–35°)

R SB = Right side bending (0–35°)

Quadrant

When Indicated

Correct deformity where it occurs

Overpressures

Repeated movements

Sustained movements

Neurological examination: S1 myotome

Supine

Neurodynamic Testing

Passive neck flexion (PNF)

Straight-leg raise (SLR)

When Indicated

Implicate or clear (sacroiliac joint, hip, knee, ankle)

Muscle length (hamstring)

MMT: transverse abdominis, rectus abdominis, internal oblique and external oblique

Quadratus lumborum

Repeated flexion in lying

Neurological examination: L2–S2 myotomes, L4–S1 reflexes, L2–S2 dermatomes

Side Lying

Stability Testing

Prone

Neurodynamic Testing

Prone knee bend (PKB)

When Indicated

Repeated extension in lying

Neurological examination: S1–S2 myotomes

MMT

Palpation

Skin (temperature, sweating, scratch test, skin rolling)

Soft tissue

Muscle

- Tone (feel for areas of thickness, swelling, tightness, spasm, or muscle guarding)
- Tenderness
- Presence of trigger points
- Ligaments (tenderness, density)

Bony alignment (tenderness, swelling, stiffness)

- Spinous process L1–L5 (thickening)
- Articular process L1–L5 (relative depth)

PAIVMs

- Central PAIVM
- Unilateral PAIVM

Clinical Syndromes

With the spine, offering complete guidelines for differential diagnosis is not feasible. The clinician must always keep in mind that any pathology in the upper extremity or lower extremity could be of spinal origin or could have some relationship to spinal dysfunction.

The Clinical Syndromes table on page 110 lists common musculoskeletal disorders of the lumbar spine. The clinical responses listed for each disorder represent possible responses rather than absolute responses. Use this table as a guideline to form a hypothesis of the nature of the problem. The patient may exhibit only partial components of a disorder or may be affected by a combination of disorders. This listing does not include all possible disorders. For example, several pathological disorders must be considered. Abbreviated treatment suggestions are included.

Clinical Syndromes

Description	Location and behavior of symptoms	History	Tests and measures, diagnostics	Intervention
DDD				
Common in males, fourth or fifth decade of life. Occupation that involves lifting or sitting, or past history of contact sports	Constant low-grade LS ache, rare to have leg symptoms. Overuse. Aggravation: bending, half bending, sitting, sitting to standing, lifting, coughing or sneezing, sudden EOR motions.	Repeated annular tears or one tear of significant magnitude to produce disc narrowing, bone spur formation, possible hyper- versus hypomobility of involved segment.	ROM: May have normal ROM except in acute episode. Provoke symptoms with sustained movements and may have difficulty returning to neutral. SLR: Negative or only LBP. Palpation: minimally painful. Diagnostics: X rays—bone spur formation; disc space narrowing; sclerosis of facets and vertebral margins; discography, MRI.	McKenzie protocol. Manual therapy techniques (central PAIMVs and rotation techniques). May require movement through range with many different techniques (spondylosis). Traction. Body mechanics. Spinal stabilization exercises. Stretches. Medical management: pain medications; intradiscal therapy; surgery: (fusion, disc replacement).
HNP				
Common in those 20–55 years of age, common in those who sit a lot.	+/– low back stiffness. Acute low back pain, +/– leg pain, +/– muscle spasm. +/– signs of nerve root compression. Aggravation: flexion, sitting, sitting to standing, standing, walking, coughing and sneezing; ambulation may be limited because of pain with WB and cramping. Ease: lying down, unloading.	Patient reports sudden onset but usually because of repetitive bending, lifting, or frequent lifting activities. Episodes are recurrent.	ROM: May have total restriction in ROM when acute or pain with hyper extension and occasionally flexion. Lumbar spine flexion may be limited. SLR: +/–. Neuro: positive responses if nerve root compression. Diagnostics: MRI, CT, myelography and CT myelography used to diagnose HNP. Plain radiographs may reveal preexisting degenerative changes.	McKenzie protocol. Manual therapy techniques. Traction. Body mechanics. Spinal stabilization exercises. Stretches. Medical management: epidural steroid injection and surgery.

Description	Location and behavior of symptoms	History	Tests and measures, diagnostics	Intervention
DERANGEMENT (MCKENZIE SYNDROME)				
Usually 20–50 years old. Pathology present.	Pain can be local, referred, or radicular. Pain can be constant or intermittent.	Pain of spinal origin associated with displacement within motion segment or intervertebral disc.	Deformity is present. ROM loss is usually present. Pain during movement. End range pain. Repeated movements can worsen symptoms or improve symptoms (centralization or peripheralization—making a change with movement testing).	Reduce derangement, maintain reduction with procedure that centralizes or abolishes pain, and prevent dysfunction through the use of exercise, patient education, including posture instruction.
SPINAL STENOSIS				
Also known as neurogenic claudication. Condition involving narrowing of the central spinal canal, lateral recesses, or the intervertebral foramina. Spinal stenosis is more common in males than females.	Back and leg symptoms, can be bilateral. Can be asymmetrical extremity symptoms. Extrasegmental. Aggravation: extension postures, prolonged standing and walking, lying flat, walking downhill (extension). Ease: flexing spine (sitting or squatting), walking uphill (flexion).	Congenital (seen in younger populations) or degenerative (sixth or seventh decade of life). Neural compromise because of obstruction of blood flow to the dural sleeve or nerve.	ROM: extension limited and painful. Peripheral pulses: present. Two-stage treadmill test: earlier onset of symptoms during level ambulation, longer total walking time during inclined ambulation, and prolonged recovery time after level walking. Diagnostics: • Plain radiographs: significant for the exclusion of conditions associated with spinal stenosis • CT scan: narrowing of the spinal canal • Myelography: show the actual amount of constriction of the thecal sac • MRI: assessment of the thecal sac and contents.	ADL instruction with neutral spine. Spinal stabilization exercises. Stretching tight structures (hip flexors, adductors, ant. hip capsule). Collar or binder. Manual therapy techniques (rotation). Intermittent traction. Medical management: pain medications; epidural steroid injections; surgery (laminectomy, fusion).

» continued

» continued

Description	Location and behavior of symptoms	History	Tests and measures, diagnostics	Intervention
VASCULAR CLAUDICATION				
Produced by PVD in which a compromised circulatory system is unable to meet the increased physiological demands of muscle activity.	Rarely have back symptoms. LE cramping or tightness especially in calf muscle. Aggravation: initial complaint of buttock or calf pain on walking a set distance on level surface, walking uphill (increased muscle effort). Ease: stop walking for a set period of time, supine lying, flexion does not ease symptoms, symptoms remain same or decrease when walking downhill.	Caused by plaque buildup along arterial walls leading to decrease in circulation to the LE muscles.	Trophic changes: skin color changes, loss of hair over digits, discoloration of tissues, temperature changes. Peripheral pulses: absent. Reflexes: normal. Two-stage treadmill test: unaffected by spinal posture and worse with inclined walking because of increased muscle effort. Diagnostics: Circulation studies and arteriograph may be required.	Acute: surgical intervention. Improve circulation.
ACUTE FACET				
	Unilateral pain— sharp over joint. Increased symptoms with stretch or compression of joint.	Sudden unguarded movement (flexion or rotation).	Palpation: local tenderness. Diagnostics: Plain radiographs may show decreased facet joint space, sclerosis, and osteophytes at joint margins.	Manual therapy: local rotation, unilateral PAIVMs. Traction at the specific level.
CHRONIC FACET				
	Unilateral pain— less sharp over joint. Increased symptoms with stretch of joint.	History of past acute facet; never entirely symptom free.	Palpation: local tenderness, stiff, thick. Diagnostics: Plain radiographs may show decreased facet joint space, sclerosis, and osteophytes at joint margins.	Manual therapy: local rotation, unilateral PAIVMs, transverse pressures. Traction at the specific level.

Description	Location and behavior of symptoms	History	Tests and measures, diagnostics	Intervention
ACUTE NERVE ROOT				
	Dermatomal (patchy); distal symptom > proximal. Severely limits activity.		ROM: very limited motion, can be latent. Neuro: responses at level involved. Can begin with ache proximally, symptom more severe distally. Diagnostics: MRI, CT, and myelography.	Manual traction supine or side lying. Manual therapy: lumbar rotations. Modalities. Medical management: epidural steroid injection and surgery.
CHRONIC NERVE ROOT				
	Dermatomal; proximal symptom > distal. Minimal limitation of activity.	History of acute nerve root injury, can be gradual, insidious onset.	Neuro: minor neuro responses. Palpation: stiff at involved segment. Diagnostics: MRI, CT, and myelography.	Manual therapy: unilateral PAIVMs and rotation techniques. Traction. Treatment of neurodynamic signs.
INSTABILITY, SPONDYLOLYSIS, OR SPONDYLOLISTHESIS				
	LBP; may refer; severe after vigorous activity; may have nerve root involvement—more likely if spondylolisthesis. Describe catch pain, severely fluctuating symptoms. Aggravation: Usually will take vigorous activity (swimming, running, lifting, and so on). Ease: Rest usually alleviates symptoms.	Usually occurs in teenagers but can occur from trauma or repeated stress factors in some adults. May have history of laminectomy. Flexion or extension injuries.	ROM: EOR movements may provoke symptoms. May have hesitation in flexion at 30-40°. May have difficulty with lumbar flexion—walk up legs, LS extension tends to hinge at one segment. Tight hamstrings. Neuro: +/– signs. Diagnostics: plain radiographs.	Rest. Avoid aggravating activities. Spinal stabilization exercises. External support. Recognize that another level may be cause of symptoms and may benefit from intervention of these levels with protection of the unstable segments. Medical management: bracing, pain medications, epidural steroid injections, surgery (fusion).

» continued

» continued

Description	Location and behavior of symptoms	History	Tests and measures, diagnostics	Intervention
STRAIN OR SPRAIN				
	LBP. Increase symptoms with stretch and resistance.	Acute trauma, usually lasts a few weeks.	ROM: painful. Palpation: soft tissue thickening, possible muscle spasm. Neuro: negative. Diagnostics: Plain radiographs may reveal defects in the pars interarticularis.	Modalities: heat and ultrasound. Massage, soft tissue. Spinal stabilization exercises.
POSTURAL DYSFUNCTION (MCKENZIE SYNDROME)				
Under age 30, usually female.	Pain is located adjacent to spine, usually intermittent.	Pain of spinal origin associated with prolonged stress of normal tissue. No underlying pathology.	No deformity. No ROM loss. No effect with repeated movements. Needs sustained position to reproduce symptoms.	Reeducate; postural retraining.
DYSFUNCTION (MCKENZIE SYNDROME)				
Usually over age 30, usually male.	Pain is located adjacent to spine, usually intermittent.	Pain of spinal origin associated with end range stress of adaptively shortened tissue.	No deformity. Loss of ROM. End range pain. Repeated movements: reproduction of symptoms, not worsened.	Remodel or stretch shortened structures; patient education, including posture instruction.

Adapted from C. Wadsworth, 1988, *Manual examination and treatment of the spine and extremities* (Baltimore, MD: Lippincott, Williams, and Wilkins).

Pelvis

This chapter addresses the pelvis, or sacroiliac, region. The sacroiliac region is a controversial area of the spine. Isolated sacroiliac dysfunction is rare; thus the clinician must not only perform a thorough assessment of the region but also address any lumbar spine or peripheral joint problems that could be contributing to the patient's complaints. The clinician should be suspicious of lumbar involvement whenever a patient complains of lower-extremity pain, tingling, or weakness of unknown etiology. The spine is often overlooked in these cases, but when it is correctly identified as the problem source, it may be very responsive to physical therapy interventions.

Joint Basics

Articulation Formed between the auricular surface of the sacrum and the auricular
surface of the ilium.

Type of Joint Amphiarthrodial joint.

Degrees of Freedom

Nutation occurs in a sagittal plane about a coronal axis of rotation that crosses the interosseous ligament.

  Counternutation occurs in a sagittal plane about a coronal axis of rotation that crosses the interosseous ligament.

Active Range of Motion

  Rotation: 0.2–2°

  Translation: 1–2 mm

Trunk Forward Bend

Patient position: Standing.

Clinician position: Standing or kneeling behind the patient. The clinician palpates the inferior aspect of both PSIS.

Method: The patient is instructed to bend forward (lumbar flexion). The clinician moves the thumbs with the PSIS and assesses symmetry of motion of the PSIS.

Normal response: The PSIS should move superiorly with equal timing and for an equal distance. The sacrum should nutate (flex) through the full range.

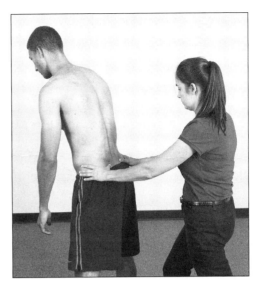

Positive response: Asymmetrical movement or timing of ilium. Tightness in the soft tissues may cause the sacrum to extend toward end range of trunk forward bending. The earlier the occurrence of the extension of the sacrum in the forward-bending range, the more problematic is this counternutation (extension) of the sacrum. Watch for early extension of the sacrum that suggests hypermobility.

Trunk Backward Bend

Patient position: Standing.

Clinician position: Standing or kneeling behind the patient. The clinician palpates the inferior aspect of both PSIS.

Method: The patient is instructed to bend back (lumbar extension). The clinician moves the thumbs with the PSIS and assesses symmetry of motion of the PSISs.

Normal response: Bilateral innominate rotates posteriorly and the sacrum remains in nutation.

Positive response: Asymmetrical movement or timing of ilium; counternutation of the sacrum.

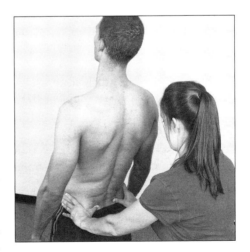

Hip Extension and Unilateral Innominate Anterior Rotation

Patient position: Standing.

Clinician position: Standing or kneeling behind the patient. The clinician places the thumb of the left hand over the inferior aspect of the left PSIS and the thumb of the right hand over the sacral base directly parallel.

Method: The clinician instructs the patient to extend the right leg, keeping the knee straight (left hip extension).

Normal response: The clinician notes the superior lateral displacement of the PSIS, checking both sides for symmetry and timing.

Positive response: Asymmetrical movement or timing of ilial anterior rotation.

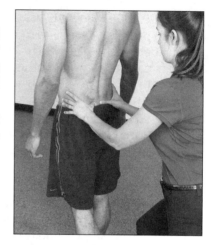

Hip Flexion or Unilateral Innominate Posterior Rotation

Patient position: Standing.

Clinician position: Standing or kneeling behind the patient. The clinician places the thumb of the left hand over the inferior aspect of the left PSIS and the thumb of the right hand over the sacral base directly parallel.

Method: The clinician instructs the patient to raise the left leg off the ground (left hip flexion).

Normal response: The clinician evaluates the inferomedial displacement of the PSIS on the sacrum, checking both sides for symmetry and timing.

Positive response: Asymmetrical movement or timing of ilial posterior rotation.

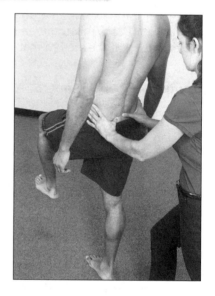

Pain Provocation Tests: Anterior Gapping (Distraction)

Patient position: Supine.

Clinician position: Standing in a walk-stance position on side of patient facing the head of the patient. The clinician crosses his or her arms and places the heel of each hand on the medial aspect of each ASIS.

Method: Apply a slow, steady posterior-lateral force, distracting the anterior aspect of the SIJ. Hold the force for 20 seconds or until pain is reproduced.

Positive response: Assess end feel and complaints of pain.

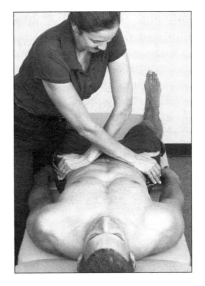

Pain Provocation Tests: Posterior Gapping

Patient position: Side lying with pillow under head and knees bent in comfortable position.

Clinician position: Standing behind patient. With elbows bent approximately 30°, the clinician places both hands over the patient's superior aspect of the ilium.

Method: Apply a slow, steady medial force, distracting the posterior aspect of the SIJ. Hold the force for 20 seconds.

Positive response: Assess end feel and complaints of pain.

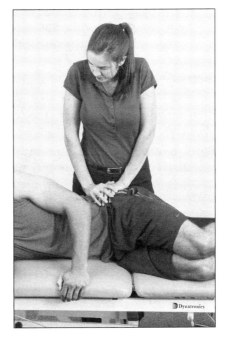

Pain Provocation Tests: Posterior Shear

Patient position: Hook lying in supine.

Clinician position: Standing in a walk-stance position on the right side of the patient facing the head of the patient. The clinician places the third and fourth fingertips of the left hand over the sacral sulcus and the soft palm of the right hand over the patient's ASIS.

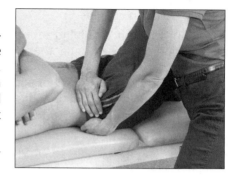

Method: Apply a gentle anterior-to-posterior force and compare sides.

Positive response: Assess the end feel, quantity and quality of movement between each ilium and the sacrum, and reproduction of symptoms.

Pain Provocation Tests: Superior Shear

Patient position: Hook lying in supine.

Clinician position: Standing in a walk-stance position on the right side of the patient facing the head of the patient. The clinician places the third and fourth fingertips of the left hand over the sacral sulcus and the right hand on the patient's right knee.

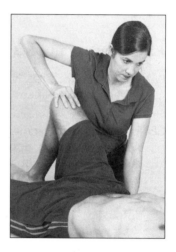

Method: Apply an inferior-to-superior force through the distal end of the femur and compare sides.

Alternative method: Apply the force through the ischial tuberosity.

Positive response: Assess the end feel, quantity and quality of movement, and symptoms.

Ilial Rotation

Patient position: Side lying.

Clinician position: Standing in a squat-stance position facing the patient. The clinician places the third and fourth fingertips of the left hand over the sacral sulcus and the right hand on the patient's right ASIS.

Method: With the right hand, gently move the right ilium into posterior rotation with a superior-posterior force (see figure *a*). For anterior rotation, the right hand wraps around the superior aspect of the iliac crest and with an anterior and inferior force moves the ilium into anterior rotation (see figure *b*).

Positive response: Increased or decreased mobility or reproduction of symptoms, asymmetrical movement.

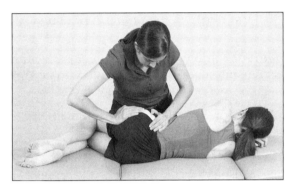

a

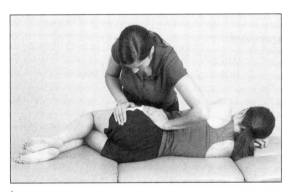

b

End Feel

Not described.

Capsular Pattern

Not described.

Close-Packed Position

Not described.

Loose-Packed Position

Not described.

Stability

Anterior Sacroiliac Ligament   A thickening of the anterior and inferior parts of the joint capsule.

Interosseous Ligament   Strong set of multiple fibers. Fills most of the open space along the posterior and superior margin of the SI joint. Forms the most substantial bond between the sacrum and the ilium.

Short and Long Posterior Sacroiliac Ligaments   Helps reinforce the posterior side of the SI joint.

Short: from the posterior-lateral sacrum superiorly and laterally to the ilium

Long: from the third and fourth sacral segments to the posterior-superior iliac spine

Sacrotuberous Ligament   From posterior-superior iliac spine, lateral sacrum, and coccyx distally to the ischial tuberosity.

Sacrospinous Ligament   Deep to the sacrotuberous ligament. From the lateral and caudal end of the sacrum and coccyx distally to the ischial spine.

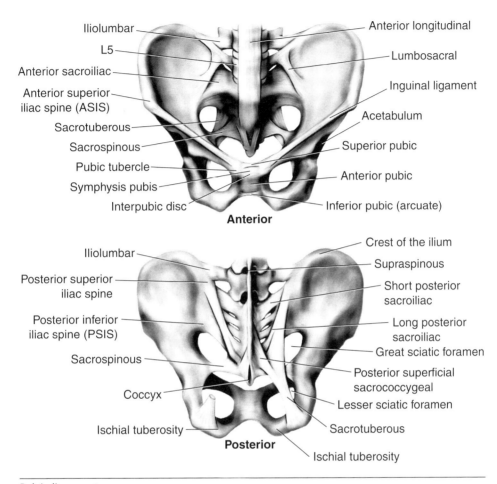

Iliolumbar
L5
Anterior sacroiliac
Anterior superior iliac spine (ASIS)
Sacrotuberous
Sacrospinous
Pubic tubercle
Symphysis pubis
Interpubic disc

Anterior longitudinal
Lumbosacral
Inguinal ligament
Acetabulum
Superior pubic
Anterior pubic
Inferior pubic (arcuate)

Anterior

Iliolumbar
Posterior superior iliac spine
Posterior inferior iliac spine (PSIS)
Sacrospinous
Coccyx
Ischial tuberosity

Crest of the ilium
Supraspinous
Short posterior sacroiliac
Long posterior sacroiliac
Great sciatic foramen
Posterior superficial sacrococcygeal
Lesser sciatic foramen
Sacrotuberous
Ischial tuberosity

Posterior

Pelvic ligaments.

Reprinted, by permission, from R. Behnke, *Kinetic anatomy*, 2nd ed. (Champaign, IL: Human Kinetics), 174.

Force Closure

Assessment: Force closure requires external forces to act across the joint surface to increase the compression of the joint and decrease the shear forces. This increased stability will assist in efficient and safe load transference. Muscle contraction of the anterior oblique (supine) or posterior oblique (prone) systems increases compression across the SIJ. Changes in ease of movement or decreased pain suggest that strengthening of the muscular group involved may be helpful.

Patient position: Supine.

Clinician position: Standing on the right side of the patient facing the head of the patient. The clinician places his or her right hand on the patient's left shoulder and instructs the patient to perform a right straight leg raise (SLR) (see figure *a* and *b*). The clinician notes compensatory motions, ease of movement, or reproduction of symptoms.

Method: Provide resistance (isometric contraction) to trunk flexion and right rotation through the shoulder. Then ask the patient to perform a SLR.

Alternative method: Prone.

Positive response: Change in movement or pain.

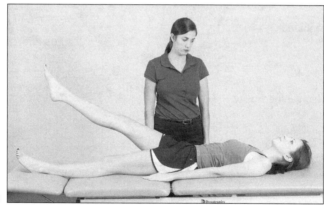

a

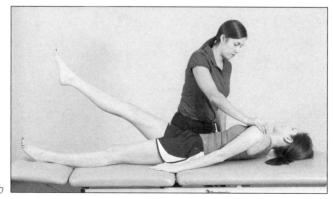

b

Form Closure

Assessment: Panjabi described the interaction between the components of the spinal system that provides stability. These components are the passive system of joint and ligamentous stability, the active system of the myofascia, and the neural control system. Form closure describes an intact joint with joint surfaces that articulate so that mechanical stability is inherent. The shape of the joint surface, the ligamentous integrity, and the friction coefficient of the joint all contribute to form closure. During this test, the clinician's hands provide external fixation of the pelvis. Improved function or decreased pain suggests that use of an external support may be helpful.

Patient position: Supine.

Clinician position: Standing on the right side of the patient facing the head of the patient. The clinician places his or her hands over the patient's iliac crests and instructs the patient to perform a right SLR (see figure *a* and *b*). The clinician notes compensatory motions, ease of movement, or reproduction of symptoms.

Method: The clinician gently and evenly compresses the patient's iliac crests in a corsetlike manner and then asks the patient to perform a right SLR.

Alternative method: Prone.

Positive response: Change in movement or pain.

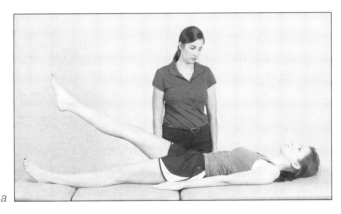

a

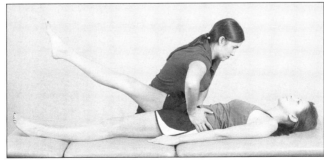

b

Patrick Test (FABER)

(Refer to Hip Special Tests)

Leg Length Tests

Patient position: Supine, lying with legs 15–20 cm (4–8 in.) apart and parallel to each other.

Clinician position: Standing on the side of the table facing the side of the patient. The clinician properly aligns both lower limbs with the pelvis.

Method: Using a measuring tape, compare the length of both limbs from the ASIS to either the lateral or medial malleoli (see figure *a*).

Alternative method:

- Leg length test: hook lying. The patient is hook lying with the legs together. The clinician observes the height of the tibia in the frontal plane (see figure *b*) and the length of the femur in the sagittal plane (see figure *c*).

- Leg length test: prone knee-bend test. The patient is lying in the prone position with the legs straight. The clinician assesses the leg length with the legs straight, looking at the heels, and then passively bends the patient's knees to 90°. The clinician assesses leg length again. The test is considered positive if a change in length occurs between positions.

Examination: To distinguish true length discrepancy from functional shortening. Clinical syndromes: hip adduction syndrome.

Positive response: A difference in limb length.

Biomechanics: ASIS to malleoli on either limb suggests proper alignment of the pelvis, hip, and lower limbs and equal lengths of the femur and tibia bones. A leg length difference of less than 1/4 in. (.6 cm) is usually nonpathological. Apparent or functional shortening has no anatomical or structural difference in bone lengths and the converse is true for real bone length differences.

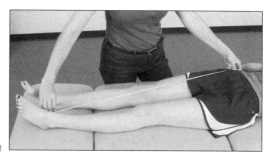

a

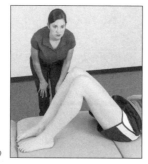

b

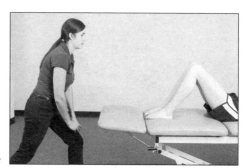

c

Arthrokinematics

Flexion Sacroiliac Joint Nutation

The relative anterior tilt of the top of the sacrum on the ilium

Can also occur if the ilium rotates posteriorly on the sacrum

Sacroiliac Joint Counternutation

The relative posterior tilt of the top of the sacrum on the ilium

Can also occur if the ilium rotates anteriorly on the sacrum

Neurology

Refer to chapter 6, "Lumbar Spine."

Surface Palpation

Standing
Iliac crest

Posterior superior iliac spine

Anterior superior iliac spine

Greater trochanter

Sitting
Posterior landmarks

Supine
Abdominal quadrants

Inguinal region

Iliac crest

Anterior superior iliac spine

Symphysis pubis

Greater trochanter

Prone
Lumbar spinous process

Lumbar facets, transverse processes

Sacral spine

Iliac crest

Posterior superior iliac spine

Coccyx

Ischial tuberosity

Sciatic nerve

Piriformis

Supraspinous ligament

Paraspinal muscles

Inferior lateral angles

Sacral sulcus

Anterior
Abdominal quadrants

Inguinal region

Iliac crest

Anterior superior iliac spine

Symphysis pubis

Greater trochanter

Muscle Origin and Insertion

Refer to chapter 6, "Lumbar Spine."

EXAMINATION SEQUENCE

HISTORY

Location of Symptoms

Unilateral

Rare referral superior to L5

May or may not be over the involved joint

Pain in the buttock, lower abdomen, groin, anteromedial or posterior thigh, possibly extending below the knee, coccydynia

Fortain's point—one and one-quarter inferior and medial to PSIS is a positive sign

Types of Symptoms

Dull ache or sharp catches

Heaviness of buttock or leg (feels "dead")

Hip or back feels "out of place"

Clicking or a deep "clunk" or "thunk"

Subjective paresthesias

Aggravating Factors

Single-leg stance, gait (variable phases will be painful depending on the patient's dysfunction), stepping up or down on affected side, turning over in bed, twisting on stance leg, sitting (particularly if WB is unequal), rising to stand, sexual intercourse, crossing legs, asymmetrical stresses

Ease Factors

Tight pants or back support, sitting for short periods

Special Questions

24 hours

- Night pain: metastatic disease versus twisted or asymmetrical sleeping position
- General health: inflammatory disease, hypermobility syndrome, post-partum

TESTS AND MEASURES

Standing

Observation

General appearance, affect, visual cues of symptoms

Willingness to move

Body structure, level of fitness

Posture

Changes of body contour (atrophy, swelling, spasm)

Skin (scars)

Implicate or Clear Lumbar Spine

Neurological Examination, as Indicated

Functional Tests

Walking, single-leg stance, single-leg hopping, single-leg twist, sitting with legs crossed at knee; others per SE

AROM: Sacrum or Ilium

Trunk forward bend

Trunk backward bend

Hip flexion

Hip extension

Surface Palpation

Iliac crest

PSIS

ASIS

Greater trochanter

Special Tests

Leg length tests

Sitting

Surface Palpation of Posterior Landmarks

Supine

Observation

Surface Palpation of Anterior Landmarks

Implicate or Clear Hip

Neurological Examination

Muscle Length or Strength Tests

Special Tests

Leg length tests

Form closure or force closure

Stability tests (posterior shear, superior shear, anterior gapping)

Side Lying

PAM: Ilial Rotation

Muscle Length or Strength Tests

Special Test: Provocation and Stability Test—Posterior Gapping

Observation

Surface Palpation: Prone Landmarks, Soft Tissue, Spine

Neurological Examination

PAM: PA Over Sacrum (Base and Apex)

Muscle Length or Strength Tests

Pelvic floor

Transverse abdominis

Rectus abdominis

Internal oblique and external oblique

Quadratus lumborum

Special Tests: Form Closure or Force Closure

Clinical Syndromes

The Clinical Syndromes table on page 131 lists common musculoskeletal disorders of the pelvis, or SI, seen by clinicians. The clinical responses listed for each disorder represent possible responses rather than absolute responses. Use this table as a guideline to form a hypothesis of the nature of the problem. The patient may exhibit only partial components of a disorder or may be affected by a combination of disorders. This listing does not include all possible disorders. For example, several pathological disorders must be considered. Abbreviated treatment suggestions are included.

Clinical Syndromes

Description	Location and behavior of symptoms	History	Tests and measures, diagnostics	Intervention
HYPERMOBILE PELVIC GIRDLE				
Instability in one of the pelvic joints, usually SI.	Deep clunk or shift in pelvis with position changes.	Pregnancy—hormonal influences, breastfeeding and return to normal hormone levels. Trauma (macro or micro).	Pelvis: generalized hypermobility. SIJ: Increased range or soft end feel with PAM or stability test, with or without clunking. Pain with provocation testing, difficulty or pain with SLR. Pubic symphysis: Increased range with PAM of pubic bone. Difficulty and weakness with SLR. Adductors tender to palpation and tender during adductor contraction.	Medical management: rare surgical fixation.
HYPOMOBILE PELVIC GIRDLE				
Ilium	Local pain in buttock or over SIJ that can refer into posterior leg; dull ache in anterior thigh.	Posterior rotation: stepping off curb, fall on buttock. Anterior rotation: back leg slips posterior. Upslip with posterior rotation. Downslip with anterior rotation. Pubic symphysis: Superior pubis, running downhill, inferior pubis sitting on one side with the inferior side off chair.	Palpation: asymmetry in pelvic landmarks after leg length has been accounted for, mobility tests may be stiff or painful. Diagnostics: unable to detect on X ray.	Mobilization, manipulation, muscle energy to restore normal movement.
Sacrum	Pain over the SIJ or LS junction or along lateral border of sacrum.	Rotation: twisting on fixed leg. Side bend: fall on coccyx.	Palpation: asymmetry in pelvic landmarks. Mobility tests may be stiff or painful.	Mobilization, manipulation, muscle energy to restore normal movement.

Upper Extremity

The focus of part III is to provide detailed information to the clinician on the major joints of the upper extremity along with the objective sequence. Part III contains four chapters related to the upper extremity. Chapter 8 describes the shoulder joint complex, including the glenohumeral, sternoclavicular, acromioclavicular, and scapulothoracic joints. Chapter 9 covers the elbow and forearm, including the humeroulnar, humeroradial, superior radioulnar, and distal radioulnar joints. Chapter 10 deals with the wrist and hand, including the many joints of the fingers and thumb. The last chapter of part III is a synopsis of functional tests for the upper extremity.

The chapters follow a consistent format. First, the joint articulation is described, followed by a description of type of joint and degrees of freedom. Next, arthrokinematics are described as well as joint open- and close-packed positions, end feel, and capsular pattern. The remainder of each chapter describes stability of the joint, special tests, neurological assessment, surface palpation, muscle origins and insertions, and actions and innervations. Finally, a clinical syndrome table is presented to help the clinician perform musculoskeletal differential diagnoses.

Shoulder Joint Complex

The shoulder joint complex consists of many different types of joints. Included in this myriad of joints are the glenohumeral joint, sternoclavicular joint, acromioclavicular joint, and scapulothoracic joint (figure 8.1). When evaluating the arthrokinematics of the shoulder, the clinician must assess the movements of each of these joints. For this reason, arthrokinematics are listed after the description of all individual joints. The shoulder complex has a great range of motion and is a common area for upper-extremity pathology of various kinds. As always, any shoulder assessment should include a cervical spine assessment.

GLENOHUMERAL JOINT (GH)

The glenohumeral joint is the true shoulder joint (see figure 8.1). Its anatomical makeup allows for multiplanar motion, important for functional use of the hand.

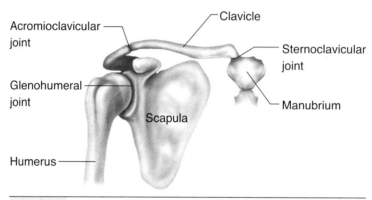

Figure 8.1 Bones and joints of the shoulder girdle.

Joint Basics

Articulation   Convex humeral head and the concave glenoid fossa.

Type of Joint   Diarthrosis, spheroidal, ball-and-socket joint.

Degrees of Freedom

- Flexion and extension in sagittal plane about a coronal axis through the humeral head
- Abduction and adduction in coronal plane about a sagittal axis through the humeral head
- Internal and external rotation in transverse plane about a longitudinal axis through the humeral head

In addition, circumduction and horizontal abduction and adduction occur at the glenohumeral joint.

Active Range of Motion

Flexion: 0–180°

Extension: 0–60°

Abduction: 0–180°

Internal rotation: 0–70°

External rotation: 0–90°

Horizontal adduction: 0–40°

Horizontal abduction: 0–90°

Flexion (Right)

Examination: Shoulder AROM.

Patient position: Supine with the arms to the sides.

Clinician position: Standing beside the patient for AROM. After the patient has achieved the available range of motion (without deviations), the clinician stands to the right side of the patient and places the left hand over the patient's right scapula and grasps the patient's right anterior arm with the right hand.

Method: The clinician stabilizes the scapula with the left hand and gently applies overpressure into flexion with the right hand oscillating into the end range.

Positive response: Limited range of motion or reproduction of symptoms.

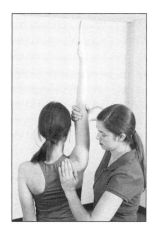

Abduction (Right)

Examination: Shoulder AROM.

Patient position: Standing with the arms to the sides.

Clinician position: Standing behind the patient for AROM. After the patient has achieved the available range of motion (without deviations), the clinician stands to the right side of the patient, places the left hand over the patient's right scapula, and grasps the patient's right lateral arm with the right hand.

Method: The clinician stabilizes the scapula with the left hand and gently applies overpressure into abduction with the right hand oscillating into the end range.

Positive response: Limited range of motion or reproduction of symptoms.

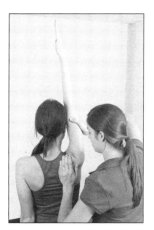

Horizontal Adduction (Right)

Examination: Shoulder AROM.

Patient position: Supine with the arms to the sides.

Clinician position: Standing beside the patient for AROM. After the patient has achieved the available range of motion (without deviations), the clinician stands to the left side of the patient and places the left hand over the patient's right elbow and grasps the patient's left posterior shoulder with the right hand.

Method: The clinician gently applies overpressure into horizontal adduction oscillating into the end range.

Positive response: Limited range of motion or reproduction of symptoms.

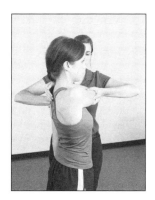

Internal Rotation—Hand Behind Back (Right)

Examination: Shoulder AROM.

Patient position: Supine with the arms to the sides.

Clinician position: Standing beside the patient for AROM. After the patient has achieved the available range of motion (without deviations), the clinician stands to the right side of the patient and places the left hand over the patient's right scapula and grasps the patient's right posterior forearm with the right hand.

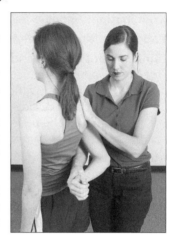

Method: The clinician stabilizes the patient's right scapula with the left hand and gently applies overpressure into internal rotation with the right hand oscillating into the end range.

Alternative method: Combine overpressure into shoulder internal rotation, adduction, and extension.

Positive response: Limited range of motion or reproduction of symptoms.

External Rotation (Right)

Examination: Shoulder AROM.

Patient position: Supine with the arms to the sides.

Clinician position: Standing beside the patient for AROM. After the patient has achieved the available range of motion (without deviations), the clinician stands to the right side of the patient and places the left hand over the patient's right elbow and grasps the patient's right anterior forearm with the right hand.

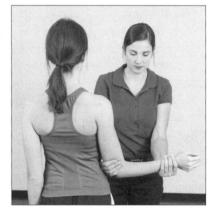

Method: The clinician gently applies overpressure into external rotation oscillating into the end range.

Positive response: Limited range of motion or reproduction of symptoms.

Internal Rotation—Glenohumeral Joint (Right)

Examination: Shoulder PROM.

Patient position: Supine at the edge of the right side of the table.

Clinician position: Standing in a walk-stance position facing the end of the table. The clinician rests the patient's right arm on the clinician's left thigh. The clinician grasps the patient's right wrist with the right hand and stabilizes the patient's right anterior shoulder or humeral head with the left forearm while holding on to the patient's distal arm with the left hand.

Method: The clinician moves the patient's arm into internal rotation with the right hand while stabilizing the humeral head with the left forearm.

Positive response: Limited range of motion or reproduction of symptoms.

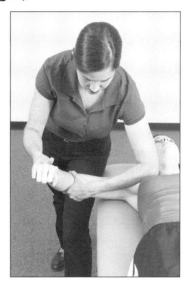

External Rotation

Examination: Shoulder PROM.

Patient position: Supine at the edge of the right side of the table.

Clinician position: Standing in a walk-stance position facing the head of the table. The clinician rests the patient's right arm on the clinician's right thigh. The clinician grasps the patient's right wrist with the left hand and stabilizes the patient's right shoulder or humeral head with the right forearm while holding on to the patient's distal arm with the right hand.

Method: The clinician moves the patient's arm into external rotation with the left hand while stabilizing the humeral head with the right hand.

Alternative method: Perform at 0° of shoulder abduction.

Positive response: Limited range of motion or reproduction of symptoms.

Internal Rotation—Glenohumeral Joint (Right)

Examination: Shoulder PROM.

Patient position: Supine at the edge of the right side of the table.

Clinician position: Standing in a walk-stance position facing the end of the table. The clinician rests the patient's right arm on the clinician's left thigh. The clinician grasps the patient's right wrist with the right hand and stabilizes the patient's right anterior shoulder or humeral head with the left forearm while holding on to the patient's distal arm with the left hand.

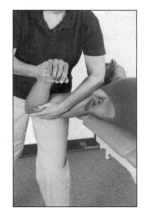

Method: The clinician moves the patient's arm into internal rotation with the right hand while stabilizing the humeral head with the left forearm.

Positive response: Limited range of motion or reproduction of symptoms.

External Rotation

Examination: Shoulder PROM.

Patient position: Supine at the edge of the right side of the table.

Clinician position: Standing in a walk-stance position facing the head of the table. The clinician rests the patient's right arm on the clinician's right thigh. The clinician grasps the patient's right wrist with the left hand and stabilizes the patient's right shoulder or humeral head with the right forearm while holding on to the patient's distal arm with the right hand.

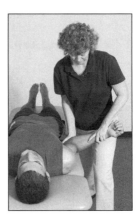

Method: The clinician moves the patient's arm into external rotation with the left hand while stabilizing the humeral head with the right hand.

Alternative method: Perform at 0° of shoulder abduction.

Positive response: Limited range of motion or reproduction of symptoms.

Glenohumeral Joint Anterior Glide (Right)

Assessment: External rotation, extension, horizontal abduction. The clinician can assess anterior glide in a variety of abducted positions.

Patient position: Prone with the arm relaxed, the neck in a comfortable position, and a pillow under the abdomen (if needed for comfort).

Clinician position: Standing in a walk-stance position on the right side of the patient facing the head of the table. The clinician supports the weight of the patient's right arm in 90° of abduction with the right hand. The clinician places the ulnar border of the left hand along the glenohumeral joint line; the clinician's left elbow should be in slight flexion (30°).

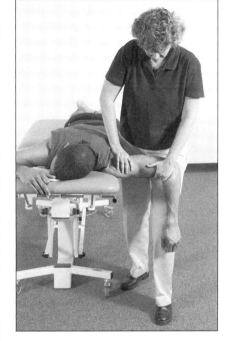

Method: The clinician applies a posterior-to-anterior force, bringing the humerus anterior in relationship to the glenoid while moving the arm as a unit. Apply first pressures gently; increase amplitude and depth of the movement if no pain response occurs. Assess quality of movement through the range and end feel; compare with the other side.

Alternative method: The clinician can assess the anterior glide in a variety of abducted positions.

Intervention: Use appropriate grade of movement (I–IV) to treat pain or resistance. Anterior glide increases shoulder external rotation, extension, and horizontal abduction.

Biomechanics: According to the convex–concave rule, the convex glides anteriorly on the concave glenoid during ER, extension, and horizontal abduction.

Glenohumeral Joint Posterior Glide (Right)

Assessment: Internal rotation, flexion, horizontal adduction.

Patient position: Supine with the arm relaxed.

Clinician position: Standing in a walk-stance position on the right side of the patient facing the head (or end) of the table. The clinician supports the weight of the patient's right arm in 90° of abduction with the right hand (*a*). The clinician places the ulnar border of the right hand along the humeral head; the clinician's left elbow should be in slight flexion (30°).

Method: The clinician applies an anterior-to-posterior force, bringing the humerus posterior in relationship to the glenoid while moving the arm as a unit. Apply first pressure gently; increase amplitude and depth of the movement if no pain response occurs. Assess quality of movement through the range and end feel; compare with the other side.

Alternative method: The clinician can assess the posterior glide in a variety of abducted and internal rotated positions.

Intervention: Use appropriate grade of movement (I–IV) to treat pain or resistance. Posterior glide increases internal rotation, flexion, and horizontal adduction (*b*).

Biomechanics: According to the convex–concave rule, the convex humerus glides posteriorly on the concave glenoid during internal rotation, flexion, and horizontal adduction.

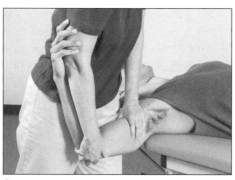

a

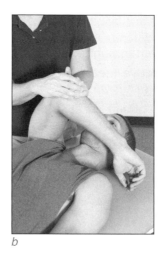

b

Glenohumeral Joint Inferior Glide (Right)

Assessment: Abduction, flexion.

Patient position: Supine with the arm relaxed.

Clinician position: Standing in a walk-stance position on the right side of the patient facing the end of the table. The clinician supports the weight of the patient's right arm in 90° of abduction with the right hand (*a*). The clinician places the web space of the left hand on the superior humerus, distal to the acromion.

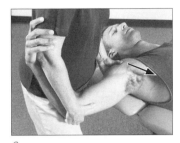
a

Method: The clinician applies an inferior force through the humeral head. Apply first pressures gently; increase amplitude and depth of the movement if no pain response occurs. Assess quality of movement through the range and end feel (*b-c*); compare with the other side.

Alternative method: The clinician can assess the anterior glide in a variety of positions.

Intervention: Use appropriate grade of movement (I–IV) to treat pain or resistance. Inferior glide increases elevation.

Biomechanics: According to the convex–concave rule, the convex humerus glides inferiorly during abduction and flexion.

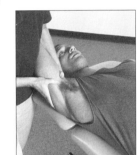
b

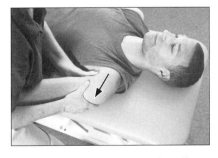
c

Lateral Glide

Assessment: General mobility.

Patient position: Supine with the arm relaxed.

Clinician position: Standing in a walk-stance position on the right side of the patient facing the head of the table. The clinician supports the weight of the patient's right arm in 45° of abduction with the left hand. The clinician places the web space of the right hand superiorly just below the axilla with the right elbow perpendicular to the patient's arm.

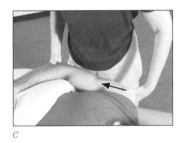

Method: The clinician applies a lateral force through the humeral head. Apply first pressures gently; increase amplitude and depth of the movement if no pain response occurs. Assess quality of movement through the range and end feel; compare with the other side.

End Feel

Flexion: Firm from tissue stretch; posterior and inferior capsules become tight.

Extension: Firm from tissue stretch; anterior capsule becomes tight.

Abduction: Hard from humerus contacting acromial arch; firm from tissue stretch; inferior capsule becomes tight.

Adduction: Soft from tissue approximation.

Internal rotation: Firm from tissue stretch; posterior capsule, infraspinatus, or teres minor becomes tight.

External rotation: Firm from tissue stretch; anterior and inferior capsules become tight.

Horizontal abduction: Firm from tissue stretch; anterior capsule becomes tight.

Horizontal adduction: Soft from tissue approximation or firm from tissue stretch; posterior capsule, infraspinatus, or teres minor becomes tight.

Capsular Pattern

Restriction in external rotation followed by abduction followed by internal rotation.

Close-Packed Position

Maximal shoulder abduction and external rotation

Internal rotation and extension

Loose-Packed Position

60° abduction, 30° horizontal adduction.

Stability

Glenohumeral Ligaments   The glenohumeral ligaments attach to the upper and anterior edge of glenoid to anterior and inferior humeral head (figure 8.2).

Superior: provides anterior stabilization of humerus at 60° of elevation

Middle: provides anterior stabilization of humerus at 90° of elevation

Inferior: provides anterior stabilization of humerus at 120° of elevation

All portions of the ligament are taut in humeral external rotation and abduction.

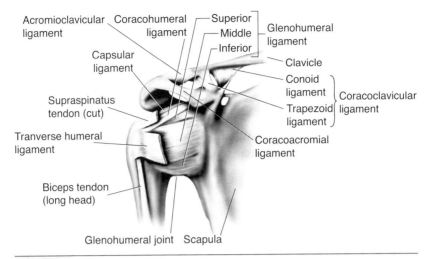

Figure 8.2 Glenohumeral ligaments.

Reprinted, by permission, from R. Behnke, *Kinetic anatomy*, 2nd ed. (Champaign, IL: Human Kinetics), 43.

Coracohumeral Ligament From the root of the coracoid process, the coracohumeral ligament passes laterally and downward to the greater tubercle blending with the supraspinatus tendon. It checks external rotation and extension and strengthens the superior capsule.

Capsule The capsule attaches medially around glenoid fossa proximal to the labrum, extends to the root of the coracoid process enclosing the proximal attachment of the long head of the biceps, and attaches laterally at the anatomical neck of the humerus, extending a sleeve along the bicipital groove.

Glenoid Labrum This fibrocartilaginous rim deepens the glenoid cavity and makes the joint articulation more congruent.

Transverse Humeral Ligament This ligament bridges the gap between the greater and lesser tuberosity and strengthens the shoulder capsule.

Coracoacromial Ligament This ligament blends with the trapezius and deltoid to form a roof over the humeral head, closes the coracoacromial arch, and prevents superior dislocation of the humeral head.

Thoracic Outlet (Inlet) Syndrome Tests: Adson Maneuver

Assessment: Scaleni compression of subclavian artery.

Patient position: Sitting.

Clinician position: Standing to the side of the patient, grasping the arm, and monitoring radial pulse.

Method: Abduct, retract, and externally rotate the arm. Turn the patient's head and hyperextend the neck toward the test side. The patient takes a deep breath.

Positive response: Diminution or disappearance of pulse or reproduction of neurological symptoms.

Thoracic Outlet (Inlet) Syndrome Tests: Pectoralis Minor Syndrome Test

Assessment: Constriction of middle portion of axillary artery by pectoralis minor.

Patient position: Sitting.

Clinician position: Standing to the side of the patient, grasping the arm, and monitoring radial pulse.

Method: Hyperabduction of the shoulder girdle. Have the patient hold breath and rotate the neck away from the arm.

Positive response: Diminution or disappearance of pulse or reproduction of neurological symptoms.

Thoracic Outlet (Inlet) Syndrome Tests: Costoclavicular Syndrome Test (Adson's Test)

Assessment: Compression of the subclavian artery by the first rib and clavicle.

Patient position: Sitting.

Clinician position: Standing to the right of the patient.

Method: Locate the radial pulse with the right index finger of the patient's right arm. Instruct the patient to turn his or her head to the right. After the patient is in position, ask the patient to extend his or her head while using the right hand to laterally rotate and extend the patient's shoulder. Instruct the patient to take a deep breath and hold it.

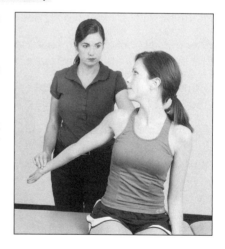

Positive response: Disappearance of pulse.

Biomechanics: The patient's position of the arm and neck with breath holding can occlude the subclavian artery.

Hawkins-Kennedy Impingement Test (Right)

Assessment: Impingement of the supraspinatus tendon.

Patient position: Sitting or standing with the arm resting comfortably to the side.

Clinician position: Standing in front of the patient. The clinician grasps the patient's right wrist with the right hand. The clinician flexes the patient's right arm to 90° of shoulder flexion and 90° of elbow flexion.

Method: The clinician medially rotates the patient's shoulder.

Alternative method: Perform the test in different degrees of forward flexion or horizontal adduction.

Positive response: Reproduction of symptoms.

Sensitivity: .92, specificity: .44 (MacDonald et al, 2000).

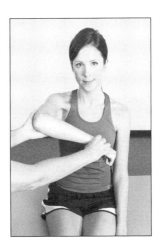

Neer's Test

Assessment: Impingement of the supraspinatus tendon.

Patient position: Sitting or standing.

Clinician position: Standing in front of the patient.

Method: The clinician passively elevates the patient's arm overhead in the scapular plane with the arm medially rotated.

Alternative method: Perform the test with the patient's arm laterally rotated to check the AC joint.

Positive response: Pain.

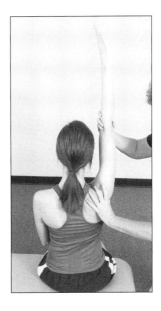

Crossover Impingement Test

Assessment: Impingement.

Patient position: Standing.

Clinician position: Standing, grasping the patient's arm.

Method: The clinician applies overpressure into horizontal adduction.

Positive response: Anterior pain—subscapularis, supraspinatus, long head of biceps; superior pain—acromioclavicular joint; posterior pain—infraspinatus, teres minor, posterior capsule.

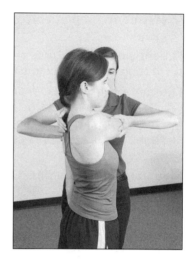

Supraspinatus "Empty Can" Test

Assessment: Supraspinatus tendonitis.

Patient position: Standing or sitting with the shoulder elevated to 90° in the scapular plane with the thumb pointed down.

Clinician position: Standing in front of the patient.

Method: The clinician applies resistance (isometric) to abduction through the patient's forearm.

Positive response: Weakness or pain in the supraspinatus region.

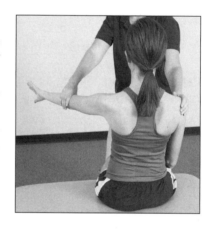

Rotator Cuff Tears: Rotator Cuff Rupture Test (Drop Arm Test)

Assessment: Rotator cuff rupture.

Patient position: Sitting.

Clinician position: Standing in front of the patient.

Method: Passively move the arm to 90° abduction. The patient should hold the arm as the clinician applies slight pressure.

Positive response: Inability to hold the arm in test position.

Sensitivity: .08, specificity: .97 (Calis et al., 2000).

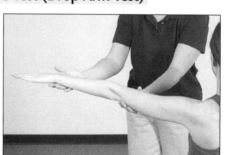

Instability Tests: Glenohumeral Load and Shift (Right)

Assessment: Anterior and posterior stability of GH joint.

Patient position: Sitting with the arm supported on the thigh; the shoulder and neck are relaxed.

Clinician position: Standing behind the patient. The clinician places the left hand over the patient's shoulder with the thumb across the posterior glenohumeral joint line and humeral head, the index finger across the anterior glenohumeral joint line and humeral head, and the long finger over the coracoid process. Using the right hand, the clinician grasps the head of the humerus with the thumb over the posterior humeral head and the fingers over the anterior humeral head.

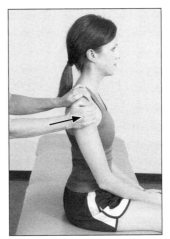

Method: The clinician compresses the humeral head medially to center it within the glenoid fossa. The clinician then applies an anteromedial force to assess anterior stability and applies a posterior force to assess posterior stability.

Alternative method: Perform the test in the supine position.

Positive response: Increased amount of translation (see Glenohumeral Translation Grades table) compared with the uninvolved side, reproduction of symptoms.

Glenohumeral Translation Grades

Trace	<5 mm
I	5–10 mm; humeral head rides up glenoid slope but not over the rim.
II	10–15 mm; humeral head rides up and over the glenoid rim but spontaneously reduces when stress is removed.
III	>15 mm; humeral head rides up and over the glenoid rim and remains dislocated when stress is removed.

Apprehension or Relocation Test (Right)

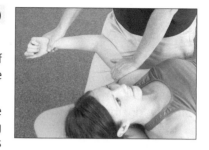

Assessment: Anterior GH stability.

Patient position: Supine on the right side of the table with the glenoid at the edge of the table.

Clinician position: Standing in a walk-stance position on the right side of the table facing the head of the table. The clinician abducts the patient's right arm to 90°. The clinician cradles the patient's right arm with the right arm, resting the patient's arm on the clinician's right thigh. The clinician holds the patient's right forearm with the left hand.

Method: Laterally rotate the patient's shoulder slowly (apprehension test). If the test produces pain or apprehension, apply a posteriorly directed force to the humeral head with the right hand (relocation test).

Positive response: Apprehension test: pain or apprehension. Relocation test: pain or apprehension relief with the posteriorly directed force and can tolerate maximum external rotation with the humeral head maintained in the reduced position.

Sensitivity: .44, specificity: .87 (Guanche & Jones., 2003).

Posterior Glide 90° Flexion and Internal Rotation

Assessment: Posterior instability.

Patient position: Supine. The shoulder is in 90° of flexion and relaxed into internal rotation with the elbow in 90° of flexion; allow posterior capsule to tighten.

Clinician position: Alongside the patient.

Method: Place one hand behind the shoulder across the posterior humeral head. The other hand applies an axial compressive force through the humerus.

Positive response: Pain, apprehension, and instability.

Multidirectional Instability Test (Sulcus Sign, Right)

Assessment: Multidirectional instability, especially inferior.

Patient position: Sitting or standing with the arm at the side in neutral and relaxed position.

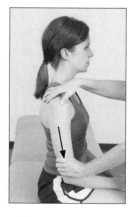

Clinician position: Standing on the right side of the patient facing the patient. The clinician's left hand grasps the anterior-medial aspect of patient's right arm. The clinician palpates the acromiohumeral space anteriorly, laterally, and posteriorly with the thumb, index finger, and middle finger of the right hand, respectively.

Method: Apply an inferior distraction force to the patient's arm through the humerus.

Alternative method: Perform the test in the supine position.

Positive response: Excessive inferior translation with sulcus defect at acromion (gapping or dimpling of skin).

Labral Tests: Glenoid Labrum Test (Clunk Test)

Assessment: Torn glenoid labrum.

Patient position: Supine, with the arm overhead in full abduction.

Clinician position: Place one hand on the posterior aspect of the humeral head; the other hand holds the humerus just proximal to the elbow.

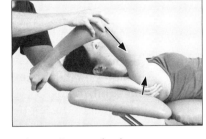

Method: Apply an anterior force to the humeral head while applying compression and rotation to the humerus.

Positive response: Pain, clunk, grinding, pseudolocking.

G-H Joint Tests: Quadrant Test

Assessment: Articulating surface of the GH joint.

Patient position: Supine.

Clinician position: The clinician's caudal arm slides palmar surface up, under the scapula so that the fingers can drape over the upper trapezius. The clinician then grasps the elbow with the other hand, keeping the elbow flexed.

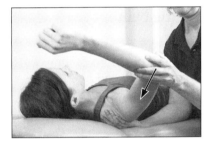

Method: Abduct the shoulder through an arc of motion within the GH joint.

Positive response: Pain, crepitus, limitation of range of motion.

G-H Joint Tests: Locking Test

Assessment: Glenohumeral dysfunction.

Patient position: Supine.

Clinician position: The clinician's caudal arm slides palmar surface up, under the scapula so that the fingers can drape over the upper trapezius. The clinician then grasps the elbow with the other hand, keeping the elbow flexed.

Method: Move the arm from abduction toward full flexion, until it reaches a stopping point where it becomes locked.

Positive response: Pain, joint grinding, reproduction of symptoms.

Biceps Tendon Tests: Transverse Humeral Ligament Test (for Subluxation of Long Head of Biceps)

Assessment: Integrity of the transverse humeral ligament.

Patient position: Sitting with the elbow flexed.

Clinician position: Resist elbow flexion or passive external rotation.

Positive response: Tendon subluxates medially, which may cause pain.

Biceps Tendon Tests: Biceps Brachii Test (Speed's Test)

Assessment: Biceps tendinitis.

Patient position: Sitting or standing with the elbow in extension and the forearm supinated.

Clinician position: Standing in front of the patient. The clinician places the right hand on the patient's right wrist and lightly palpates the bicipital groove with the index finger of the left hand.

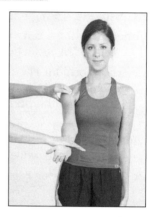

Method: The clinician resists shoulder forward flexion in supination from 0–90°.

Positive response: Increased tenderness in the bicipital groove.

Sensitivity: .18, **Specificity:** .87 (Guanche & Jones, 2003).

Muscle Length Tests: Pectoralis Minor Length Test

Patient position: Supine.

Clinician position: Standing at the head of the table facing the end of the table.

Method: The clinician measures the distance between the posterior acromion and the table for each shoulder.

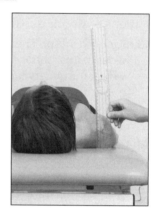

Positive response: A distance greater than 1 in. (2.5 cm) is considered tight.

Biomechanics: Tightness in the pectoralis minor will cause an anterior tilt of the scapula because of its attachment to the coracoid. An anterior tilt of the scapula will cause malpositioning between the humerus and glenoid, especially with elevation.

Muscle Length Tests: Latissimus Dorsi Muscle Length

Patient position: Supine.

Clinician position: Standing alongside the patient to observe the patient's movement.

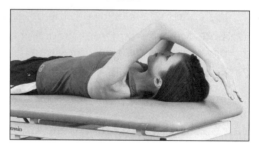

Method: The patient brings the forearms together so that the palms face her or him. The patient then lifts the arms overhead to touch the fingertips behind the head.

Positive response: The patient should achieve full shoulder elevation without arch in the back or separation of the forearms.

Biomechanics: Tightness in the latissimus dorsi can cause excessive internal rotation of the humerus, leading to poor humeral position with elevation.

STERNOCLAVICULAR JOINT (SC)

Articulation   The clavicle articulates with the manubrium of the sternum and cartilage of the first rib; the clavicle is convex cephalocaudally and concave antero-posteriorly; the manubrium and first costal cartilage are concave cephalocaudally and convex anteroposteriorly. An articular disc divides the joint into two separate compartments.

Type of Joint   Diarthrodial, sellar joint.

Degrees of Freedom

- Elevation and depression in a coronal plane about a sagittal axis that passes through the medial end of the clavicle
- Protraction and retraction in a sagittal plane about a coronal axis that passes longitudinally through the manubrium
- Rotation in a transverse plane about a longitudinal axis that passes length-wise through the clavicle

Active Range of Motion

None.

SC Joint Anterior Glide

Assessment: Clavicular movement during shoulder girdle protraction.

Patient position: Supine with the arm relaxed.

Clinician position: Standing in a walk-stance position on the right side of the patient facing the head of the table. The clinician grasps the midproximal clavicle with the fingertips on the posterior surface of the clavicle and the thumb tips on the anterior surface of the clavicle.

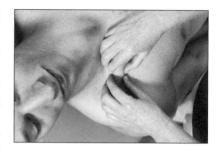

Method: The clinician applies an anterior force through the midproximal clavicle. Apply first pressures gently; increase amplitude and depth of the movement if no pain response occurs. Assess quality of movement through the range and end feel; compare with the other side.

Alternative method: Prone position with varying degrees of shoulder abduction.

Intervention: Use appropriate grade of movement (I–IV) to treat pain or resistance.

Biomechanics: According to the convex–concave rule, the concave clavicle glides anteriorly during protraction.

SC Joint Posterior Glide

Assessment: Clavicular movement during shoulder girdle retraction.

Patient position: Supine with the arm relaxed.

Clinician position: Standing in a walk-stance position on the right side of the patient facing the head of the table. The clinician places the tips of the thumbs along the proximal anterior surface of the clavicle.

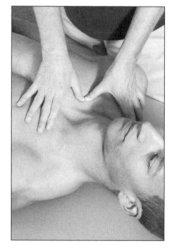

Method: The clinician applies a posterior force through the proximal clavicle. Apply first pressures gently; increase amplitude and depth of the movement if no pain response occurs. Assess quality of movement through the range and end feel; compare with the other side.

Intervention: Use appropriate grade of movement (I–IV) to treat pain or resistance.

Biomechanics: According to the concave–convex rule, the concave clavicle glides posteriorly with retraction.

Dorsal Glide

Assessment: Clavicular retraction

Patient position: Supine.

Clinician position: The clinician places the thumb on the anterior surface of the proximal end of the clavicle and places the middle phalanx along the caudal surface of the clavicle to support the thumb.

Method: Push with the thumb in a posterior direction.

Superior Glide

Assessment: Clavicular depression.

Patient position: Supine.

Clinician position: The clinician grasps the clavicle with the fingers and thumbs.

Method: Apply a superior glide to the clavicle.

Inferior Glide

Assessment: Clavicular elevation.

Patient position: Supine.

Clinician position: The clinician grasps the clavicle with the fingers and thumbs.

Method: Apply a caudal glide to the clavicle.

End Feel

Not applicable; no active range of motion.

Capsular Pattern

Pain only at extremes of range.

Close-Packed Position

Maximal shoulder elevation.

Loose-Packed Position

Shoulder in anatomical neutral.

Stability

Articular Disc   Attached to the clavicle and first costal cartilage; prevents medial dislocation of the clavicle.

Interclavicular Ligament   Extends from one clavicle to another; limits depression of the clavicle and supports the weight of the upper extremity.

Costoclavicular Ligament   Extends from the inferior surface of the medial end of the clavicle to the first rib; limits protraction, retraction, and elevation of the clavicle.

Anterior Ligament   Extends from the anterior manubrium of the sternum to the anteromedial end of the clavicle; reinforces the joint capsule and limits the posterior movement of the medial end of the clavicle associated with retraction and protraction.

Posterior SC Ligament   Extends from the posterior sternum to the posterior medial end of the clavicle; reinforces the joint capsule and limits the anterior movement of the medial end of the clavicle associated with retraction and protraction.

Special Tests

No special tests for this joint.

ACROMIOCLAVICULAR JOINT (AC)

Articulation   Acromion of the scapula and distal end of the clavicle. Concave acromion and convex clavicular joint. Fibrocartilaginous disc separates articulation.

Type of Joint   Diarthrodial, plane synovial joint.

Degrees of Freedom

- Tipping in a sagittal plane about a coronal axis that passes lengthwise through the clavicle
- Abduction and adduction in a transverse plane about a longitudinal axis that passes through the lateral end of the clavicle
- Upward and downward rotation in a coronal plane about a sagittal axis that passes through the lateral end of the clavicle

Active Range of Motion

None.

AC Joint Anterior Glide

Assessment: Anterior motion of the distal clavicle.

Patient position: Supine with the arm relaxed.

Clinician position: Kneeling at the head of the table facing the end of the table. The clinician places the tips of the thumbs along the distal posterior surface of the clavicle.

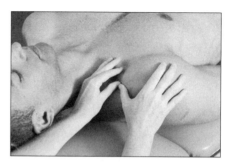

Method: The clinician applies an anterior force through the distal clavicle. Apply first pressures gently; increase amplitude and depth of the movement if no pain response occurs. Assess quality of movement through the range and end feel; compare with the other side.

Alternative method: Prone position with varying degrees of shoulder abduction.

Intervention: Use appropriate grade of movement (I–IV) to treat pain or resistance.

Biomechanics: The distal clavicle must rotate during shoulder elevation.

AC Joint Posterior Glide

Assessment: Posterior movement of the distal clavicle.

Patient position: Supine with the arm relaxed.

Clinician position: Standing in a walk-stance position on the right side of the patient facing the head of the table. The clinician places the tips of the thumbs along the distal anterior surface of the clavicle.

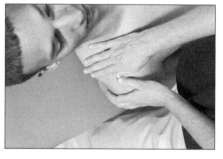

Method: Apply a posterior force through the distal clavicle. Apply first pressures gently; increase amplitude and depth of the movement if no pain response occurs. Assess quality of movement through the range and end feel; compare with the other side.

Intervention: Use appropriate grade of movement (I–IV) to treat pain or resistance.

Biomechanics: The distal clavicle must rotate during shoulder elevation.

End Feel

Not applicable; no active range of motion.

Capsular Pattern

Pain at extremes of range of horizontal adduction.

Close-Packed Position

Arm abducted to 90°.

Loose-Packed Position

Shoulder in anatomical neutral.

Stability

Coracoclavicular Ligament   This ligament holds the clavicle to the coracoid process; the trapezoid runs in an anterolateral direction and pulls the clavicle into backward rotation. It also checks overriding or lateral movement of the clavicle on the acromion. The conoid portion runs in a posteromedial direction and checks superior movement of the clavicle on the acromion. It also prevents excessive widening of the scapuloclavicular angle.

Acromioclavicular Ligament   This ligament runs from the acromion process to the clavicle. It maintains apposition of the joint and prevents posterior dislocation of the clavicle on the acromion.

Coracoacromial Ligament   This ligament blends with the trapezius and deltoid to form a roof over the humeral head. It closes the coracoacromial arch and prevents superior dislocation of the humeral head.

Acromioclavicular Shear Test

Assessment: Injury to the AC joint.

Patient position: Sitting with the arm relaxed at the side.

Clinician position: The clinician cups the hands together and compresses them over the AC joint.

Method: The compression creates a posterior-to-anterior glide of the joint.

Positive response: Pain with compression.

Horizontal Adduction

Assessment: AC joint stability.

Patient position: Sitting.

Method: The patient horizontally adducts the arm. The clinician may apply slight overpressure.

Positive response: Pain with movement.

SCAPULOTHORACIC JOINT (ST)

Articulation   Anterior surface of the scapula and posterior surface of the thorax.

Type of Joint   Not a true synovial joint, the scapulothoracic joint consists of the scapula and muscles covering the posterior thoracic wall.

Degrees of Freedom

- Elevation and depression in the frontal plane either cranially (elevation) or caudally (depression).

- Abduction and adduction following the contour of the thoracic cage; abduction is movement away from the spine, and adduction is movement toward it.

- Upward and downward rotation about a sagittal axis in which the inferior angle moves laterally for upward rotation and medially for downward rotation. Lateral and superior glide are required for upward rotation, and medial and inferior glide are required for downward rotation.

- Anterior tilting about a coronal axis in which the inferior angle moves posteriorly.

- Winging of the scapula around the vertical axis.

Active Range of Motion

None.

Scapulothoracic Joint: Scapular Alignment

Patient position: Standing with the arms resting at the sides.

Clinician position: Standing behind the patient.

Method: The clinician observes scapular position, distance from the spine, height symmetry, and scapulohumeral rhythm with shoulder abduction.

Positive response: Scapula should sit 2 to 3 in. (5 to 7.5 cm) from the spine; scapulohumeral rhythm: 2:1 ratio.

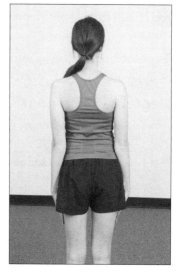

Scapulothoracic Joint: Scapular Mobility (Right)

Superior glide: To assess scapular elevation.

Inferior glide: To assess scapular depression.

Lateral glide: To assess abduction or protraction of the scapula.

Medial glide: To assess adduction or retraction of the scapula.

Patient position: Left side lying, facing the clinician. The patient's right arm is draped over the clinician's left forearm.

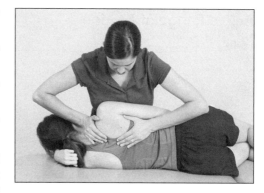

Clinician position: Standing in a squat-stance position facing the patient. The clinician places the right hand on top of the scapula, and the clinician's left hand cups the axilla under the medial border and inferior angle of the right scapula.

Method: Move the scapula in the direction to be assessed. Apply first pressures gently; increase amplitude and depth of the movement if no pain response occurs. Assess quality of movement through the range and end feel; compare with the other side.

Positive response: Limited range of motion or reproduction of symptoms.

Glide Test (Kibler Slide Test)

Examination: Symmetry of the scapulae.

Patient position: Standing with the arms at the sides.

Clinician position: Standing behind the patient with a measuring tape.

Method: The clinician measures the distance in centimeters between the inferior border of the scapula and the spinous process (*a*). Perform this measurement on both sides. Take the same measurement with the patient's hands on the hips (*b*) and with the patient's arms in 90° of shoulder flexion (*c*).

Positive response: A difference of 1.5 cm or greater between sides represents pathology on the side with greater scapular abduction.

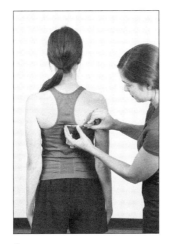

a

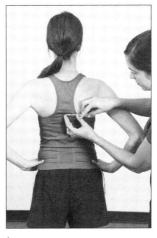

b

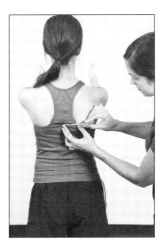

c

End Feel

Not applicable; no active range of motion.

Because this joint has no active movement associated with it and is not a true synovial joint, information in the other categories does not apply to it.

Arthrokinematics

Flexion

ST: The scapula abducts and upwardly rotates in rhythm with GH movement to maintain muscle length–tension relationship.

AC: The clavicle glides superiorly.

SC: The clavicle glides inferiorly and rotates laterally.

GH: The humeral head glides inferiorly and posteriorly on the glenoid. The humerus undergoes lateral distraction while spinning internally.

Thoracic spine: Extends.

Extension

ST: The scapula adducts and downwardly rotates.

AC: The clavicle glides inferiorly and anteriorly.

SC: The clavicle glides superiorly and medially rotates.

GH: The humeral head glides superiorly and anteriorly.

Abduction

ST: Initial 30°—the scapula is set against the thorax 30° to full abduction; the scapula rotates upwardly and forward around the rib cage.

AC: The clavicle glides inferiorly and anteriorly.

SC: The clavicle inferiorly glides from 90° to 120°; the clavicle then rotates backward along its long axis.

GH: The humeral head glides inferiorly and rolls superiorly on the glenoid (the rotator cuff muscles counteract the superior rolling of the head of the humerus). The humerus spins into lateral rotation on its long axis as it elevates above 90°.

Thoracic spine: Extends.

Unilateral elevation: The upper thoracic spine must side bend and rotate toward the side of elevation; the lower thoracic side bends away from the side of motion.

Adduction

ST: The scapula rotates downwardly with minimal to no winging.

AC: The clavicle glides superiorly and posteriorly.

SC: The clavicle glides superiorly.

GH: The humeral head glides superiorly and rolls inferiorly on the glenoid.

External Rotation

ST: The scapula adducts as the arm retracts.

SC: The clavicle rotates about the long axis.

GH: The humeral head glides anteriorly.

Internal Rotation

ST: The scapula abducts as the arm protracts.

SC: The clavicle rotates about the long axis.

GH: The humeral head glides posteriorly.

Horizontal Abduction

ST: The scapula adducts.

AC: Distraction of the joint occurs.

SC: The clavicle glides posteriorly.

GH: The humeral head glides anteriorly.

Horizontal Adduction

ST: The scapula abducts.

AC: Compression of the joint occurs.

SC: The clavicle glides anteriorly.

GH: The humeral head glides posteriorly.

Scaption   Similar to abduction, but the humerus elevates in the same plane as the scapula.

Circumduction   Combined movement of flexion, abduction, extension, and adduction.

Force Couples

1. Scapular upward rotation: the upper and lower trapezius and the serratus anterior, with the center of rotation within the scapula.

2. Humeral force couple: the deltoid pulling up and the rotator cuff pulling down, with the center of rotation between the greater tuberosity and the deltoid tubercle.

Neurology

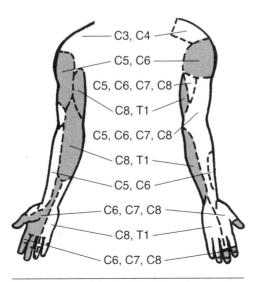

C3, C4

C5, C6

C5, C6, C7, C8

C8, T1

C5, C6, C7, C8

C8, T1

C5, C6

C6, C7, C8

C8, T1

C6, C7, C8

Dermatomes of the upper extremity.

Nerve root	Reflex	Motor	Sensory
C5	Biceps reflex	Deltoid Biceps	Lateral arm
C6	Brachioradialis reflex	Wrist extensors Biceps	Lateral forearm
C7	Triceps reflex	Wrist flexors Finger extensors Triceps	Middle finger
C8	Abductor digiti minimi	Finger flexors Hand intrinsics	Medial forearm
T1		Hand intrinsics	Medial arm

Peripheral Nerves

Nerve	Motor	Sensory
Axillary	Teres minor: shoulder external rotation	Lateral deltoid
Median	Abductor pollicis brevis (ape hand)	DIP area of first finger
Radial	Extensor carpi radialis brevis (wrist drop)	Dorsal web space
Ulnar	Flexor carpi ulnaris (claw hand)	Dorsal and palmar fifth digit

Surface Palpation

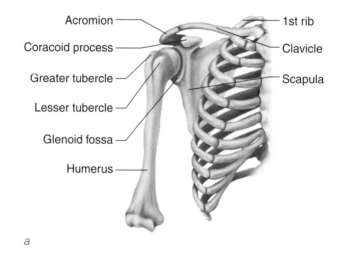

Acromion — 1st rib
Coracoid process — Clavicle
Greater tubercle — Scapula
Lesser tubercle
Glenoid fossa
Humerus

a

» continued

Shoulder bones: (*a*) anterior view; (*b*) posterior view.

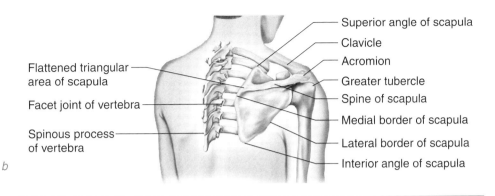

Superior angle of scapula

Clavicle

Acromion

Greater tubercle

Spine of scapula

Medial border of scapula

Lateral border of scapula

Interior angle of scapula

Flattened triangular area of scapula

Facet joint of vertebra

Spinous process of vertebra

b

» continued

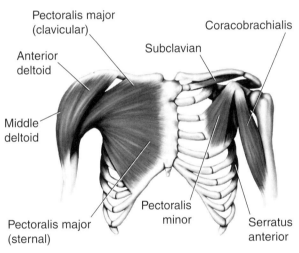

Pectoralis major (clavicular)

Coracobrachialis

Subclavian

Anterior deltoid

Middle deltoid

Pectoralis major (sternal)

Pectoralis minor

Serratus anterior

Anterior

a

Trapezius:
- Upper
- Upper middle
- Lower middle
- Lower

Levator scapulae

Supraspinatus

Rhomboids

Teres minor

Teres major

Infraspinatus

Posterior deltoid

Latissimus dorsi

b **Posterior**

Shoulder muscles.

Reprinted, by permission, from R. Behnke, *Kinetic anatomy*, 2nd ed. (Champaign, IL: Human Kinetics), 47.

Anterior

Suprasternal notch

Sternum (manubrium)

Costal cartilage

Xiphoid process

SC joint

Clavicle

AC joint

Humerus (greater tubercle, lesser tubercle, bicipital groove)

Coracoid process

First rib

Posterior (Levels)

Scapula (acromion process, spine, medial border, inferior angle)

Spinous process of lower cervical and thoracic spine

Supraclavicular fossa

Infraclavicular fossa

Muscle Origin and Insertion

Muscle	Origin and insertion
Biceps	Short head: apex of coracoid process of scapula Long head: supraglenoid tubercle to radial tuberosity and aponeurosis of biceps brachii
Coracobrachialis	Coracoid process of scapula to medial surface adjacent to deltoid tuberosity
Deltoid	Lateral third of clavicle, acromion process, spine of scapula to deltoid tubercle on humerus
Infraspinatus	Infraspinatus fossa to greater tubercle on humerus
Latissimus dorsi	Spinous process of thoracic vertebrae 6–12 and lumbar 1–5 lower 3–4 ribs, iliac crest, inferior angle of scapula to intertubercular groove on humerus
Levator scapulae	Transverse process of cervical vertebrae 1–4 to superior angle of scapula
Rhomboids	Spinous process of C7 and T1–T5 to medial border of scapula
Serratus anterior	Ribs 1–8 to underside of scapula along medial border
Subscapularis	Subscapular fossa of scapula to lesser tubercle on humerus
Supraspinatus	Supraspinous fossa to superior facet of greater tubercle of humerus
Trapezius	Upper: external occipital protuberance, medial one third of superior nuchal line, ligamentum nuchae, spinous process of C7 Middle: spinous processes of T1–T5 Lower: spinous processes of T6–T12 Upper: lateral one-third of clavicle and acromion process Middle: medial margin of acromion and superior lip of spine of scapula Lower: tubercle at apex of spine of scapula
Teres major	Posterior surface of scapula at inferior angle to lesser tubercle of humerus
Teres minor	Lateral border of posterior scapula to greater tubercle on humerus

Adapted, by permission, from J. Hamill and K. Knudzen, 1995, *Biomechanical basis of human movement* (Baltimore, MD: Lippincott, Williams, and Wilkins), 498, 499.

Muscle Action and Innervation

Action	Muscle involved	Nerve supply	Nerve root
Forward flexion	1. Deltoid (anterior fibers)	Axillary	C5, C6 (post. cord)
	2. Pectoralis major (clavicular fibers)	Lateral pectoral	C5, C6 (lat. cord)
	3. Coracobrachialis	Musculocutaneous	C5, C6, C7
	4. Biceps	Musculocutaneous	C5, C6, C7
Extension	1. Deltoid (posterior fibers)	Axillary	C5, C6 (post. cord)
	2. Teres major	Subscapular	C5, C6 (post. cord)
	3. Teres minor	Axillary	C5, C6 (post. cord)
	4. Biceps	Thoracodorsal	C6, C7, C8
	5. Pectoralis major (clavicular fibers)	Lateral pectoral	C5, C6 (lat. cord)
	6. Triceps (long head)	Radial	C5, C6, C7, C8, T1
Horizontal adduction	1. Deltoid (anterior fibers)	Axillary	C5, C6 (post. cord)
	2. Pectoralis major (clavicular fibers)	Lateral pectoral	C5, C6 (lat. cord)
Horizontal abduction	1. Deltoid (posterior fibers)	Axillary	C5, C6 (post. cord)
	2. Teres major	Subscapular	C5, C6 (post. cord)
	3. Teres minor	Axillary	C5, C6 (post. cord)
	4. Infraspinatus	Suprascapular	C5, C6, (brachial plexus)
Abduction	1. Deltoid	Axillary	C5, C6
	2. Supraspinatus	Suprascapular	C5, C6
	3. Infraspinatus	Suprascapular	C5, C6
	4. Subscapularis	Subscapular	C5, C6
	5. Teres minor	Axillary	C5, C6
Adduction	1. Pectoralis major	Lateral pectoral	C5, C6
	2. Latissimus dorsi	Thoracodorsal	C6, C7, C8
	3. Teres minor	Axillary	C5, C6
Internal rotation	1. Pectoralis major	Lateral pectoral	C5, C6
	2. Latissimus dorsi	Thoracodorsal	C6, C7, C8
	3. Teres major	Axillary	C5, C6
	4. Deltoid (anterior fibers)	Axillary	C5, C6
	5. Subscapularis	Subscapular	C5, C6
External rotation	1. Infraspinatus	Suprascapular	C5, C6
	2. Teres minor	Axillary	C5, C6
	3. Deltoid	Axillary	C5, C6

» continued

Action	Muscle involved	Nerve supply	Nerve root
Elevation of scapula	1. Trapezius (upper fibers)	Accessory cranial nerve XI	C4, C5
	2. Levator scapulae	Dorsal scapular cervical 3 and 4	C4, C5
	3. Rhomboid major	Dorsal scapular	C4, C5
	4. Rhomboid minor	Dorsal scapular	
Depression of scapula	1. Serratus anterior	Long thoracic	C5, C6
	2. Pectoralis major	Lateral pectoral	C5, C6
	3. Latissimus dorsi	Thoracodorsal	C6, C7, C8
	4. Pectoralis minor	Medial pectoral	C8, T1
	5. Trapezius (low fibers)	Accessory cranial nerve XI	C3, C4 nerve roots
Scapular protraction	1. Serratus anterior	Long thoracic	C5, C6
	2. Pectoralis major	Lateral pectoral	C5, C6
	3. Latissimus dorsi	Thoracodorsal	C6, C7, C8
	4. Pectoralis minor	Medial pectoral	C8, T1
Scapular retraction	1. Trapezius	Accessory	Cranial nerve XI
	2. Rhomboid major	Dorsal scapular	C5
	3. Rhomboid minor	Dorsal scapular	C5
Scapular upward rotation	1. Trapezius (upper fibers)	Accessory	Cranial nerve XI C3, C4 nerve roots
	2. Serratus anterior	Long thoracic	C5, C6
Scapular downward rotation	1. Levator scapulae	C3, C4 Dorsal scapular	C3, C4
	2. Rhomboid major	Dorsal scapular	C5
	3. Rhomboid minor	Dorsal scapular	C5
	4. Pectoralis minor	Medial pectoral	C8, T1

Adapted from *Orthopedic Physical Assessment*, 2nd ed., D. J. Magee, pg. 104. Copyright 1992, with permission from W. B. Saunders.

EXAMINATION SEQUENCE

HISTORY

Location of Symptoms

Common patterns of referral from the spine: triceps or medial to the scapula (could be scapulothoracic joint), supraspinatus fossa (could be supraspinatus tendinitis or tear).

The clinician may need to question popping, catching, locking, and slipping out of joint if not offered spontaneously.

Check symptom-free areas—CS, TS, scapula, AC joint, elbow, wrist, and hand.

Glenohumeral joint: deep in the shoulder joint (can be anterior or posterior), pain near deltoid insertion with no local pain, "arm band" pain—frequently worse laterally but all around arm, referred along the entire C5 dermatome (typically less severe distally), paresthesia in the index finger and thumb, spread into the supraspinatus fossa or to neck (not common).

AC joint: always local pain over the joint (anterior more common than posterior); may refer to clavicle, neck, thin line into the deltoid or biceps (rare) and C4 dermatome.

SC joint: local joint pain, spread up and lateral but not down.

Scapulothoracic joint: underneath shoulder blade, often from a trauma that affects the neck.

Aggravating Factors

GH: reach up (flexion or abduction—combing hair, removing undershirt or slip, reaching for high object), HBB (IR—putting arm into coat or shirt sleeve, putting hand into back pocket, donning belt or tucking in shirt, fastening bra, toileting), HBH (ER—combing hair, washing upper back, side lying with affected side down), lying on side (ER—compression of GH joint), pushing up (compression of GH joint)

AC or SC joint: HF (reaching for seatbelt or alarm, applying deodorant, side lying with affected side up and arm across body, side lying on affected side)

Biceps: lift, HBB

Ease Factors

Movement versus rest

Bracing or supports

TESTS AND MEASURES

Standing

Observation—General Posture, Alignment, Glide Test, Step Sign, Scapular Position

AROM With OP

Flexion: 0–180° (stabilize scapula)

Extension: 0–60°

Abduction: 0–180° (stabilize scapula)

HAC (hand across chest): 130°

ER: 0–90°

IR: HBB (hand behind back): T5–T10—normal (stabilize scapula)

HBB combination (ext, add, IR)—stabilize scapula

Functional Tests

Dependent on aggravating factors; includes HBB, overhead reach, HAC, lying on side, push-up, and so on

Special Tests

Hawkins-Kennedy impingement test

Supraspinatus test—"empty can test"

Neer's test—impingement

Drop arm test—rotator cuff rupture

Speed's test—biceps tendinitis

Sulcus sign—inferior instability

Sitting

Implicate or Clear Cervical Spine

Neurological Examination When Indicated

MMT

Scapular abduction and upward rotation: serratus anterior

Scapular elevation: upper trapezius

Shoulder flexion: anterior deltoid, supraspinatus, coracobrachialis (test in side lying if less than fair)

Shoulder scaption: deltoids, supraspinatus (test in side lying if less than fair)

Shoulder abduction: middle deltoid, supraspinatus (test in supine if less than fair)

Elbow flexion: biceps, brachialis, brachioradialis

Special Tests

Load and shift—anterior and posterior stability of GH joint

Supine

Palpation

Skin quality (temperature, sweating, skin rolling), soft tissue, bony structures

Implicate or Clear the Elbow

Neurological Examination When Indicated

Muscle Length Tests

Pectoralis minor length, latissimus dorsi length, humeral rotation

PROM

Flexion (stabilize scapula)

Abduction (stabilize scapula)

IR at 90° of shoulder abduction: 0–70° (stabilize head of humerus)

ER at 90° of shoulder abduction (stabilize head of humerus)

ER at 0°

HAC (stabilize scapula)

PAMs

GH joint: posterior (abduction), inferior (0° abduction, 90° abduction, and full flexion)

SC and AC joints: posterior, anterior glides

MMT

Shoulder horizontal adduction: pectoralis major

Special Tests

Apprehension and relocation test—instability and dislocation

Clunk test—torn glenoid labrum

Neurodynamic testing

Side Lying

PAM: Scapulothoracic Glides

Prone

Palpation (Include the Cervical Spine to Finish the Clearing Process)

PAMs—Anterior Glide

MMT

Scapular adduction: middle trapezius

Scapular depression and adduction: lower trapezius

Scapular adduction and downward rotation: rhomboids

Shoulder extension—latissimus dorsi, teres major, posterior deltoid (test in side lying if less than fair)

Shoulder horizontal abduction—posterior deltoid (test in sitting if less than fair)

Shoulder external rotation—infraspinatus, teres minor

Shoulder internal rotation—subscapularis

Elbow extension—triceps brachii

Clinical Syndromes: Acromioclavicular Joint

Description	Location and behavior of symptoms	History	Tests and measures, diagnostics	Intervention
AC SPRAIN OR SEPARATION				
Type I: incomplete tear of acromio-clavicular (AC) ligament. Type II: tear of AC ligament, partial tear of coracocla-vicular (CC) ligament. Type III–VI: complete tear of AC and CC ligaments.	Point tenderness over AC joint. Aggravating factors for all: functional activities such as lifting objects, combing hair, washing opposite axilla, reaching back to retrieve a wallet. Occupational or recreational activities such as pushing or overhead work, weightlifting, golfing, swimming, throwing, athletics, and so on.	AC sprain or sep-aration: direct force applied to acromion with the arm in an adducted position, which drives the acromion medially. Can also occur from indirect force to the acromion (fall onto out-stretched arm).	Positive HAC test. Painful arc 160–180° of shoulder abduc-tion; HBB may cause pain. PAM: abnormal mobility osteolysis. Diagnostics: X rays (+) for OA and separation. MRI. AC sprain or separa-tion. Type I: • No deformity. • No instability. • Pain on elevation and abduction past 90°. • Pain or spasm on HAC. Type II: • Widening of joint to palpation. • Palpable gap or minor step defor-mity. • Swelling, bruising, some instability. Type III–VI: • Swelling, bruising, step deformity. • Demonstrable instability. • Wider area of tenderness. • Tearing of deltoid and trapezius.	Education: activity modification. Modalities: NSAIDs, ice, later US, HMP, interfer-ential therapy. Manual therapy: joint mobilization. Therapeutic exercise: restore normal flexibil-ity, strengthen the rotator cuff muscles. Assistive devices: support for comfort. Home instruction. Medical manage-ment: Sprain or dislocation: primary AC fixation, primary coracoclavicular ligament fixation, dynamic muscle transfer, excision of distal clavicle.
OA OF AC JOINT				
Degenerative joint disease of the AC joint.	Stiffness, pain over the AC joint.	Repetitive over-head lifting.	Positive HAC test. Painful arc 160-180 degrees of shoulder abduction, HBB may cause pain. PAM: abnormal mobility.	Open resection of the distal clavicle, arthroscopic resection.
OSTEOLYSIS OF AC JOINT				
Softening, absorp-tion, or dissolu-tion of bone at the AC joint.	Stiffness, pain over the AC joint of distal clavicle.	Several theories to the cause. May be due to pre-existing trauma.	Pain with PAM but no instability.	Open resection of the distal clavicle, arthroscopic resection.

Clinical Syndromes: Glenohumeral Joint

Description	Location and behavior of symptoms	History	Tests and measures, diagnostics	Intervention
ADHESIVE CAPSULITIS				
Onset between 40 and 60 years old, F > M. Frozen shoulder, loss of glenohumeral range of motion.	Stage I: pain in and around the GH joint, increases with shoulder movement, no complaint of stiffness. Stage II: pain felt deeply or in area of deltoid insertion—may radiate down arm to elbow, disturbs sleep, pain with most movements, increasing stiffness. Inability to perform ADLs. Loss of ROM perceived as weakness. Stage III: minimal pain at rest. Stage IV: gradual resolution of stiffness.	Usually spontaneous and gradual but may be sudden or overnight. Stage I–III: may last for a few weeks to several months. Stage IV is usually entered by the 4th or 5th month and may last from 6 to 12 months.	Stage I: • Active and passive movements near full range (end range—pain with OP). • Resisted tests strong and painless. Stage II: • Lateral drift with flexion, forward drift with abduction, hitching of shoulder with flexion and abduction (reverse scapulohumeral rhythm). • Active movements more limited and painful in all directions. • Resisted movements remain painless. Stage III: • Marked limitation of active and passive movement in all directions. Movement substituted by scapula, trunk. • Regional muscle atrophy. Stage IV: • Gradual return of motion. Diagnostics: X ray—negative. Arthrography: decreased capsular size (6–8 ml of contrast allowed in joint instead of 20–30 ml normally).	Spontaneous resolution over time. Stage I and II: • Modalities: meds. • Manual therapy: massage and forcible movements contraindicated; mobilization techniques for pain. • Therapeutic exercise: exercise, massage, and forcible movements contraindicated. • Assistive devices: sling. • Home instruction: rest, positions that ease. Stage III and IV: • Manual therapy: mobilization techniques (accessory and physiological movements), manipulation. • Therapeutic exercise: stretching. • Assistive devices: none. • Home instruction.

» continued

» continued

Description	Location and behavior of symptoms	History	Tests and measures, diagnostics	Intervention
GH DISLOCATIONS: ANTERIOR				
Complete subluxation of humerus from glenoid, may be single trauma or repetitive.	Apprehension to mechanical shifting limits activities. Anterior or posterior pain present. Complaints of slipping, popping, or sliding.	Direct force: force applied directly to the posterior aspect of the humeral head, driving it anteriorly. Indirect force: indirect force via the externally rotated and abducted limb (football player attempting to block high pass).	• Hollow underneath the acromion, patient supports arm in adducted position across trunk. • Apprehension with horizontal abduction and lateral rotation, weak scapular stabilizers.	• Modalities: ice and NSAIDS. • Assistive devices: immobilization 2 days to 8 weeks. • Therapeutic exercise: up to 3 weeks—avoid ER and ABD past 45°, isometrics, gentle pendular exercises, 3–6 weeks—ER to neutral, maintain fitness, 6 weeks—progress all exercises, avoid ABD or ER until 8 weeks, do not work ROM unless signs of stiffness. Medical management: reduction by modified Stimson technique—gentle traction on the arm over a period of time—spontaneous reduction or gentle rotation of arm allows shoulder to relocate. May need open reduction if irreducible, large glenoid fragment displaced, instability after reduction, fractured humerus, vascular damage.

Description	Location and behavior of symptoms	History	Tests and measures, diagnostics	Intervention

GH INSTABILITY

Description	Location and behavior of symptoms	History	Tests and measures, diagnostics	Intervention
Increased movement of humerus relative to glenoid. • Anterior • Posterior • Multidirectional	Anterior: Apprehension to mechanical shifting limits activities. Anterior or posterior pain present. Complaints of slipping, popping, or sliding. Posterior: Anterior or posterior pain present. Multidirectional: Pain may or may not be present. May be pronounced while carrying luggage or turning over while sleeping.	• History of dislocation. • History of overuse with underlying muscular imbalance or incoordination of GH or scapulothoracic complex. • Altered structural integrity of capsule or ligaments.	Anterior: • Apprehension with horizontal abduction and lateral rotation. • Weak scapular stabilizers. • Positive load and shift. Multidirectional: • Looseness of shoulder in all directions. • Positive sulcus sign. In general: • May have pain with F, HAC, HBB. • Abduction: may have painful arc—manual stabilization may eliminate painful arc. • Positive impingement signs. • Poor scapulohumeral movement. • PROM: end feel often loose with less of ligamentous tightening than normal. • IR and horizontal flexion (HAC)—limited because of tight posterior capsule. • Resisted movements: pain free and full strength. • May have positive instability tests.	• Reduce inflammation. • Manual therapy: restore passive accessory movements. • Therapeutic exercise: restore normal muscle length. Strengthening (endurance, concentric and eccentric strength, coordination, scapular stabilization). • Taping of glenohumeral joint or scapula.

» continued

» continued

Description	Location and behavior of symptoms	History	Tests and measures, diagnostics	Intervention
IMPINGEMENT				
Pain with overhead activities secondary to encroachment of soft-tissue structures and acromioclavicular arch.	Intermittent superficial pain—may be local at the site of lesion. Typically pain is in the anterior shoulder. Pain with overhead movements. Pain with lying on side.			• Modalities: anti-inflammatory. • Manual therapy: joint mobilization to posterior capsule if appropriate. Deep friction massage.
Primary: older professional (>35 years) or recreational athlete or older, nonathletic individual.		Primary: direct compression by encroachment of the subacromial compartment. (Type III hooked acromion, degenerative changes on undersurface of acromion or AC joint.)	Primary: • Negative stability tests. • Positive impingement tests. • Painful arc between 60 and 120°. • Abnormal scapulohumeral rhythm. • Restricted internal rotation and horizontal flexion because of tight posterior capsule.	Primary: therapeutic exercise: normalize ROM (especially IR), rotator cuff strengthening and stretching (pectoralis major, pectoralis minor, rhomboids, upper trapezius).
Secondary	Young overhead.	Instability.	• Positive impingement tests and stability tests. • Increased external rotation. • Weak scapular muscles.	• Therapeutic exercise: focus on dynamic stability (scapular and rotator cuff strengthening). • Home instruction: rest, avoid offending sport.

Description	Location and behavior of symptoms	History	Tests and measures, diagnostics	Intervention
ROTATOR CUFF TEAR, TENDINITIS, OR TENDINOSIS				
Intermittent superficial pain—may be local at the site of lesion; deep anterior ache after use of the arm may radiate. • Supraspinatus • Infraspinatus • Biceps • Subscapularis	Supraspinatus: outer aspect of the shoulder to the deltoid insertion and if severe enough may radiate as far as the elbow. Infraspinatus: posterior aspect of the shoulder—can radiate down posterior arm. Biceps: anterior shoulder—can radiate down anterior aspect of upper arm. Subscapularis: local discomfort.	New use or overuse. Exacerbation and remissions over several years.	• ROM: +/– painful arc; HF—no pain with OP; HBB—pain with OP, poor scapulohumeral rhythm. • Positive impingement tests. • Resisted movements strong and painful if minor lesion, weak and painful if severe (ABD = supra, ER = infra, teres minor, IR = subscap, biceps = Speeds test). • Tenderness, thickening of affected tendon.	• Education: postural instruction, ergonomic advice. • Modalities: ice, US, iontophoresis. • Manual therapy: mobilization, soft-tissue techniques including deep friction massage. • Therapeutic exercise: muscle stretching, strengthening. • Assistive devices: none. • Home instruction: rest from activities that aggravate the condition, instruction in sleeping positions.
ROTATOR CUFF				
Partial rupture: usually middle-aged or older unless trauma Intermittent, superficial, anterior shoulder; deep anterior shoulder ache after use of arm. Night pain.	May describe similar distinct incident as complete rupture with great pain that does not settle quickly. (Fall onto elbow or hand with arm in abducted and extended position, sudden jarring or sharp movement).	• Active movements: full range with pain with OP, painful arc with abduction. HBB—anterior shoulder pain. • Drop arm test—can hold with increase pain. • Stability tests—negative. • Resisted static tests: weak and painful, palpation of affected tendons.	MRI. See tendinitis.	Progressive strengthening.

» continued

» continued

Description	Location and behavior of symptoms	History	Tests and measures, diagnostics	Intervention
Complete rupture: feeling of weakness. Night pain.	See partial rupture.	• Limited active movement with little pain. Full passive range—may have pain at EOR. • Positive drop arm test. • Negative stability tests. • Resisted static tests: weak and painless. • Palpation—negative as free ends retract. Diagnostics: may show increased space between acromion and humerus. May need MRI or arthrogram to confirm.	Elderly—usually do not repair. Goal is to maintain adequate ROM for ADLs. Young—surgical repair. MRI.	• Initial PROM. • Progressive strengthening.

Miscellaneous Shoulder Syndromes

Description	Location and behavior of symptoms	History	Tests and measures, diagnostics	Intervention
SUBACROMIAL BURSITIS				
Inflammation of the bursa located between deltoid and capsule.	Pain with elevation of arm.	May have history of prolonged overhead activity the previous day. Episodes resolve spontaneously over 4–6 weeks.	Acute: gross limitation of ABD without limitation of rotation. Greater range of passive ABD than active. Resisted testing: negative unless severe and irritable.	• Education: activity modification. • Modalities: ice, NSAID, bursal injections. • Manual therapy: mobilization. • Home instruction: rest.
SPINE REFERRAL				
C4, 5, 6.	See cervical spine clinical syndrome table.	Comparable sign with palpation to specific spinal levels. Comparable sign with CS clearing tests.	See cervical spine clinical syndrome table.	

Adapted, by permission, from C. Wadsworth, 1988, *Manual examination and treatment of the spine and extremities* (Baltimore, MD: Lippincott, Williams, and Wilkins), 106.

Elbow and Forearm

Elbow and forearm motions are important for positioning of the hand for function. Loss of elbow motion will severely limit activities of daily living, as well as sporting activities. The elbow and forearm consist of the humeroulnar, humeroradial, and superior and inferior radioulnar joints. The complex arthrokinematics make this joint a challenge for the clinician. This chapter covers osteology, arthrokinematics, range of motion, muscle origin and insertion, muscle action, neurology, and special tests for the four joints. Clinical syndromes are presented in a table at the end of the chapter. A recommended sequence for the subjective and objective exam is also included.

HUMEROULNAR JOINT (HU)

Articulation   Convex trochlea of the humerus and concave trochlear notch on proximal ulna.

Type of Joint   Diarthrodial hinge joint.

Degrees of Freedom

- Flexion and extension in a sagittal plane about a coronal axis through the humeral epicondyles
- Abduction and adduction in a frontal plane about a sagittal axis through the humeral epicondyles

Active Range of Motion

Elbow flexion: 0–150°

Elbow extension: 0–10° of hyperextension

Joint Distraction

Assessment: General mobility.

Patient position: Supine, elbow bent beyond 90°, may use a stabilization belt to hold the humerus down.

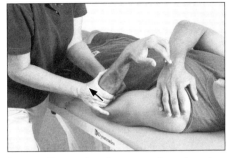

Clinician position: Standing on the side of the table in a walk-stance position facing the patient. The clinician places interlaced fingers over the proximal ulna on volar surface.

Method: The clinician applies a scoop and then a distraction force against the ulna at 45° to the shaft. Apply first pressures gently; increase amplitude and depth of the movement if no pain response occurs. Assess quality of movement through the range and end feel; compare with the other side.

Biomechanics: This technique will distract the ulna from the humerus.

Medial Glide of Ulna

Assessment: Elbow extension.

Patient position: Supine with the elbow flexed to 30° and the forearm supinated.

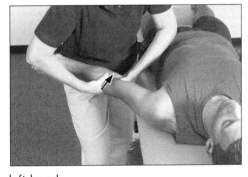

Clinician position: Standing on the side of the table in a walk-stance position facing the patient. The clinician stabilizes the distal humerus with the web space of the right hand and holds the forearm proximally near the elbow with the web space of the left hand.

Method: The clinician applies a medially directed force. Apply first pressures gently; increase amplitude and depth of the movement if no pain response occurs. Assess quality of movement through the range and end feel; compare with the other side.

Biomechanics: The concave ulna glides medially on the convex trochlea for elbow extension.

Lateral Glide of Ulna

Assessment: Elbow flexion.

Patient position: Supine with the elbow flexed to 30° and the forearm supinated.

Clinician position: Standing on the side of the table in a walk-stance position facing the patient. The clinician stabilizes the distal humerus with the web space of the left hand holds the forearm proximally near the elbow with the web space of the right hand.

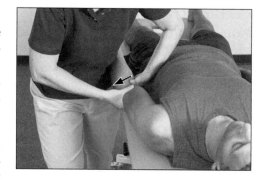

Method: The clinician applies a lateral force. Apply first pressures gently; increase amplitude and depth of the movement if no pain response occurs. Assess quality of movement through the range and end feel; compare with the other side.

Intervention: Use appropriate grade of movement (I–IV) to treat pain or resistance. A lateral glide to the humeroradial joint helps increase elbow flexion.

Biomechanics: The concave ulna glides laterally on the convex trochlea for elbow flexion.

End Feel

Flexion: Soft due to muscle bulk of anterior forearm and anterior arm.

Flexion: Hard due to minimal muscle bulk; coronoid process contacts coronoid fossa.

Flexion: Firm due to tension in the posterior joint capsule and the triceps.

Extension: Hard due to olecranon process contacting the olecranon fossa.

Extension: Firm due to tensions in the anterior joint capsule, collateral ligaments, and biceps.

Capsular Pattern

Greater limitation in flexion than extension.

Close-Packed Position

Full extension with forearm supination.

Loose-Packed Position

70–90° of flexion, 10° of supination.

Stability

Medial (Ulnar) Collateral Ligament

Anterior band (see figure 9.1): runs from anterior aspect of medial epicondyle to medial coronoid process

Posterior band: runs from posterior medial epicondyle to medial olecranon

Oblique cord: connects anterior and posterior band; restricts medial angulation of the ulna on the humerus

Capsule   Encloses humeroulnar joint, radiohumeral joint, and proximal radio-ulnar joint. Anteriorly and above, it is attached to the humerus along the upper margins of the coronoid and radial fossa and to the front of the medial and lateral epicondyles; below, it is attached to the margin of the coronoid process of the ulna and to the annular ligament. Posteriorly and above, it is attached to the margins of the olecranon fossa of the humerus; below, it is attached to the upper margin and sides of the olecranon process of the ulna and to the annular ligament.

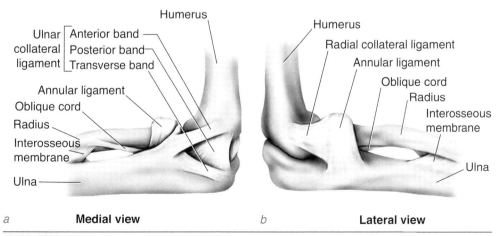

a   **Medial view**   *b*   **Lateral view**

Figure 9.1   Elbow ligaments.

Reprinted, by permission, from R. Behnke, *Kinetic anatomy*, 2nd ed. (Champaign, IL: Human Kinetics), 65.

Medial Collateral Stress Test

Assessment: Integrity of medial collateral ligament.

Patient position: Sitting with the arm relaxed, the forearm supinated and cradled in the clinician's hands, and the elbow flexed to 20°.

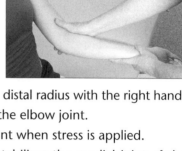

Clinician position: Standing in front of the patient. The clinician holds the elbow at the medial joint with the left hand and grasps the distal radius with the right hand.

Method: The clinician applies a valgus stress to the elbow joint.

Positive Response: Abnormal gapping of the joint when stress is applied.

Biomechanics: The medial collateral ligament stabilizes the medial joint of the elbow.

Sensitivity: .65, specificity: .50 (O'Driscoll, Lawton, and Smith 2005).

Tinel's Sign

Assessment: Involvement of the ulnar nerve.

Patient position: Sitting with the arm relaxed and supported by the table.

Clinician position: Standing in front of the patient.

Method: Tap along the ulnar nerve where it travels along the groove between the olecranon and the medial epicondyle.

Positive response: Tingling sensation that reproduces the patient's symptoms

Sensitivity: .70, specificity: .98 (Novak et al., 1994).

Medial Epicondylitis Test

Assessment: Medial epicondylitis.

Patient position: Sitting with the arm relaxed.

Clinician position: Standing in front of the patient. The clinician stabilizes and palpates the medial epicondyle with the right hand.

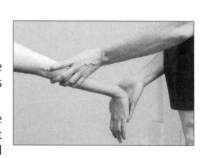

Method: The clinician passively supinates the patient's forearm with the elbow and wrist in extension while palpating the medial epicondyle.

Alternative method: Resist wrist flexion.

Positive response: Pain over the medial epicondyle.

Biomechanics: This test places maximal strain on the flexor muscles of the wrist.

Pinch Test

Assessment: Entrapment of the anterior interosseous nerve as it passes between the two heads of the pronator teres.

Patient position: Sitting.

Method: The patient pinches the tip of the index finger and thumb with a tip-to-tip pinch.

Positive response: Abnormal tip-to-tip pinch; must pinch pulp to pulp.

Elbow Quadrant Test

Assessment: Joint integrity.

Patient position: Supine with the arm relaxed.

Clinician position: One hand grasps the distal forearm and the other hand stabilizes the distal humerus, slightly flexing the patient's elbow.

Method: Take the forearm through a small arc of motion.

Positive response: Reproduction of symptoms or crepitus.

Elbow Flexion Test

Assessment: Ulnar nerve involvement.

Patient position: Sitting or standing; elbow is fully flexed with the wrist in neutral and shoulder girdle abduction and depression.

Clinician position: The clinician observes the patient for signs and symptoms.

Method: The clinician asks the patient to hold this position for 3 to 5 minutes.

Positive response: A tingling or paresthesia in ulnar nerve distribution of the forearm and hand. Sensitivity: .75, specificity: .99 (Novak et al, 1994).

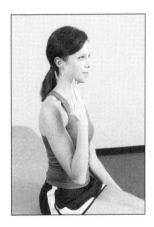

HUMERORADIAL JOINT (HR)

Articulation   Convex capitulum of the humerus and concave radial head.

Type of Joint   Diarthrodial sellar joint.

Degrees of Freedom

- Flexion and extension in sagittal plane about a coronal axis
- Abduction and adduction in coronal plane about a sagittal axis
- Internal and external rotation in transverse plane about a vertical axis

Active Range of Motion

Active range of motion for the elbow is the same as for the humeroulnar joint.

Humeroradial Distraction

Assessment: Joint mobility.

Patient position: Sitting.

Clinician position: Standing on the side of the table facing the side of the patient. The clinician stabilizes the humerus by grasping the patient's distal arm with the right hand while palpating the humeroradial joint. The clinician grasps the distal radius (not the ulna) with the thenar eminence and fingers of the left hand.

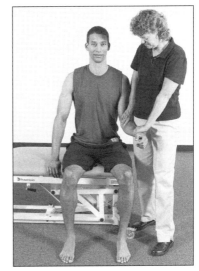

Method: The clinician pulls the radius along its long axis. A slight trunk rotation may facilitate the mobilizing force. Apply first pressures gently; increase amplitude and depth of the movement if no pain response occurs. Assess quality of movement through the range and end feel; compare with the other side.

Alternative method: This technique can be performed in the supine position.

Intervention: Use appropriate grade of movement (I–IV) to treat pain or resistance.

Biomechanics: This technique creates a distraction between the humerus and radius.

Volar Glide (*Right*)

Assessment: Flexion (volar glide).

Patient position: Supine with the elbow extended and supinated to the end range of the available range (with a pillow under the arm).

Clinician position: Standing on the side of the table in a walk-stance position facing the patient. The clinician stabilizes the humerus by grasping the medial forearm with the right

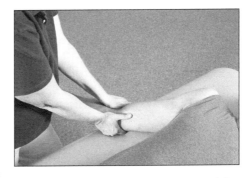

hand and places the palmar surface of the left hand on the volar aspect of the forearm with the fingers on the dorsal aspect of the radial head.

Method: The clinician moves the radial head volarly with the fingers. Apply first pressures gently; increase amplitude and depth of the movement if no pain response occurs. Assess quality of movement through the range and end feel; compare with the other side.

Intervention: Use appropriate grade of movement (I–IV) to treat pain or resistance.

Biomechanics: The radial head glides volarly with elbow flexion.

Dorsal Glide

Assessment: Extension (dorsal glide).

Patient position: Supine with the elbow extended and supinated to the end range of the available range (with a pillow under the arm).

Clinician position: Standing on the side of the table in a walk-stance position facing the patient. The clinician stabilizes the humerus by grasping the medial forearm with the right hand and places the palmar surface of the left hand on the volar aspect of the forearm with the fingers on the dorsal aspect of the radial head.

Method: The clinician moves the radial head dorsally with the palm of the hand. Apply first pressures gently; increase amplitude and depth of the movement if no pain response occurs. Assess quality of movement through the range and end feel; compare with the other side.

Intervention: Use appropriate grade of movement (I–IV) to treat pain or resistance.

Biomechanics: The radial head glides dorsally with elbow extension.

End Feel

Flexion: Soft due to soft-tissue block or bony block in thin individual

Extension: Firm due to soft tissue

Forearm pronation: Firm due to muscular end feel

Forearm supination: Firm due to ligament

Capsular Pattern

Flexion, extension, supination, pronation.

Close-Packed Position

90° flexion and 5° supination.

Loose-Packed Position

70° flexion and 35° supination.

Stability

Lateral (radial) collateral ligament: attached by its apex to the lateral epicondyle of the humerus and by its base to the upper margin of the annular ligament.

Lateral Collateral Stress Test

Assessment: Integrity of the lateral collateral ligament.

Patient position: Sitting with the arm relaxed, the forearm supinated and cradled in the clinician's hands, and the elbow slightly flexed.

Clinician position: Standing in front of the patient. The clinician holds the elbow at the medial joint with the right hand and grasps the distal radius with the left hand.

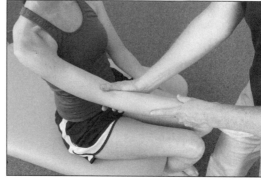

Method: The clinician applies a varus stress to the elbow joint.

Positive response: Abnormal gapping of the joint when stress is applied.

Biomechanics: The lateral collateral ligament stabilizes the lateral joint of the elbow.

Tennis Elbow Test

Assessment: Lateral epicondylitis.

Patient position: Sitting.

Clinician position: Move the patient's arm to approximately 70° of flexion with the fist clenched and wrist extended (a).

Method: Apply resistance against wrist extension (b).

Positive response: Pain along lateral epicondyle.

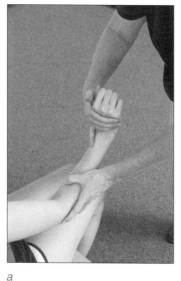

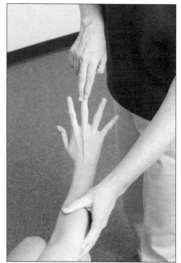

a   b

SUPERIOR RADIOULNAR JOINT (SRU)

Articulation   Concave radial notch and annular ligament and convex head of the radius.

Type of Joint   Diarthrodial pivot joint.

Degrees of Freedom

Supination and pronation in transverse plane about a vertical axis.

Active Range of Motion

Pronation: 0–80°

Supination: 0–80°

Anterior or Volar Glide

Assessment: Glides for supination.

Patient position: Sitting with the forearm supported by the table.

Clinician position: Positioned so that both thumbs are anterior to the radial head. The clinician rests the fingers down on the patient's forearm (*a*).

Method: The clinician applies a volar force to the radial head by pushing with both thumbs (*b*). Apply first pressures gently; increase amplitude and depth of the movement if no pain response occurs. Assess quality of movement through the range and end feel; compare with the other side.

Intervention: Use appropriate grade of movement (I–IV) to treat pain or resistance.

Biomechanics: Because the radial head is convex, an anterior or volar glide will facilitate supination on the concave radial notch of the ulna.

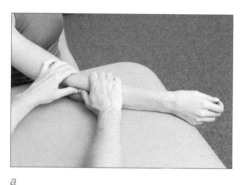

a

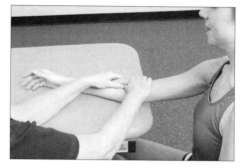

b

Posterior or Dorsal Glide

Assessment: Glide for pronation.

Patient position: Sitting with the forearm supported by the table.

Clinician position: Positioned so that both thumbs are posterior to the radial head. The clinician rests the fingers down on the patient's forearm.

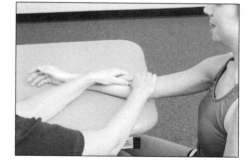

Method: The clinician applies a dorsal force to the radial head by pushing with both thumbs. Apply first pressures gently; increase amplitude and depth of the movement if no pain response occurs. Assess quality of movement through the range and end feel; compare with the other side.

Intervention: Use appropriate grade of movement (I–IV) to treat pain or resistance.

Biomechanics: Because the radial head is convex, a posterior or dorsal glide will facilitate pronation on the concave radial notch of the ulna.

End Feel

Pronation: Hard (the ulna contacts the radius).

Pronation: Firm (due to tension in the radioulnar ligament, supinator, interosseous membrane).

Supination: Firm (due to tension in the palmar radioulnar ligament of the distal radioulnar joint, interosseous membrane, pronator quadratus, quadrate ligament).

Capsular Pattern

Equal limitation of supination and pronation.

Close-Packed Position

Full pronation and full supination.

Loose-Packed Position

70° flexion, 35° supination.

Stability

Annular Ligament   Runs from the anterior margin of the radial notch of the ulna around the radial head to the posterior margin of the radial notch; blends with capsule and lateral ligament, protects the radial head, and stabilizes the radial head next to the ulna.

Quadrate Ligament   Runs from the inferior edge of the radial notch to the neck of radius; reinforces inferior joint capsule and limits supination.

Oblique Cord   Runs from just inferior to the radial notch on the ulna to inferior portion of bicipital tuberosity of radius; resists distal displacement of the radius during pulling movements.

Interosseous Membrane   Runs between the radius and ulna to provide transmission of forces.

Special Tests

No special tests for this joint.

DISTAL RADIOULNAR JOINT (DRU)

Articulation   Convex ulnar head and concave ulnar notch of the radius.

Type of Joint   Diarthrodial pivot joint.

Degrees of Freedom

Supination and pronation in transverse plane about a vertical axis.

Active Range of Motion

Pronation: 0–80°

Supination: 0–80°

Distal Radioulnar Volar Glide

Assessment: Glide for pronation.

Patient position: Sitting with the arm on the treatment table in resting position and the wrist off the edge of the table.

Clinician position: Standing or sitting perpendicular to the dorsal surface of the patient's hand. The clinician stabilizes the distal ulna by placing the fingers of the right hand on the dorsal surface and the thenar eminence and thumb on the volar surface. The clinician places the left hand in the same manner around the distal radius.

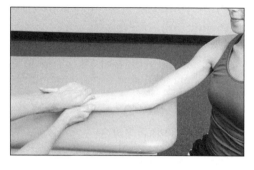

Method: Glide the distal radius volarly parallel to the ulna. Apply first pressures gently; increase amplitude and depth of the movement if no pain response occurs. Assess quality of movement through the range and end feel; compare with the other side.

Intervention: Use appropriate grade of movement (I–IV) to treat pain or resistance.

Biomechanics: According to the convex–concave rule, the radius glides volarly for pronation.

Distal Radioulnar Dorsal Glide

Assessment: Glide for supination.

Patient position: Sitting with the arm on the treatment table in resting position and the wrist off the edge of the table.

Clinician position: Standing or sitting perpendicular to the volar surface of the patient's hand. The clinician stabilizes the distal ulna by placing the fingers of the left hand on the dorsal surface and the thenar eminence and thumb on the volar surface. The clinician places the right hand in the same manner around the distal radius.

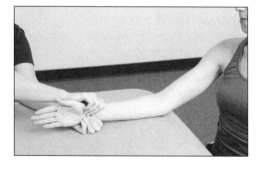

Method: Glide the distal radius dorsally parallel to the ulna. Apply first pressures gently; increase amplitude and depth of the movement if no pain response occurs. Assess quality of movement through the range and end feel; compare with the other side.

Intervention: Use appropriate grade of movement (I–IV) to treat pain or resistance.

Biomechanics: According to the convex–concave rule, the radius glides dorsally for supination.

End Feel

Supination: Firm due to ligamentous restraints

Pronation: Firm due to muscular end feel

Capsular Pattern

Full range with pain at extreme ranges.

Close-Packed Position

5° of supination.

Loose-Packed Position

10° of supination.

Stability

Interosseous Membrane   Consists of a broad sheet of collagenous tissue.

Articular Disc   Proximally articulates with the ulnar head and distally with the lunate and triquetrum; holds the radius and ulna together and helps transfer forces.

Anterior Radioulnar Ligament   Attaches above the ulnar head to the ulnar notch and stabilizes the anterior aspect of the joint.

Posterior Radioulnar Ligament   Posterior aspect of the head of the ulna to the posterior ulnar notch; stabilizes the posterior aspect of the joint.

Special Tests

No special tests for this joint.

Arthrokinematics

Extension

HU: The ulna slides posteriorly, superiorly, and medially on the trochlea until the ulnar olecranon process enters the olecranon fossa; the ulna deviates laterally and internally rotates.

HR: The concave surface of the radial head slides posteriorly on the capitulum.

Flexion

HU: The trochlear ridge of the ulna slides anteriorly, superiorly, and laterally along the trochlear groove until the coronoid process reaches the floor of the coronoid fossa; the ulna deviates medially and externally rotates.

HR: The rim of the radial head slides anteriorly in the capitulotrochlear groove to enter the radial fossa.

Pronation

SRU: The convex rim of the head of the radius spins posteriorly within the annular ligament and the concave radial notch. The ulnar head moves distally and dorsally.

Supination

SRU: The convex rim of the head of the radius spins anteriorly within the annular ligament and the concave radial notch. The ulnar head moves proximally and volarly.

Neurology

Nerve root	Reflex	Muscle	Sensory
C5	Biceps	Biceps	Lateral arm
C6	Brachioradialis	Wrist extensors	Lateral forearm
C7	Triceps	Triceps	Index and middle finger
C8	Abductor digiti minimi	Thumb extensors	Medial forearm
T1	None	Finger abductors	Medial arm

Peripheral Nerves

Nerve	Motor	Sensory
Anterior interosseous	Flexor pollicis longus, radial half of flexor digitorum profundus, pronator quadratus	
Median	Abductor pollicis brevis (ape hand)	DIP area of first finger
Radial	Extensor carpi radialis brevis (wrist drop)	Dorsal web space
Ulnar	Flexor carpi ulnaris (claw hand)	Dorsal or palmar fifth digit

Surface Palpation

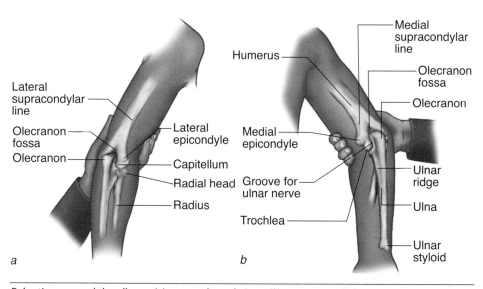

Palpation around the elbow: (*a*) posterolateral view; (*b*) posteromedial view.

Anterior

- Medial epicondyle
- Lateral epicondyle
- Medial supracondylar line
- Lateral supracondylar line
- Cubital fossa (lateral to medial): biceps tendon, brachial artery, median nerve
- Brachioradialis, pronator teres, tendon of biceps, bicipital aponeurosis, brachialis
- Median nerve
- Cubital vein
- Ulnar styloid
- Radial styloid
- Flexor carpi ulnaris
- Palmaris longus
- Flexor carpi radialis
- Pronator teres

Posterior

- Olecranon process
- Olecranon fossa
- Triceps tendon
- Ulnar nerve in cubital tunnel
- Head of the radius
- Anconeus

Muscle Origin and Insertion

Muscle	Origin and insertion
Anconeus	Lateral epicondyle of humerus to olecranon process on ulna
Biceps	Short head: apex of coracoid process of scapula Long head: supraglenoid tubercle to radial tuberosity and aponeurosis of biceps brachii
Brachialis	Anterior surface of lower humerus to coronoid process on ulna
Brachioradialis	Lateral supracondylar ridge of humerus to styloid process of radius
Extensor carpi radialis brevis	Lateral epicondyle of humerus to base of third metacarpal
Extensor carpi radialis longus	Lateral supracondylar ridge of humerus to base of second metacarpal
Extensor carpi ulnaris	Lateral epicondyle to base of fifth metacarpal
Flexor carpi ulnaris	Medial epicondyle to pisiform, hamate, base of fifth metacarpals
Flexor carpi radialis	Medial epicondyle to base of second and third metacarpals
Pronator quadratus	Distal anterior surface of ulna to distal anterior surface of radius
Pronator teres	Medial epicondyle and coronoid process on ulna to midway down on the lateral surface of radius
Supinator	Lateral epicondyle to upper, lateral side of radius
Triceps	Long head: infraglenoid tubercle of scapula Lateral head: lateral and posterior surfaces of proximal one-half of body of humerus, and lateral intermuscular septum Medial head: distal two-thirds of medial and posterior surfaces of humerus below the radial groove and from medial intermuscular septum to olecranon process and antebrachial fascia

Adapted from J. Hamill and K. Knudzen, 1995, *Biomechanical basis of human movement* (Baltimore, MD: Lippincott, Williams, and Wilkins), 500, 501.

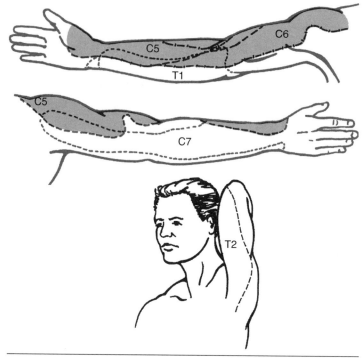

Dermatomes around the elbow.

Muscle Action and Innervation

Action	Muscle involved	Nerve supply	Nerve root
Elbow flexion	Brachialis	Musculocutaneous	C5–C6 (C7)
	Biceps brachii	Musculocutaneous	C5–C6
	Brachioradialis	Radial	C5–C6
	Pronator teres	Median	C6–C7
	Flexor carpi ulnaris	Ulnar	C7–C8
Elbow extension	Triceps	Radial	C6–C8
	Anconeus	Radial	C7–C8
Forearm supination	Supinator	Radial	C5–C6
	Biceps brachii	Musculocutaneous	C5–C6
Forearm pronation	Pronator quadratus	Median	C5–C6
	Pronator teres	Median	C6–C7
	Flexor carpi radialis	Median	C6–C7
Wrist flexion	Flexor carpi radialis	Median	C6–C7
	Flexor carpi ulnaris	Ulnar	C7–C8
Wrist extension	Extensor carpi radialis longus	Radial	C6–C7
	Extensor carpi radialis brevis	Radial	C7–C8
	Extensor carpi ulnaris	Radial	C7–C8

Adapted from *Orthopedic Physical Assessment*, 2nd ed., D.J. Magee, pg. 104. Copyright 1992, with permission from W. B. Saunders.

EXAMINATION SEQUENCE

HISTORY

Profile

Occupation and recreational activities—consider effect of elbow pain on level of function or disability (repetitive wrist flexion and extension or pronation and supination, sporting activities, overuse or abuse)

Location of Symptoms

Common patterns of referral from the C-spine nerve root: C6, C7, C8.

May need to question popping, catching, locking, and slipping out of joint if not offered spontaneously.

Check symptom-free areas—CS, TS, scapula, AC joint, GH joint, wrist, and hand.

Lateral joint: consider lateral epicondylitis, radial head fracture, supracondylar fracture, osteochondritis of capitellum.

Medical joint: consider medial epicondylitis, ulnar collateral sprain, Panner's disease in the young throwing athlete, ulnar nerve.

Anterior: consider biceps tendon injury, osteochondritis dissecans.

Posterior joint: consider olecranon bursitis, triceps tendon strain.

Aggravating Factors

Biceps: lift, HBB

Triceps: pushing, pressing

Wrist flexion, extension

Pronation and supination (opening a door): proximal radioulnar joint

Ease Factors

Movement versus rest

Bracing or supports

Medication

History

Fall on outstretched hand (FOOSH)

Repetitive

TESTS AND MEASURES

Standing

Observation

Posture or structure (carrying angle: males = 5–10°; females = 15°)

Implicate or Clear Shoulder

Functional Tests

Observation—Posture, Atrophy or Deformities, Edema in UE

Palpation—Bony or Soft Tissue (Anterior, Posterior, Lateral, Medial)

Girth

Implicate or Clear Cervical Spine

Neurological Examination (Segmental, Peripheral, or Central as Indicated)

AROM With OP

Elbow flexion (0–150°)

Elbow extension (0°)—note hyperextension

Forearm pronation (0–80°)

Forearm supination (0–80°)

PAMs

Humeroulnar joint—medial glide

Humeroradial joint—distraction, lateral glide

Proximal radioulnar joint—anterior (volar) glide, posterior (dorsal) glide

Distal radioulnar joint—volar glide, dorsal glide

MMT

Elbow flexion (biceps)

Forearm pronation and supination

Special Tests

Varus or valgus stress test

Lateral epicondylitis test

Medial epicondylitis test

Tinel's test of ulnar nerve

Elbow flexion test

Neurological Examination as Indicated

Implicate or Clear Wrist

PAMs

Humeroulnar joint—distraction

Humeroradial joint—volar glide, dorsal glide

Neurodynamic Testing

Implicate or Clear Cervical Spine With Palpation

MMT: Elbow Extension (Test in Sitting Position if Less Than Fair)

Clinical Syndromes

Description	Location and behavior of symptoms	History	Tests and measures, diagnostics	Intervention
LATERAL EPICONDYLITIS				
Tendinitis of wrist extensor at common origin on lateral epicondyle.	Dull ache at rest; sharp pain with lifting activity at lateral epicondyle.	Gradual onset usually involving repetitive wrist extension.	Resisted wrist extension causes pain; tenderness over lateral epicondyle. + lateral epicondylitis test; rule out C-spine.	Check radial nerve, ergonomic assessment, check radial head mobility, soft-tissue mobilization.
MEDIAL EPICONDYLITIS				
Tendinitis of wrist flexors at common origin on medial epicondyle.	Pain with wrist and finger flexion at medial epicondyle.	Gradual onset usually involving repetitive wrist flexion.	Resisted wrist flexion; tenderness over medial epicondyle. + medial epicondylitis test.	Biomechanics, check joint mobility, soft-tissue mobilization.
LITTLE LEAGUER'S ELBOW				
Epiphysitis of medial epicondyle.	Pain or tenderness of medial epicondyle.	Gradual onset, throwing in baseball (curveballs), forceful pronation.	Loss of full extension, pain with resisted flexion. Diagnostics: Radiograph is positive for widening of medial physis.	Decrease inflammation, gentle ROM, may immobilize, throwing technique and pitch selection.
OSTEOCHONDRITIS DISSECANS				
Broken pieces of cartilage in joint.	Common in the capitellum. Pain or swelling, 12 to 15 years old, pain lateral or anterior.	Gradual onset (1 or 2 years), throwing curveball, gymnastics, wrestling. Trauma, changes in circulation.	Limited ROM (ext), clicking, locking. Diagnostics: X ray, bone scan, MRI.	Rest from stress. Good prognosis if diagnosed early. Surgery: curettage or drilling.
PANNER'S DISEASE				
Osteochondrosis of capitellum; variant in ossification.	90% male, dominant UE, 7 to 10 years old, pain lateral.	Atraumatic.	Swelling, tenderness, clicking, dec extension. Diagnostics: X ray.	Rest, gentle ROM.

» continued

» continued

Description	Location and behavior of symptoms	History	Tests and measures, diagnostics	Intervention
OLECRANON BURSITIS				
Inflammation of the olecranon bursa.	Obvious swelling posterior elbow.	Continuous pressure on olecranon; or acute trauma.	Swelling; limited range of motion; pain to palpation of bursa.	RICE, padding, iontophoresis.
BICEPS MUSCLE RUPTURE				
Disruption of biceps from attachment (usually distal).	Pain at area of biceps.	Quick forceful biceps contraction.	Discontinuity of biceps with bulge, loss of elbow flexion strength.	May need surgical intervention.
RADIAL HEAD FRACTURE				
	One-third of all elbow fractures, males > females, 30 to 40 years old, pain over radial head.	FOOSH: forearm supinated and elbow flexed, loading of radiocapitellar joint.	Stiff joint, unable to fully flex or extend, pain with supination–pronation. Diagnostics: X ray.	Immobilization for short period, ROM, strengthening.
MYOSITIS OSSIFICANS				
Calcification of muscle.		Trauma.	Decreased ROM. Palpation of mass.	Rest. Gentle ROM. Medical management: symptoms.
COMPLEX REGIONAL PAIN SYNDROME				
Hypovascular-ity caused by increased sympathetic activity.	Sensitive to touch, hesitation to move arm, exquisitely painful.	Gradual onset after period of immobilization.	Pitting edema, tenderness, skin changes, bluish skin, restricted movement.	Desensitization, medication, sympathetic blocks.
VOLKMANN'S ISCHEMIC CONTRACTURE				
Compartment syndrome resulting in decreased circulation and nerve distur-bance.	Severe pain in forearm muscles.	Following fracture or dislocation of the elbow, arterial ischemia.	Purple discolor-ation of hand loss of radial pulse, clawed fingers, limited finger motion.	Medication.
PULLED ELBOW				
Radial head slippage through annular ligament.	Children, 2 to 3 years old, traction with arm supinated and extended.	Pull of elbow.	Limited exten-sion, guarding of arm.	Joint manipulation.

Description	Location and behavior of symptoms	History	Tests and measures, diagnostics	Intervention
PRONATOR TERES SYNDROME				
Median nerve compression at pronator teres.	Paresthesia in thumb, index finger, middle finger aggravated with activity, pain volar aspect of forearm, not nocturnal.	Dislocation, entrapment.	Weakness in muscles of forearm and hand innervated by median nerve (FCR, PL, FD). Phalen's (–). Diagnostics: EMG.	Rule out cervical; relative rest, splinting, check neurodynamics and joint mechanics.
ANTERIOR INTEROSSEOUS SYNDROME				
Median nerve compression.	Sudden severe arm pain that resolves in a few hours, no loss of sensation.	Trauma, entrapment.	Weakness of FPL, PQ, FDP; unable to pinch tip to tip.	Rule out cervical; relative rest, splinting, check neurodynamics and joint mechanics.
RADIAL TUNNEL SYNDROME				
Radial nerve compression at elbow.	Pain over lat hum epicondyle, tender radial head, numb radial nerve.	Trauma, entrapment.	Resisted middle finger extension. Diagnostics: EMG.	Rule out cervical; relative rest, splinting, check neurodynamics and joint mechanics.
POSTERIOR INTEROSSEOUS SYNDROME				
Radial nerve compression at arcade of Frohse.	Tender to palpation distal from lateral epicondyle.	Trauma, entrapment, history of lateral epicondylitis.	Symptoms with resisted wrist ext, unable to extend thumb or fingers at MCP. Diagnostics: EMG.	Rule out cervical; rule out lateral epicondyle; relative rest, splinting, check neurodynamics and joint mechanics.
CUBITAL TUNNEL SYNDROME				
Ulnar nerve compression.	Paresthesia radiating to dorsal fourth and fifth digits.	Trauma, entrapment.	Weak pinch, grasp. Claw hand. Froment's (+). Tinel's (+).	Rule out cervical; relative rest, splinting, check neurodynamics and joint mechanics.
SPINE REFERRAL				
	C5, 6, 7.	See cervical spine clinical syndromes table.	Comparable sign with CS clearing tests and palpation to specific spinal levels.	See cervical spine clinical syndromes table.

Adapted, by permission, from C. Wadsworth, 1988, *Manual examination and treatment of the spine and extremities* (Baltimore, MD: Lippincott, Williams, and Wilkins), 106.

Wrist and Hand

The wrist and hand make up 90% of the use of the upper extremity. The wrist and hand complex consists of the radiocarpal and midcarpal joints at the wrist and the carpometacarpal, metacarpal, and interphalangeal joints of the digits. Although the shoulder, elbow, and wrist and hand are listed in separate chapters, the clinician needs to assess the entire upper-extremity chain. This chapter covers osteology, arthrokinematics, range of motion, muscle origin and insertion, muscle action, neurology, and special tests for all these joints. A table at the end of the chapter presents clinical syndromes. A recommended sequence for the subjective and objective exam is also included.

RADIOCARPAL JOINT

Articulation   A biconcave surface formed by the radial facet and radioulnar disc with a biconvex surface consisting of the scaphoid, lunate, and triquetrum.

Type of Joint   Diarthrodial ellipsoid joint.

Degrees of Freedom

- Flexion and extension in sagittal plane about a coronal axis through the head of the capitate
- Ulnar and radial deviation in coronal plane about a sagittal axis through the capitate

Active Range of Motion
(American Academy of Orthopedic Surgeons)

Flexion: 0–80°

Extension: 0–70°

Ulnar deviation: 0–30°

Radial deviation: 0–20°

Distraction

Assessment: Joint mobility of the wrist.

Patient position: Sitting with the arm on the treatment table, the palm down, and the wrist over the edge of the table.

Clinician position: Standing in a walk-stance position perpendicular to the patient's hand. The clinician stabilizes the distal radioulnar joint

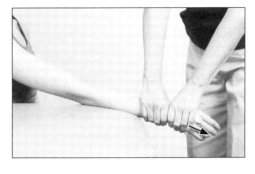

by grasping the dorsal aspect of the styloid processes of the radius and ulna with the web space of one hand and places the other hand in the same manner around the distal and proximal rows of the carpals.

Method: Apply a gentle longitudinal pull, distracting the carpals from the radius. Apply first pressures gently; increase amplitude and depth of the movement if no pain response occurs. Assess quality of movement through the range and end feel; compare with the other side.

Biomechanics: Distraction of the radiocarpal joint is caused by separation of the carpals from the radius.

Volar Glide

Assessment: Wrist extension.

Patient position: Sitting with the arm on the treatment table, the palm down, and the wrist over the edge of the table.

Clinician position: Standing in a walk-stance position perpendicular to the patient's hand. The clinician stabilizes the distal radioulnar joint by grasping the dorsal aspect of

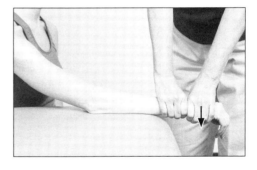

the styloid processes of the radius and ulna with the web space of one hand and places the other hand in the same manner around the distal and proximal rows of the carpals.

Method: Apply a force directed in a volar direction. Apply first pressures gently; increase amplitude and depth of the movement if no pain response occurs. Assess quality of movement through the range and end feel; compare with the other side.

Intervention: Use appropriate grade of movement (I–IV) to treat pain or resistance.

Biomechanics: According to the convex–concave rule, the carpals glide volarly for wrist extension.

Dorsal Glide

Assessment: Wrist flexion.

Patient position: Supine with arm overhead, the forearm supported on a towel roll, the palm up, and the wrist over the edge of the table.

Clinician position: Standing in a walk-stance position perpendicular to the patient's hand. The clinician stabilizes the distal radioulnar joint by grasping the dorsal aspect of the styloid processes of the radius and ulna with the web space of one hand and places the other hand in the same manner around the distal and proximal rows of the carpals.

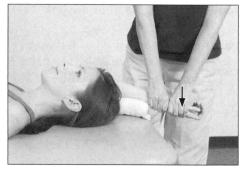

Method: Apply a force directed in a dorsal direction. Apply first pressures gently; increase amplitude and depth of the movement if no pain response occurs. Assess quality of movement through the range and end feel; compare with the other side.

Intervention: Use appropriate grade of movement (I–IV) to treat pain or resistance.

Biomechanics: According to the convex–concave rule, the carpals glide dorsally for wrist flexion.

Radial Glide

Examination: Glide associated with ulnar deviation.

Patient position: Seated with the forearm supported on a towel roll (optional), and the wrist in a neutral position and over the edge of the table.

Clinician position: Standing in a walk-stance position perpendicular to the patient's dorsal aspect of the patient's hand. The clinician stabi-

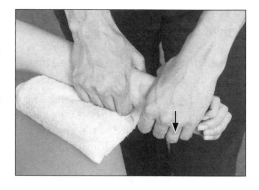

lizes the distal radioulnar joint by grasping the dorsal aspect of the styloid processes of the radius and ulna with the web space of one hand and places the other hand in the same manner around the distal and proximal rows of the carpals.

Method: Apply a force directed toward the radial border perpendicular to line of forearm. Apply first pressures gently; increase amplitude and depth of the movement if no pain response occurs. Assess quality of movement through the range and end feel; compare with the other side.

Positive response: Limited range of motion or reproduction of symptoms.

Biomechanics: According to the convex–concave rule, the carpals glide radially for ulnar deviation.

Ulnar Glide

Assessment: Radial deviation.

Patient position: Sitting with the forearm in neutral and supported with a towel roll (optional) on the table.

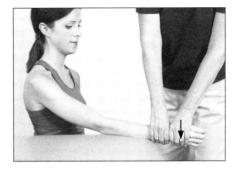

Clinician position: Standing in a walk-stance position perpendicular to the patient's dorsal aspect of the patient's hand. The clinician stabilizes the distal radioulnar joint by grasping the dorsal aspect of the styloid processes of the radius and ulna with the web space of one hand and places the other hand in the same manner around the distal and proximal rows of the carpals.

Method: Apply a force directed toward the ulnar border perpendicular to line of forearm. Apply first pressures gently; increase amplitude and depth of the movement if no pain response occurs. Assess quality of movement through the range and end feel; compare with the other side.

Intervention: Use appropriate grade of movement (I–IV) to treat pain or resistance.

Biomechanics: According to the convex–concave rule, the carpals glide ulnarly for radial deviation.

End Feel

Flexion: Firm due to tension in the dorsal radiocarpal ligament and dorsal joint capsule.

Extension: Firm due to tension in the palmar radiocarpal ligament and palmar joint capsule.

Extension: Hard (the radius contacts carpal bones).

Radial deviation: Hard (the radial styloid contacts the scaphoid).

Radial deviation: Firm due to tension in the ulnar collateral ulnocarpal ligament and ulnar portion of the joint capsule.

Ulnar deviation: Firm due to tension in the radial collateral ligament and radial portion of the joint capsule.

Capsular Pattern

Equal limitation of flexion and extension.

Close-Packed Position

Extension with radial deviation.

Loose-Packed Position

Loose-packed position is the resting position of the hand; 10° of wrist flexion and slight ulnar deviation.

Stability

Palmar Radiocarpal Ligament From the anterior edge of the distal radius to the proximal carpal row and capitate; checks supinatory movement between joint surfaces and maintains joint integrity (includes the radiocapitate, radiotriquetral, radioscaphoid ligaments).

Palmar Ulnocarpal Ligament From the anterior edge of the articular disc and base of the ulnar styloid to carpal—reinforces the ulnar side of the wrist dorsal radiocarpal ligament; from the posterior edge of the distal radius to the triquetrum and lunate—checks supinatory movement between joint surfaces and maintains joint integrity (includes the ulnolunate, ulnotriquetral, ulnocapitate ligaments).

Radial Collateral Ligament Radial styloid to the scaphoid, trapezium, first metacarpal; limits ulnar deviation.

Ulnar Collateral Ligament Ulnar styloid process to the medial triquetrum, pisiform, and articular disc; limits radial deviation.

Dorsal Radiocarpal Ligament Posterior border of the distal radius to the scaphoid, lunate, and triquetrum; reinforces dorsal structures.

Fibrous Capsule Strong but loose; attaches close to articulation and proximally, just distal to the inferior epiphyseal line of the radius and ulna (figure 10.1, *a–c*).

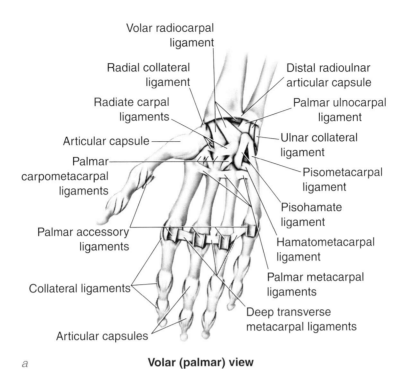

Volar radiocarpal ligament

Radial collateral ligament

Radiate carpal ligaments

Articular capsule

Palmar carpometacarpal ligaments

Palmar accessory ligaments

Collateral ligaments

Articular capsules

Distal radioulnar articular capsule

Palmar ulnocarpal ligament

Ulnar collateral ligament

Pisometacarpal ligament

Pisohamate ligament

Hamatometacarpal ligament

Palmar metacarpal ligaments

Deep transverse metacarpal ligaments

a   **Volar (palmar) view**

Distal radiocarpal articular capsule

Palmar ulnocarpal ligament

Dorsal radiocarpal ligaments

Radiocarpal collateral ligament

Dorsal intercarpal ligaments

Articular capsule

Dorsal carpometacarpal ligaments

Dorsal metacarpal ligaments

Collateral ligaments

Articular capsules

b   **Dorsal view**

» continued

Figure 10.1   (*a*) Palmar view of the wrist and hand ligaments; (*b*) dorsal view of the ligaments of the wrist; (*c*) volar aspect of the triangular fibrocartilage complex.

Reprinted from R. Behnke, *Kinetic anatomy*, 2nd ed. (Champaign, IL: Human Kinetics), 78.

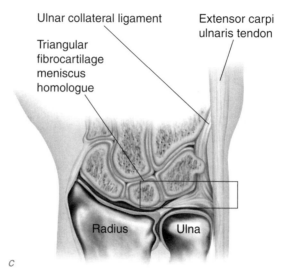

Ulnar collateral ligament

Triangular
fibrocartilage
meniscus
homologue

Extensor carpi
ulnaris tendon

Radius

Ulna

c

Figure 10.1 continued

Triangular Fibrocartilage Complex The triangular fibrocartilage complex consists of a fibrocartilage disc (meniscus homologue) interposed between the triquetrum carpal and the distal ulna. The function of this complex is to enhance joint congruity and cushion against compressive forces.

Phalen's Test

Assessment: Median nerve compression, carpal tunnel syndrome.

Patient position: Sitting. The patient places the dorsum of both hands together with the fingers pointing down (*a*).

Clinician position: Sitting in front of the patient.

Method: The patient is instructed to maintain this position for 60 seconds. The clinician notes the time of onset of symptoms and stops the test when symptoms are reproduced (*b*).

Alternative method: Reverse Phalen's test—same as Phalen's test except the hands are reversed (*b*).

Positive response: Increase in the patient's symptoms in the medial nerve distribution.

Biomechanics: These maneuvers place maximal compression or distraction of the median nerve.

Sensitivity: .68, specificity: .91 (Ahn 2001).

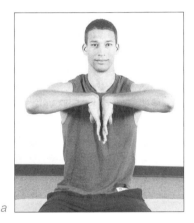
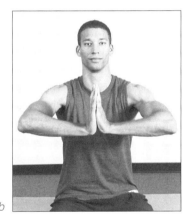

a

b

Median Nerve Tinel's Sign

Assessment: Median nerve.

Patient position: Sitting with the forearm supinated.

Clinician position: Standing alongside the patient

Method: The clinician taps over the patient's volar carpal ligament with the fingertip.

Positive response: Pain or paresthesia distal to the wrist.

Sensitivity: .68, specificity: .90 (Ahn 2001).

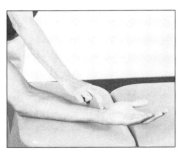

Finkelstein's Test

Assessment: Tenosynovitis of the thumb (de Quervain's).

Patient position: Sitting.

Method: The patient makes a fist with the thumb inside the fingers.

Clinician position: The clinician stabilizes the forearm and ulnarly deviates the wrist.

Positive response: Pain over the abductor pollicis longus and extensor pollicis brevis.

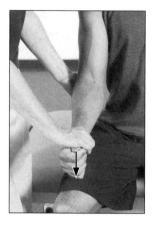

Allen Test

Assessment: Patency of the radial and ulnar arteries.

Patient position: Sitting with the forearm free to move. The elbow is bent with the fingers pointing up toward the ceiling.

Method: The clinician compresses the radial and ulnar arteries at the wrist; one thumb is on the ulnar artery and one thumb is on the radial artery (*a*). The patient should open and close his or her fist quickly. The clinician releases the pressure on one artery and observes the filling pattern of the vessels in the palm (*b*). The same is repeated for the other artery.

Positive response: Blanching remains in the palm after pressure is released from the artery. The test can also be used to test individual fingers.

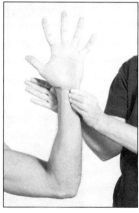
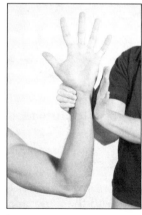

a   b

MIDCARPAL JOINT

Articulation   Proximally scaphoid, lunate, and triquetrum and distally trapezium, trapezoid, capitate, and hamate.

Type of Joint   Diarthrodial plane joint.

Degrees of Freedom

Primarily glide occurs.

Active Range of Motion

None.

Volar Glide

Assessment: Extension.

Patient position: Sitting with the forearm in pronated position.

Clinician position: Facing the patient. The proximal hand is on the proximal row of carpal bones to be stable; the other hand is on the distal row of carpal bones.

Method: Apply force through the distal hand in volar direction.

Dorsal Glide

Assessment: Flexion.

Patient position: Sitting with the forearm in supinated position.

Clinician position: Facing the patient. The proximal hand is on the proximal row of carpal bones to be stable; the other hand is on the distal row of carpal bones.

Method: Apply force through the distal hand in dorsal direction.

End Feel

Same as with movements for radiocarpal joints.

Capsular Pattern

None.

Close-Packed Position

Extension with ulnar deviation.

Loose-Packed Position

Neutral or slight flexion with ulnar deviation.

Stability

Palmar Intercarpal Ligament   Connects carpal on palmar side, reinforces the palmar arch.

Dorsal Intercarpal Ligament   Connects dorsal proximal and distal row of carpals.

Special Tests

None.

CARPOMETACARPAL JOINT (CMC, 2 TO 5)

Articulation   Distal carpal and proximal metacarpals; second metacarpal with the trapezium, trapezoid, capitate; third metacarpal with the capitate; fourth with the capitate and hamate; fifth with the hamate.

Type of Joint   Diarthrodial condyloid joint; the fifth CMC is referred to as sellar joint.

Degrees of Freedom

- Flexion and extension
- Abduction and adduction

Active Range of Motion

None.

Volar or Dorsal Glide

Assessment: Volar or dorsal glide of metacarpal for flexion and extension.

Patient position: Sitting with the forearm supported.

Clinician position: The clinician stabilizes the carpal with one hand, grasping with the thumb dorsally and index finger volarly. The other hand grasps around the proximal portion of the metacarpal.

Method: Apply force in a volar or dorsal direction.

Distraction

Assessment: Mobility.

Patient position: Sitting with the forearm supported.

Clinician position: The clinician stabilizes the carpal with one hand, grasping with the thumb dorsally and index finger volarly. The other hand grasps around the proximal portion of the metacarpal.

Method: Apply long-axis distraction to the metacarpal to separate the joint.

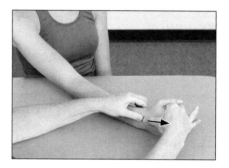

End Feel

Not applicable.

Capsular Pattern

Equal limitation in all directions.

Close-Packed Position

Not described.

Loose-Packed Position

Functional position of the wrist.

Stability

Palmar or Dorsal CMC Bands From the distal carpal bones to metacarpal bases.

Interosseous Ligament From the capitate and hamate to the third and fourth metacarpals.

Special Tests

None.

Arthrokinematics of the Wrist Complex

Extension About 45° of the movement occurs at the radiocarpal joint, and 25° occurs at the midcarpal joint.

1. Proximal carpal bones move volarly on the radius (the trapezium and trapezoid bones slide dorsally on the scaphoid).
2. The capitate and hamate bones slide volarly on the scaphoid, lunate, and triquetrum.
3. The scaphoid spins on the radius at full extension; approximation of the scaphoid and lunate to the radius and disc.

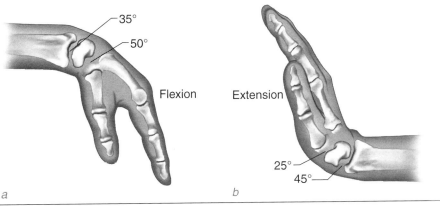

(*a*) Flexion of the wrist; (*b*) extension of the wrist.

Flexion   About 50° of the movement occurs at the midcarpal joint, and 30° of the movement occurs at the radiocarpal joint.

1. Proximal carpal bones move dorsally on the radius (the trapezium and trapezoid move volarly on the scaphoid).
2. The capitate and hamate bones slide dorsally on the scaphoid, lunate, and triquetrum; distraction of the radiocarpal joint.

Ulnar Deviation   Occurs primarily at the radiocarpal joint.

1. Proximal carpal bones glide radially; ulnar glide of hamate and capitate on the triquetrum and lunate.
2. The proximal surface of trapezoid glides radially on the scaphoid; the trapezium and trapezoid move volarly.

Radial Deviation   Occurs primarily at the midcarpal joint.

1. Proximal carpal bones move toward the ulna; the proximal scaphoid also moves volarly.
2. The proximal surface of the capitate and hamate slide ulnarly.
3. The trapezoid moves dorsally.

METACARPOPHALANGEAL JOINTS (MCP, 2 TO 5)

Articulation   Convex distal end of each metacarpal and the concave end of each proximal phalanx.

Type of Joint   Diarthrodial condyloid joint.

Degrees of Freedom

- Flexion and extension in sagittal plane through coronal axis that runs through the heads of the metacarpals
- Abduction and adduction in coronal plane through sagittal axis using the third digit as the standard

Active Range of Motion

Flexion: 0–90°

Extension: 0–30°

Abduction: 0–80°

Adduction: 0°

Distraction

Assessment: Mobility of the joint.

Patient position: Sitting with the forearm in pronated position.

Clinician position: Sitting (or standing in a walk-stance position) perpendicular to the patient's hand. The clinician stabilizes the desired MCP and holds accompanying proximal phalanx firmly.

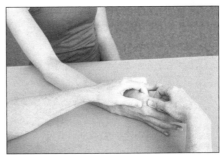

Method: Distract the proximal phalanx from metacarpals. Apply first pressures gently; increase amplitude and depth of the movement if no pain response occurs. Assess quality of movement through the range and end feel; compare with the other side.

Intervention: Use appropriate grade of movement (I–IV) to treat pain or resistance.

Biomechanics: This technique creates separation between the phalanx and metacarpal.

Glides

Volar glide: To assess flexion.

Dorsal glide: To assess extension.

Radial glide: To assess abduction.

Ulnar glide: To assess adduction.

Patient position: Sitting with the forearm supported.

Clinician position: Fixate the proximal bone with the fingers; wrap the fingers and thumb of the other hand around the distal bone close to the joint.

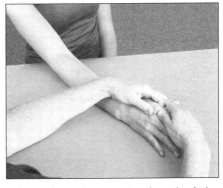

Method: Apply the glide force by the thumb against the proximal end of the bone.

End Feel

Flexion: Hard (the palmar phalanx contacts metacarpal bones).

Flexion: Firm due to tension in the dorsal joint capsule and collateral ligaments.

Extension: Firm due to tension in the palmar joint capsule and palmar ligament.

Abduction: Firm due to tension in the collateral ligaments, fascia of web space, and palmar interosseous.

Capsular Pattern

Equal restriction in flexion and extension.

Close-Packed Position

Full flexion.

Loose-Packed Position

Slight flexion.

Stability

Fibrous Capsule   Encloses the heads of metacarpals and the bases of proximal phalanx.

Collateral Ligaments   Run from the tubercle and adjacent depression on the side of the metacarpal head to the base of phalanx.

Deep Transverse Metacarpal Ligaments   Unite MCP ligaments and hold heads of MCP together.

Volar Plate   Fixed distally to the base of phalanx and proximal neck of MCP bone; attaches to deep transverse metacarpal ligament, flexor sheath, and collateral ligaments; prevents hyperextension of the joint.

Special Tests

None.

PROXIMAL INTERPHALANGEAL JOINTS (PIP, 2 TO 5)

Articulation   Convex head of the proximal phalanx and the concave base of the more distal phalanx.

Type of Joint   Diarthrodial hinge joint.

Degrees of Freedom

Flexion and extension in the sagittal plane.

Active Range of Motion

Flexion: 0–120°

Extension: 0–5°

Distraction and Glides

Distraction: To assess mobility.

Ventral glide: To assess flexion.

Dorsal glide: To assess extension.

Patient position: Sitting with the forearm supported.

Clinician position: Fixate the proximal bone with the fingers; wrap the fingers and thumb of the other hand around the distal bone close to the joint.

Method: Apply the glide force by the thumb against the proximal end of the more distal bone.

End Feel

Flexion: Hard (the palmar middle phalanx contacts the proximal phalanx).

Flexion: Soft (soft tissue contacts soft tissue).

Flexion: Firm due to tension in the dorsal joint capsule and collateral ligaments.

Extension: Firm due to tension in the palmar joint capsule and palmar ligament.

Capsular Pattern

Equal restriction in flexion and extension.

Close-Packed Position

Full extension.

Loose-Packed Position

Slight flexion.

Stability

Collateral Ligaments   Reinforce the sides of the joint.

Volar Plate   Fixed distally to the base of the phalanx and proximal neck of proximal phalangeal bone, flexor sheath, and collateral ligaments; prevents hyperextension of the joint.

Pinch Test

Assessment: Anterior interosseous nerve.

Patient position: Sitting with the forearm in pronation and resting on a table.

Method: The subject is asked to pinch the tips of the index finger and thumb together (*a*).

Positive response: The subject pinches the pulps of the digits instead of the tips (*b*).

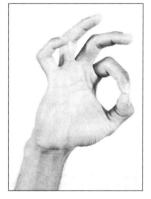
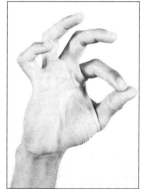

a　　　　　　　　　　*b*

Bunnel-Littler Test

Assessment: Tightness or contracture in joint capsule of PIP joint.

Patient position: Sitting.

Clinician position: Metacarpophalangeal joint held in extension (*a*).

Method: Move the PIP joint into flexion.

Positive response: The PIP does not move into flexion. If flex MCP and PIP move into more flexion, then intrinsic muscle tightens (*b*).

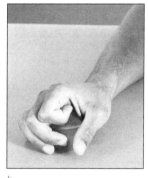

a　　　　　　　　　　*b*

Jersey Finger Sign

Assessment: Rupture of the flexor digitorum profundus.

Patient position: Sitting.

Method: The patient is asked to make a fist. The clinician assesses flexion of the distal phalanx of each finger.

Positive response: Inability of a finger to flex.

DISTAL INTERPHALANGEAL JOINTS (DIP, 2 TO 5)

Articulation   Convex head of the proximal phalanx and the concave base of the distal phalanx.

Type of Joint   Diarthrodial hinge joint.

Degrees of Freedom

Flexion and extension in the sagittal plane.

Active Range of Motion

Flexion: 0–90°

Extension: 0–10°

Distraction and Glides

Distraction: To assess mobility.

Ventral glide: To assess flexion.

Dorsal glide: To assess extension.

Patient position: Sitting with the forearm supported.

Clinician position: Fixate the proximal bone with the fingers; wrap the fingers and thumb of the other hand around the distal bone close to the joint.

Method: Apply the glide force by the thumb against the proximal end of the more distal bone.

End Feel

Flexion: Firm due to tension in the dorsal joint capsule, collateral ligaments, and oblique retinacular ligament

Extension: Firm due to tension in the palmar joint capsule and palmar ligaments

Capsular Pattern

Greater limitation in flexion than in extension.

Close-Packed Position

Maximal extension.

Loose-Packed Position

Slight flexion.

Stability

Collateral Ligaments Reinforce the sides of the joint.

Volar Plate Fixed distally to the base of the phalanx and proximal neck of proximal phalangeal bone, flexor sheath, and collateral ligaments; prevents hyperextension of the joint.

Special Tests

None.

Arthrokinematics of the Fingers

MCP

Flexion Base of the phalanx glides volarly, supination of the phalanx on the metacarpal, digits rotate radially; MCPs converge.

Extension Base of the phalanx glides dorsally, reverse of flexion; MCPs diverge.

Abduction Base of the phalanx glides toward the side that is abducting.

Adduction Base of the phalanx glides toward the side that is adducting.

PIP and DIP

Flexion Concave base of the phalanx glides palmarly.

Extension Concave base of the phalanx glides dorsally.

THUMB CARPOMETACARPAL JOINTS

Articulation   Concavoconvex trapezium (concave: anterior and posterior; convex: medial and lateral) and base of the first metacarpal (concave: medial and lateral; convex: anterior and posterior).

Type of Joint   Diarthrodial sellar joint.

Degrees of Freedom

- Flexion and extension in the frontal plane about a dorsal palmar axis through the trapezium
- Abduction and adduction in the sagittal plane about a radial ulnar axis through the base of the first CMC

Active Range of Motion

None measured.

Distraction

Assessment: Mobility of the joint.

Patient position: Forearm and hand resting on the treatment table.

Clinician position: Fixate the trapezium with the hand closer to the patient; grasp the patient's metacarpal by wrapping the fingers around it.

Method: Apply long-axis traction to separate the joint surfaces.

Glides

Ulnar glide: To assess flexion.

Radial glide: To assess extension.

Dorsal glide: To assess abduction.

Ventral glide: To assess adduction.

Patient position: Sitting with the forearm relaxed.

Clinician position: Same as with distraction.

Method: The direction of force will depend on the desired glide.

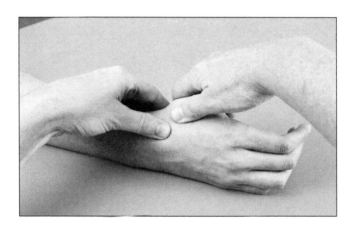

End Feel

Flexion: Soft due to muscle bulk of the thenar eminence contacting the palm

Flexion: Firm due to tension in dorsal joint capsule, short extensors, and short abductors

Extension: Firm due to tension in anterior joint capsule and dorsal interosseous

Abduction: Firm due to tension in fascia and skin of web and adductor muscle, and dorsal interosseous

Opposition: Soft due to muscle bulk of thenar eminence contacting palm

Opposition: Firm due to tension in joint capsule, short extensor of thumb, and transverse metacarpal ligament

Capsular Pattern
Abduction limited most, followed by extension.

Close-Packed Position
Full opposition.

Loose-Packed Position
Midabduction and adduction, and midflexion and extension.

Stability

Anterior and Posterior Oblique Ligaments   From the anterior and posterior surfaces of the trapezium to converge distally to ulnar side of first MCP; anterior is taut in extension and posterior is taut in flexion.

Radial CMC Ligament   From the radial surfaces of the trapezium to the first MCP.

Special Tests
None.

THUMB METACARPOPHALANGEAL JOINTS

Articulation   First metacarpal and first proximal phalanx.

Type of Joint   Diarthrodial condyloid joint.

Degrees of Freedom
- Flexion and extension in the frontal plane around an anterior-posterior axis
- Abduction and adduction in the sagittal plane around a medial-lateral axis

Active Range of Motion
None measured.

Distraction

Assessment: Mobility of the joint.

Patient position: Forearm and hand resting on the treatment table.

Clinician position: Fixate the proximal trapezii complex (trapezium and trapezoid) with the fingers; wrap the fingers and thumb of the other hand around the phalanx of the thumb.

Method: Apply long-axis traction to separate the joint surfaces.

Glides

Volar glide: To assess flexion.

Dorsal glide: To assess extension.

Patient position: Sitting with the forearm supported.

Clinician position: Fixate the trapezii complex with the fingers; wrap the fingers and thumb of the other hand around the distal bone close to the joint.

Method: Apply the glide force by the thumb against the proximal end of the bone.

End Feel

Flexion: Hard (the palmar phalanx is contacting the first metacarpal bone).

Flexion: Firm due to tension in the dorsal joint capsule, collateral ligament, and short extensor muscles of the thumb.

Extension: Firm due to tension in the palmar joint capsule, palmar ligament, and short flexor muscle of thumb.

Capsular Pattern

More limitation in flexion than extension.

Close-Packed Position

Maximal opposition.

Loose-Packed Position

Slight flexion.

Stability

Collateral Ligaments   Reinforce the sides of the joint.

Volar Plate   Fixed distally to the base of the phalanx and proximal neck of proximal phalangeal bone, flexor sheath, and collateral ligaments; prevents hyperextension of the joint.

Sesamoids   Two sesamoids located on volar surface; maintained by fibers of collateral ligaments and an intersesamoid ligament.

Froment's Sign

Assessment: Adductor pollicis weakness from ulnar nerve injury.

Patient position: Sitting.

Method: A piece of paper is placed between the thumb and the radial side of the index finger.

Clinician: The clinician attempts to remove the paper from the patient's grasp.

Positive response: The patient is unable to grasp the paper or substitutes with the thumb flexors.

Biomechanics: The adductor pollicis is innervated by the ulnar nerve. This technique tests the strength of the adductor pollicis muscle.

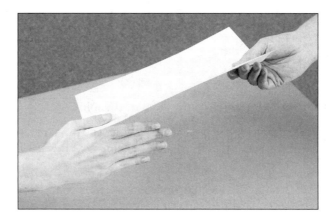

THUMB INTERPHALANGEAL JOINTS (IP)

Articulation   Convex distal end of proximal phalanx and concave proximal end of distal phalanx.

Type of Joint   Diarthrodial hinge joint.

Degrees of Freedom

Flexion and extension.

Active Range of Motion

None.

Distraction and Glides

Distraction: To assess mobility.

Ventral glide: To assess flexion.

Dorsal glide: To assess extension.

Patient position: Sitting with the forearm supported.

Clinician position: Fixate the proximal bone with the fingers; wrap the fingers and thumb of the other hand around the distal bone close to the joint.

Method: Apply the glide force by the thumb against the proximal end of the bone.

End Feel

Flexion: Firm due to tension in the collateral ligaments.

Flexion: Hard (the palmar distal phalanx contacts the proximal phalanx).

Extension: Firm due to tension in the palmar joint capsule and palmar ligament.

Capsular Pattern

Greater limitation in flexion than extension.

Close-Packed Position

Maximal extension.

Loose-Packed Position

Slight flexion.

Stability

Collateral Ligaments   Reinforce the sides of the joint.

Volar Plate   Fixed distally to the base of the phalanx and proximal neck of proximal phalangeal bone, flexor sheath, and collateral ligaments; prevents hyperextension of the joint.

Special Tests

None.

Arthrokinematics of the Thumb

CMC

Flexion   Concave surface of the first metacarpal slides ulnarly on the convex surface of the trapezium; medial rotation of the first metacarpal.

Extension   Concave surface of the first metacarpal slides radially on the convex surface of the trapezium; lateral rotation of the first metacarpal.

Abduction   Convex surface of the first metacarpal slides dorsally on the concave surface of the trapezium with medial rotation.

Adduction   Convex surface of the first metacarpal slides palmarly on the concave surface of the trapezium with lateral rotation.

MCP

Flexion   Concave base of the phalanx glides palmarly.

Extension   Concave base of the phalanx glides dorsally.

IP

Flexion   Concave base of the phalanx glides palmarly.

Extension   Concave base of the phalanx glides dorsally.

Active Range of Motion of the Wrist and Hand

Joint	Motion	Range of motion
Wrist	Flexion	0–80°
	Extension	0–70°
	Ulnar deviation	0–30°
	Radial deviation	0–20°
MCP (2–5)	Flexion	0–90°
	Extension	0–45°
	Abduction	0–30°
PIP (2–5)	Flexion	0–100°
DIP (2–5)	Flexion	0–90°
	Extension	0–10°
CMC (thumb)	Abduction	0–70°
	Flexion	0–15°
MCP (thumb)	Flexion	0–50°
DIP (thumb)	Flexion	0–80°

Neurology

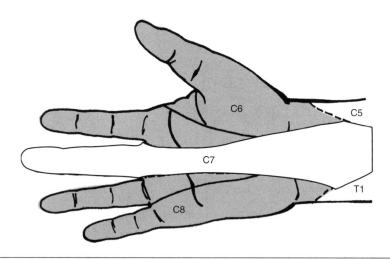

Palmar view of hand dermatomes.

Neurology

Nerve root	Reflex	Muscle	Sensory
C6	Brachioradialis	Wrist extensors	Thumb and index finger
C7	Triceps	Wrist flexors, finger extensors	Middle finger
C8	Abductor digiti minimi	Finger flexors	Fourth and fifth digits
T1	None	Finger abductors, finger adductors	Medial forearm

Peripheral Nerves

Nerve	Motor	Sensory
Axillary	Deltoid	Lateral arm, deltoid patch
Median	Thumb pinch, opposition of thumb, thumb abduction	Palmar thumb, second, third, and half of fourth
Radial	Wrist extension, thumb extension	Dorsum of thumb, second, third, and half of fourth
Ulnar	Thumb adduction, little finger abduction	Lateral half of fourth and fifth
Musculocutaneous	Biceps	Lateral forearm

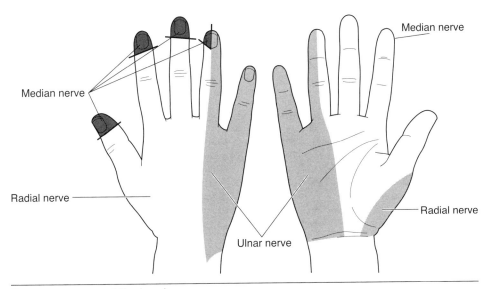

Cutaneous nerves of the hand.

Surface Palpation

Radial styloid process

Anatomical snuff box

Scaphoid

Trapezium

Lister's tubercle

Capitate

Lunate

Ulnar styloid process

Triquetrum

Pisiform

Hook of hamate

Metacarpals

First metacarpal

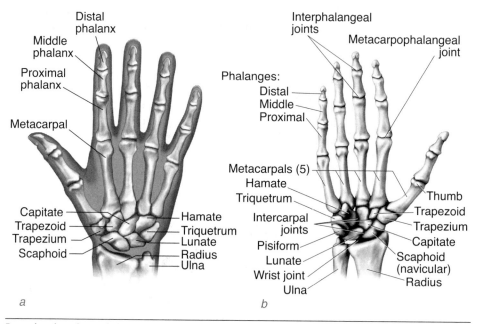

Bony landmarks and skin creases of the hand: (*a*) dorsal view; (*b*) palmar view.

Reprinted from R. Behnke, *Kinetic anatomy*, 2nd ed. (Champaign, IL: Human Kinetics), 77.

Muscle Origin and Insertion

Superficial

Deep

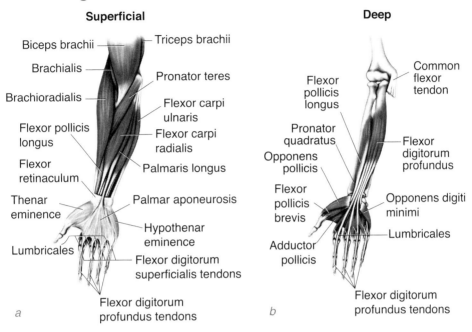

a

b

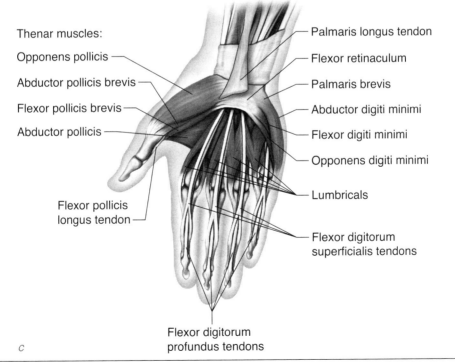

c

Muscles acting on the wrist: (*a*) superficial view; (*b*) deep view of the muscles of the lower arm and wrist; (*c*) deep view of the muscles of the hand.

Reprinted from R. Behnke, *Kinetic anatomy*, 2nd ed. (Champaign, IL: Human Kinetics), 77.

Muscle	Origin and insertion
Abductor digiti minimi	Pisiform bone to base of proximal phalanx of the little finger
Abductor pollicis brevis	Scaphoid, trapezium to base of proximal phalanx
Abductor pollicis longus	Middle of radius to radial side of base of first metacarpal
Adductor pollicis	Capitate, base of second and third metacarpal to base of proximal phalanx
Dorsal interossei	Between the metacarpals of the four fingers to the base of the proximal phalanx of second, third, and fourth fingers
Extensor carpi radialis brevis	Lateral epicondyle of humerus to base of third metacarpal
Extensor carpi radialis longus	Lateral supracondylar ridge of humerus to base of second metacarpal
Extensor carpi ulnaris	Lateral epicondyle of humerus to base of fifth metacarpal
Extensor digiti minimi	Tendon of extensor digitorum to proximal phalanx of little finger
Extensor digitorum	Lateral epicondyle of humerus to the dorsal hood of the four fingers
Extensor indicis	Lower ulna and interosseous membrane to dorsal hood of index finger
Extensor pollicis brevis	Middle of radius and ulna to base of proximal phalanx of thumb
Extensor pollicis longus	Middle third of ulna and interosseous membrane to base of distal phalanx of thumb
Flexor carpi radialis	Medial epicondyle of humerus to base of second and third metacarpals
Flexor carpi ulnaris	Medial epicondyle to pisiform, hamate, base of fifth metacarpal
Flexor digiti minimi	Hamate bone to proximal phalanx of little finger
Flexor digitorum profundus	Anterior, medial ulna to base of distal phalanx of four fingers
Flexor digitorum superficialis	Medial epicondyle to base of middle phalanx of four fingers
Flexor pollicis brevis	Trapezium, trapezoid, capitate to base of proximal phalanx of thumb
Flexor pollicis longus	Middle radius and interosseous membrane to base of distal phalanx of thumb
Lumbricales	Tendon of flexor digitorum profundus to dorsal hood of the four fingers
Opponens digiti minimi	Hamate bone to fifth metacarpal
Opponens pollicis	Trapezium to first metacarpal
Palmar interossei	Sides of second, fourth, and fifth metacarpals to base of proximal phalanx of same fingers
Palmaris longus	Medial epicondyle to palmar aponeurosis

Adapted from J. Hamill and K. Knudzen, 1995, *Biomechanical basis of human movement* (Baltimore, MD: Lippincott, Williams, and Wilkins), 501, 502.

Muscle Action and Innervation

Refer to figure 10.1 on page 213 for a dorsal view of the ligaments of the wrist.

Action	Muscle involved	Nerve supply	Nerve root
Wrist flexion	Flexor carpi radialis	Median	C6–C7
	Flexor carpi ulnaris	Ulnar	C7–C8
Wrist extension	Extensor carpi radialis longus	Radial	C6–C7
	Extensor carpi radialis brevis	Radial	C7–C8
	Extensor carpi ulnaris	Radial	C7–C8
Ulnar deviation	Flexor carpi ulnaris	Ulnar	C7–C8
	Extensor carpi ulnaris	Radial	C7–C8
Radial deviation	Flexor carpi radialis	Median	C6–C7
	Extensor carpi radialis longus	Radial	C6–C7
	Abductor pollicis longus	Radial	C7–C8
	Extensor pollicis brevis	Radial	C7–C8
Finger extension	Extensor digitorum communis	Radial	C7–C8
	Extensor indices (second digit)	Radial	C7–C8
	Extensor digiti minimi (fifth digit)	Radial	C7–C8
Finger flexion	Flexor digitorum profundus	Median	C8, T1
	Flexor digitorum superficialis	Median	C7–C8, T1
	Lumbricals	1–2 median 3–4 ulnar	C8, T1
	Interossei	Ulnar	C8, T1
	Flexor digiti minimi (fifth digit)	Ulnar	C8, T1
Finger abduction	Dorsal interossei	Ulnar	C8, T1
	Abductor digiti minimi	Ulnar	C8, T1
Finger adduction	Palmar interossei	Ulnar	C8, T1
Thumb extension	Extensor pollicis longus	Radial	C7–C8
	Extensor pollicis brevis	Radial	C7–C8
	Abductor pollicis longus	Radial	C7–C8
Thumb flexion	Flexor pollicis brevis	Superficial head: median	C8, T1
	Flexor pollicis longus	Deep head: ulnar	C8, T1
	Opponens pollicis	Median	C8, T1
		Median	C8, T1
Thumb abduction	Abductor pollicis longus	Radial	C7–C8
	Abductor pollicis brevis	Median	C8, T1
Thumb adduction	Adductor pollicis	Ulnar	C8, T1
Opposition	Opponens pollicis	Median	C8, T1
	Flexor pollicis brevis	Median	C8, T1
	Abductor pollicis brevis	Median	C8, T1
	Opponens digiti minimi	Ulnar	C8, T1

Adapted from *Orthopedic Physical Assessment*, 2nd ed., D.J. Magee, pg. 185. Copyright 1992, with permission from W. B. Saunders.

HISTORY

Ask Hand Dominance

Profile

Occupation and recreational activities—consider effect of wrist or hand pain on level of function or disability (repetitive wrist flexion and extension or pronation and supination, sporting activities, overuse/abuse)

Location of Symptoms

Common patterns of referral from the C-spine nerve root: C6, C7, C8.

May need to question popping, catching, locking, and slipping out of joint if not offered spontaneously.

Check symptom-free areas—CS, TS, scapula, AC joint, GH joint, elbow.

Palmar: consider CTS, ulnar neuritis, wrist flexor injury.

Dorsal: consider wrist and finger extensors.

Ulnar side: consider triangular fibrocartilage complex.

Radial side: consider scaphoid fracture.

Aggravating Factors

ADLs

Lifting

Pushing

Opening a door

Ease Factors

Movement versus rest

Bracing or supports

Medication

History

FOOSH

Wrist extended < 35°: radius fracture

Wrist extended > 90°: carpal bones fracture

Radial deviation: scaphoid fracture

Repetitive Stress Syndrome: Carpal Tunnel Syndrome

TESTS AND MEASURES

Sitting

Observation—Posture, Atrophy, or Deformation

Palpation—Bony (Carpals: Scaphoid, Lunate, Triquetrum, Pisiform, Trapezium, Trapezoid, Capitate, Hamate), Soft Tissue

Implicate or Clear Cervical Spine

Neurological Examination (Segmental, Peripheral, or Central as Indicated)

AROM With OP

Wrist flexion (0–80°)

Wrist extension (0–70°)

Wrist radial deviation (0–20°)

Wrist ulnar deviation (0–30°)

Finger flexion and extension

Thumb motion

Opposition

PROM with OP

PAMs

Distal radioulnar joint

- Volar glide (pronation)
- Dorsal glide (supination)

Radiocarpal joint

- Distraction
- Volar glide (extension)
- Dorsal glide (flexion)
- Ulnar glide (radial deviation)
- Radial glide (ulnar deviation)

Carpometacarpal joint

- Ulnar glide (flexion)
- Volar glide (adduction)
- Radial glide (extension)
- Dorsal glide (abduction)

MCP joint—anterior and posterior glides

IP joint—anterior and posterior glides

MMT

Elbow flexion and extension

Wrist flexion and extension

Wrist radial and ulnar deviation

Finger flexion (grip dynamometer)

Finger abduction

Special Tests

Tinel's sign (ulnar nerve and median nerve)

Finkelstein's test

Phalen's test

Froment's sign

Allen test

Bunnell-Littler

Supine

Palpation

Implicate or Clear Elbow

Neurological Examination

PAM

Radiocarpal joint: dorsal glide, radial glide

Neurodynamic Testing

Prone

Implicate or Clear the Cervical Spine With Palpation

Clinical Syndromes

Description	Location and behavior of symptoms	History	Tests and measures, diagnostics	Intervention
DE QUERVAIN'S SYNDROME				
Tendinitis of the abductor pollicis longus and extensor pollicis brevis.	Pain over the APL and EPB.	Overuse of these tendons in activities requiring repeated ulnar or radial deviation.	Pain to palpation; swelling; crepitus in tendon region. + Finkelstein's test.	Acute: PRICEM, iontophoresis. Posture, ergonomics, manual therapy.
CARPAL TUNNEL SYNDROME				
Constriction of the carpal tunnel, which houses the median nerve.	Pain, numbness, nocturnal pain along the median nerve distribution.	Overuse of wrist with activities such as wrist flexion, trauma; night pain, stiffness.	Possible atrophy of hand muscles. Innervated by the median nerve. Tinel's test; Phalen's test.	Posture, ergonomics, manual therapy, splints. Medical management: surgery.
RAYNAUD'S PHENOMENON				
Vasospasm of the distal vessels of the hand and toes.	Decreased circulation distal UE, diffuse pain in hand, pale fingers.	Trauma, idiopathic; cold may trigger.	Blanching of fingers followed by reddening, Allen's test.	Medical management: vasodilatory drugs, surgical sympathectomy for worst cases. Active range of motion.
COMPLEX REGIONAL PAIN SYNDROME				
Hypovascularity caused by increased sympathetic activity.	Extreme pain and burning in entire hand.	Posttrauma.	Hand may appear mottled, red or blue, swelling may be present.	Aggressive exercise. Desensitization. Medical management: sympathetic blocks.
DUPUYTREN'S CONTRACTURE				
Palmar fascia constriction.	Flexor tendons of fourth and fifth nodules.	Idiopathic, insidious.	Appearance, palpation of nodules, inability to straighten fingers, primarily fourth and fifth.	Stretching initially. Medical management: surgical release.
COLLES FRACTURE				
Fracture of distal radius, may or may not include ulna with or without displacement.	Distal wrist pain or deformity.	Fall on outstretched hand (FOOSH).	Dinner-fork deformity, swelling, watch for loss of circulation. Diagnostics: X ray.	Closed or open reduction, postimmobilization: ROM, strengthening.

» continued

» continued

Description	Location and behavior of symptoms	History	Tests and measures, diagnostics	Intervention
SMITH'S FRACTURE				
Fracture of the distal end of radius with volar displacement.	Distal wrist pain or deformity.	FOOSH.	Swelling, watch for loss of circulation. Diagnostics: X ray.	Closed or open reduction, postimmobilization: ROM, strengthening.
TRIANGULAR FIBROCARTILAGE INJURY				
Disruption of articular disc.	Pain over ulnar styloid.	FOOSH, repetitive ulnar deviation.	Palpation: tender over TFFC, decreased grip strength.	Joint distraction, wrist strengthening. Medical management: may require surgery.
SCAPHOID–LUNATE DISASSOCIATION				
Injury to ligament complex between scaphoid and lunate.	Pain over scaphoid–lunate articulation.	FOOSH.	Watson's test.	Immobilization. Medical management: surgery.
LUNATE DISLOCATION				
Dislocation of lunate volarly.	Pain over lunate.	FOOSH, hit by outside force.	Deformity, inability to move wrist, median neuropathy. Diagnostics: X ray.	Reduction, immobilization for 3 weeks, no extension for 5 to 6 weeks.
ULNAR NEUROPATHY				
Prolonged pressure on the ulnar nerve as it passes around the hook of the hamate.	Tingling, paresthesia of the hands and fingers along ulnar distribution.	Direct pressure from prolonged wrist extension, such as with bike riding, or repeated trauma to ulna.	Possible atrophy of hypothenar eminence, interosseous, medial two lumbricals, thumb adduction. Froment's sign, Tinel's test.	Posture, ergonomics, manual therapy, splints.
BENNETT'S FRACTURE				
Fracture of first metacarpal.	Pain along MCP shaft.	Direct force from a punch.	Swelling, deformity, tender to palpation.	Protection. Medical management: closed reduction. ORIF.
BOXER'S FRACTURE				
Neck fracture of the fifth metacarpal.	Pain over fifth MCP.	Direct force from a punch.	Swelling, deformity.	Protection. Medical management: closed reduction. ORIF.

Description	Location and behavior of symptoms	History	Tests and measures, diagnostics	Intervention
MALLET FINGER				
Extensor tendon avulsed from DIP.	Pain over DIP.	Direct force causing forced flexion of distal phalanx.	Deformity in which the DIP cannot straighten.	Volar splint 6 to 8 weeks. Medical management: surgical fixation.
KIENBOCK'S DISEASE				
Osteonecrosis or AVN of lunate.	Pain over lunate.	FOOSH.	Tenderness over lunate, local swelling, decreased grip strength. Diagnostics: X ray.	Immobilization for 2 to 3 months. Prosthetic lunate. Postop: protective splinting, scar mobilization, edema reduction, AROM, strengthening.
SCAPHOID FRACTURE				
Fracture of scaphoid bone.	Pain over anatomical snuffbox, deep, dull.	FOOSH—hand usually radially deviated, males.	Tenderness over snuffbox, limited or painful wrist movement, compression, resisted pronation may cause pain. Diagnostics: X ray after 7 to 10 days.	Immobilization with cast. Medical management: surgery.
SKIER'S THUMB, GAMESKEEPER'S THUMB				
Sprain of the ulnar collateral ligament.	Pain at base of first metacarpal, ulnar side.	Direct force causing hyperextension and abduction of the first MCP joint, may also be repeated trauma.	Possible deformity, increased laxity in first MCP joint.	Strengthening, taping. Medical management: may require surgery.
SPINE REFERRAL				
	C6, 7, 8.	See cervical spine clinical syndromes.	Comparable sign with CS clearing tests and palpation to specific spinal levels.	See cervical spine clinical syndromes.

Adapted, by permission, from C. Wadsworth, 1988, *Manual examination and treatment of the spine and extremities* (Baltimore, MD: Lippincott, Williams, and Wilkins).

Functional Assessment of the Upper Extremity

The present emphasis in health care is on functional recovery of the patient. Practitioners must therefore use valid and reliable testing tools to report progress in therapy. The chapter begins with a listing of muscle imbalances associated with the function of the upper extremity. Next, functional ranges needed for activities of daily living (ADLs) are listed for the shoulder, elbow, hand, and wrist. This chapter presents functional assessment tools that have been extensively used by orthopedic practitioners. Last in this chapter is a chart on throwing mechanics that should be helpful to practitioners dealing with athletes who throw.

Muscle Imbalances

- Tight levator scapula causes elevation of the medial border of the scapula.
- Tight rhomboids cause adducted scapulae.
- Tight upper trapezius causes elevation of the scapula.
- Tight serratus anterior causes abduction of the scapula.
- Tight pectoralis minor causes anterior tilting of the scapula.

SHOULDER

Functional Range of Motion

Reaching overhead: shoulder flexion to 160°

Reaching behind back (reaching into back pocket): full internal rotation

Placing hand behind head (combing hair): full external rotation

Wash opposite axilla: full horizontal adduction

Functional Assessment of the Shoulder

Lateral Scapular Slide Test (Kibler)

Assessment: Quantify bilateral comparison of the scapula.

Patient position: Standing.

Test position: Five test positions:

1. Arm at the side
2. Hands on the hip with the thumb posterior
3. Empty can
4. 120° of elevation in the scapular plane
5. 150° of elevation in the scapular plane

Method: Measure the distance from T7 to inferior angle of the scapula in five positions.

Positive response: Greater than 1 cm of asymmetry in a bilateral comparison.

Functional Strength Testing of the Shoulder

Starting position	Action	Functional test*
Sitting	Forward flex arm to 90°	Lift 4 to 5 lb (1.8 to 2.3 kg): functional Lift 1 to 3 lb (.5 to 1.4 kg): functionally fair Lift arm weight: functionally poor Cannot lift arm: nonfunctional
Sitting	Shoulder extension	Lift 4 to 5 lb (1.8 to 2.3 kg): functional Lift 1 to 3 lb (.5 to 1.4 kg): functionally fair Lift arm weight: functionally poor Cannot lift arm: nonfunctional
Side lying	Shoulder internal rotation (can sit and use pulley)	Lift 4 to 5 lb (1.8 to 2.3 kg): functional Lift 1 to 3 lb (.5 to 1.4 kg): functionally fair Lift arm weight: functionally poor Cannot lift arm: nonfunctional
Side lying	Shoulder external rotation (can sit and use pulley)	Lift 4 to 5 lb (1.8 to 2.3 kg): functional Lift 1 to 3 lb (.5 to 1.4 kg): functionally fair Lift arm weight: functionally poor Cannot lift arm: nonfunctional
Sitting	Shoulder abduction	Lift 4 to 5 lb (1.8 to 2.3 kg): functional Lift 1 to 3 lb (.5 to 1.4 kg): functionally fair Lift arm weight: functionally poor Cannot lift arm: nonfunctional
Sitting	Shoulder abduction with wall pulley	Lift 4 to 5 lb (1.8 to 2.3 kg): functional Lift 1 to 3 lb (.5 to 1.4 kg): functionally fair Lift arm weight: functionally poor Cannot lift arm: nonfunctional
Sitting	Shoulder elevation (shoulder shrug)	Lift 4 to 5 lb (1.8 to 2.3 kg): functional Lift 1 to 3 lb (.5 to 1.4 kg): functionally fair Lift arm weight: functionally poor Cannot lift arm: nonfunctional
Sitting	Sitting push-up (shoulder depression)	Lift 4 to 5 lb (1.8 to 2.3 kg): functional Lift 1 to 3 lb (.5 to 1.4 kg): functionally fair Lift arm weight: functionally poor Cannot lift arm: nonfunctional

*Younger patients may be able to lift more weight than listed. Use opposite side for accurate comparison.

Data from M.L. Palmer and M. Epler, 1990, *Clinical assessment procedures in physical therapy* (Baltimore, PA: Lippincott, Williams, and Wilkins).

Davies Functional Shoulder Rating Scale

Symptoms (Analogue Pain Scale) 10

Pain at rest (0–10)

Pain with activity (0–10) _____

Average score at rest; with activity,
reverse numbers for actual score on scale (i.e., 3 = 7) _____

Patient's Functional Rating 20

Return to former sport with no limitation or pain =	20	_____
Return to former sport with no limitation but pain =	17–19	_____
Return to former sport with limitation but no pain =	14–16	_____
Return to former sport with limitation and pain =	11–13	_____
Inability to return to former sport level but still plays sport =	8–10	_____
Ability to return to less competitive sports with no pain =	4–7	_____
Inability to return to any sport =	0	_____

Physical Exam 10

Each of these tests can be found in the guide to the shoulder (chapter 8). Give 1 point for each positive test; if the finding is significant, add an additional point; reverse numbers for actual score on scale.

Biceps brachii test _____

Rotator cuff rupture tests _____

Impingement tests _____

Anterior instability tests _____

Posterior instability tests _____

Multidirectional instability tests _____

Active Range of Motion (ROM) 20

(Within normal limits: bilateral comparison)

Flexion (0–180°) _____

Abduction (0–180°) _____

Internal rotation (0–70°) _____

External rotation (0–90°) _____

Scaption (0–90°) _____

All motions totaled together:

0% diff =	20	_____
<5% =	18	_____
<10% =	16	_____
<15% =	14	_____
<20% =	12	_____
<25% =	10	_____
30% =	1–7	_____

Isokinetic Testing 20

Internal rotation _____

External rotation _____

Agonist–antagonist ratio _____

All tests totaled together—peak torque, total work, average power:

0% diff =	20	_____
<5% =	18	_____
<10% =	16	_____
<15% =	14	_____
<20% =	12	_____
<25% =	10	_____
30% =	1–7	_____

Kinesthetic Testing 10

Flexion < 90°	_____
Flexion > 90°	_____
Abduction < 90°	_____
Abduction > 90°	_____
Internal rotation < 45°	_____
External rotation < 45°	_____
External rotation > 45°	_____

Absolute number comparison in degrees, all tests totaled together and divided by seven tests, ability to reproduce specified angle with eyes closed:

<5 =	10	_____
<7 =	9	_____
<9 =	8	
<11 =	7	_____
<13 =	6	_____
<15 =	5	_____
<17 =	4	_____
<19 =	3	_____
21 =	1	_____

Functional Throwing Performance Index (FTPI) 10

Test: A 1 ft × 1 ft (30 cm × 30 cm) square is displayed on a wall, 4 ft (120 cm) up from the floor; the individual stands 15 ft (460 cm) from the square and throws a 20 in. (50 cm) circumference rubber playground ball.

Protocol:

1. The patient uses the crow-hop technique. _____
2. The patient performs four warm-ups. _____
3. The patient performs five maximally controlled throws and must catch the ball on the rebound. _____
4. The patient throws as many times as she or he can in 30 s. _____
5. Three 30 s tests are performed. _____
6. Analysis: Number of throws and number within square are recorded. _____
   FTPI = accuracy in target _____
   Total number of throws × 100 _____
   Total (out of 100 points) _____

From J. Loudon, M. Swift, and S. Bell, 2008, *The clinical orthopedic assessment guide*, 2nd ed. (Champaign, IL: Human Kinetics).

Davies Functional Shoulder Rating Scale

Rating	Point range
Excellent	80–100
Good	70–84
Fair	55–69
Poor	<55

FUNCTIONAL ASSESSMENT OF THE SHOULDER

Instructions: For each portion of this assessment, circle the appropriate number of points. Add the number of points scored after each test and divide by the total points available.

Pain	*Points (select one)*
None	15
Mild	10
Moderate	5
Severe	0
(Total points available)	15
Total scored	_____

ADLs

Activity level	*Points (select all that apply)*
Full work	4
Full recreation or sport	4
Unaffected sleep	2

Positioning	
Up to waist	2
Up to xiphoid	4
Up to neck	6
Up to top of head	8
Above head	10
(Total points available)	20
Total scored	_____

Range of Motion

Abduction	*Points (select one)*
0–30°	0
31–60°	2
61–90°	4
91–120°	6
121–150°	8
151–180°	10

Flexion	*Points (select one)*
0–30°	0
31–60°	2
61–90°	4
91–120°	6
121–150°	8
151–180°	10

Internal rotation	*Points (select one)*
Dorsum of hand to lateral thigh	0
Dorsum of hand to buttock	2
Dorsum of hand to lumbosacral junction	4
Dorsum of hand to waist (L3)	6
Dorsum of hand to T12	8
Dorsum of hand to T7	10

External rotation	*Points (select all that apply)*
Hand behind head with elbow held forward	2
Hand behind head with elbow held back	2
Hand on top of head with elbow held forward	2
Hand on top of head with elbow held back	2
Full elevation from on top of head	2
(Total points available)	40
Total scored	_____
Power	25 lb (11 kg)
Amount of weight lifted	_____

From J. Loudon, M. Swift, and S. Bell, 2008, *The clinical orthopedic assessment guide,* 2nd ed. (Champaign, IL: Human Kinetics). Reprinted, by permission, from C.R. Constant and A.H.G. Murley, 1987, "A clinical method of functional assessment of the shoulder," *Clinical Orthopedics Related Research* 214:160–164.

ELBOW

Functional Range of Motion

Activity	Flexion	Pronation	Supination
Open a door	30–60°	0–35°	0–25°
Put on shoes	10–20°	10–30°	None needed
Pour a pitcher	35–55°	0–40°	0–25°
Reach sacrum	65–75°	None needed	45–75°
Lift a chair	20–95°	10–35°	None needed
Reach waist	90–105°	None needed	0–30°
Hold a newspaper	75–100°	10–50°	None needed
Reach top of head	110–125°	None needed	40–60°
Operate a knife for eating	90–110°	30–40°	None needed
Operate a fork for eating	80–125°	0–15°	0–50°
Drink from a glass	40–130°	0–10°	0–10°
Reach occiput of head	135–150°	0–15°	0–15°
Use a telephone	40–135°	0–40°	0–25°

Functional Assessment of the Elbow

Starting position	Action	Functional test
Sitting	Bring hand to mouth lifting weight (elbow flexion)	Lift 5 to 6 lb (2.3 to 2.7 kg): functional Lift 3 to 4 lb (1.4 to 1.8 kg): functionally fair Lift 1 to 2 lb (.5 to .9 kg): functionally poor Lift 0 lb (0 kg): nonfunctional
Standing 3 ft (90 cm) from wall, leaning against wall	Push arms straight (elbow extension)	5 to 6 reps: functional 3 to 4 reps: functionally fair 1 to 2 reps: functionally poor 0 reps: nonfunctional
Standing, facing closed door	Open door starting with palm down (supination)	5 to 6 reps: functional 3 to 4 reps: functionally fair 1 to 2 reps: functionally poor 0 reps: nonfunctional
Standing, facing closed door	Open door starting with palm up (pronation)	5 to 6 reps: functional 3 to 4 reps: functionally fair 1 to 2 reps: functionally poor 0 reps: nonfunctional

Data from M.L. Palmer and M. Epler, 1990, *Clinical assessment procedures in physical therapy* (Baltimore, PA: Lippincott, Williams, and Wilkins).

WRIST, HAND, AND GRIP

Functional Range of Motion The amount of motion needed to perform most activities with the hand is 10° of wrist extension and 30° of wrist flexion. Figure 11.1 illustrates different types of grips.

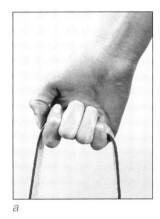

a

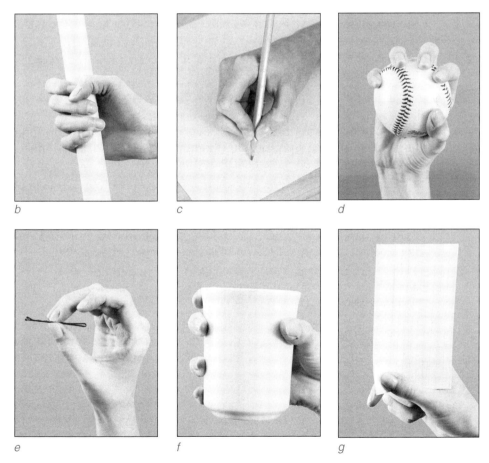

b *c* *d*

e *f* *g*

Figure 11.1 Fine motor control of the hand: (*a*) hook grasp; (*b*) fist grasp; (*c*) palmar prehension; (*d*) spherical grasp; (*e*) tip prehension; (*f*) cylindrical grasp; (*g*) lateral prehension.

Nonprehensile   Use of the hand in a nongrasp capacity; contact is with the palmar portion of the hand or hands.

Prehension   Requires grasping or taking hold of an object between two surfaces of the hand; the thumb may or may not be involved.

Power grip   A grip that is used to hold on to an object but is moved with proximal joints.

    a. Hook grip: The fingers are used as a hook as in carrying a purse or briefcase (MCPs neutral, flexion at PIP and DIP, thumb extended, use of flexor digitorum profundis [FDP] and flexor digitorum superficialis [FDS]).

    b. Cylindrical grip: The entire palmar surface surrounds a cylindrical object such as a glass. The thumb is involved (fingers adducted and flexed, thumb opposed, use of flexor pollicis longus [FPL], adductor pollicis, fourth lumbrical, FDP).

    c. Spherical grip: The grasp is adjusted to a spherical object such as a ball (fingers adducted and flexed, thumb opposed, use of finger flexors).

    d. Lateral prehension: A grip that requires two adjacent fingers to adduct to enclose the object as in holding a newspaper (thumb and index finger adducted, lumbricals).

Precision   Grips that require skillful placement of the fingers to manipulate an object.

    a. Two-point tip pinch: Tip-to-tip grip, involving the thumb and one other finger as in picking up a needle (thumb opposed and flexed; fingers flexed at MCP, PIP, DIP; use of FDP, FPL, interossei).

    b. Three-point tip pinch (three-jaw chuck): The tip of the thumb is used in conjunction with digits 2 and 3 (similar to two-point tip pinch).

    c. Two-point pad pinch: The thumb and the pad of the index finger are used to maneuver an object such as a light bulb (thumb opposed and flexed, fingers flexed at MCP and PIP, flexed or extended at DIP).

    d. Three-point pad pinch (three-jaw chuck): The thumb opposes digits 2 and 3 with the pads of the distal phalanges as in unscrewing a bottle top (similar to two-point pad pinch).

    e. Lateral pinch (lateral prehension): A thin object is grasped between the thumb and the lateral side of the index finger as when using a key (thumb adducted with IP flexion, index finger flexed and abducted).

Functional Assessment of the Wrist and Hand

Starting position	Action	Functional test
Forearm supinated, resting on table	Wrist flexion	Lift >5 lb (>2.3 kg): functional Lift 3 to 4 lb (1.4 to 1.8 kg): functionally fair Lift 1 to 2 lb (.5 to .9 kg): functionally poor Lift 0 lb (0 kg): nonfunctional
Forearm pronated, resting on table	Wrist extension lifting 1 to 2 lb (.5 to .9 kg)	>4 reps: functional 3 to 4 reps: functionally fair 1 to 2 reps: functionally poor 0 reps: nonfunctional
Forearm neutral, resting on table	Radial deviation lifting 1 to 2 lb (.5 to .9 kg)	>4 reps: functional 3 to 4 reps: functionally fair 1 to 2 reps: functionally poor 0 reps: nonfunctional
Forearm neutral, rubber band around thumb	Thumb flexion with resistance from 1 cm wide rubber band	>4 reps: functional 3 to 4 reps: functionally fair 1 to 2 reps: functionally poor 0 reps: nonfunctional
Forearm neutral, rubber band around thumb and index finger	Thumb extension against rubber band	>4 reps: functional 3 to 4 reps: functionally fair 1 to 2 reps: functionally poor 0 reps: nonfunctional
Forearm resting on table, rubber band around thumb and index finger	Thumb abduction against rubber band	>4 reps: functional 3 to 4 reps: functionally fair 1 to 2 reps: functionally poor 0 reps: nonfunctional
Forearm resting on table	Thumb adduction, lateral pinch of piece of paper	Hold 5 s: functional Hold 3 to 4 s: functionally fair Hold 1 to 2 s: functionally poor Hold 0 s: nonfunctional
Forearm resting on table	Thumb opposition, pad pinch of piece of paper	Hold 5 s: functional Hold 3 to 4 s: functionally fair Hold 1 to 2 s: functionally poor Hold 0 s: nonfunctional
Forearm resting on table	Finger flexion, grasping mug with cylindrical grip, lifting off table	>4 reps: functional 3 to 4 reps: functionally fair 1 to 2 reps: functionally poor 0 reps: nonfunctional
Forearm resting on table	Put on rubber gloves, keeping fingers straight	2 to 4 s: functional 4 to 8 s: functionally fair 10 to 20 s: functionally poor >20 s: nonfunctional
Forearm resting on table	Finger abduction against resistance of rubber band	Hold 5 s: functional Hold 3 to 4 s: functionally fair Hold 1 to 2 s: functionally poor Hold 0 s: nonfunctional
Forearm resting on table	Finger adduction of piece of paper while clinician tries to pull it out	Hold 5 s: functional Hold 3 to 4 s: functionally fair Hold 1 to 2 s: functionally poor Hold 0 s: nonfunctional

Data from M. L. Palmer and M. Epler, 1990, *Clinical assessment procedures in physical therapy* (Baltimore, MD: Lippincott, Williams, and Wilkins).

Throwing Mechanics

Shoulder and arm movements	Shoulder muscles involved	Structures under stress
Windup: Phase that prepares the pitcher for correct body posture and balance. The body rotates away from the plate.	Minimal shoulder activity.	Because acceleration and deceleration forces are minimal, potential for injury in this phase is minimal.
Cocking: The contralateral leg is placed forward, the pelvis is internally rotated, and the chest is forward. The shoulder is abducted to 90°, the humerus is externally rotated 100° to 120°, the elbow is at 90°, and the wrist is extended.	The posterior deltoid horizontally abducts the humerus. The trapezius is positioning the scapula. The supraspinatus, infraspinatus, and teres minor stabilize humeral head.	Tension is developed in anterior capsule, anterior deltoid, and pectoralis insertion. The long head of the biceps is also under tension.
Acceleration: The body is brought forward with arm trailing. The ball is accelerated forward. The shoulder moves through internal rotation. The wrist is snapped from an extended position.	The subscapularis, pectoralis major, latissimus dorsi, and teres major contract concentrically. The trapezius is firing to stabilize the scapula. The supraspinatus, infraspinatus, and teres minor work eccentrically to control horizontal adduction. The elbow flexors work eccentrically to control elbow extension.	Valgus stress is placed on the elbow. Rotational stress is placed on the humeral shaft. Impingement of supraspinatus tendon or other subacromial soft-tissue structures. Forearm flexors pull on the medial epicondyle.
Release and deceleration: Deceleration occurs following ball release to maintain the integrity of the shoulder. Initially, the humerus is internally rotating and the elbow is extending.	Subscapularis, pectoralis major, latissimus dorsi, and triceps contract concentrically up to release of ball. The trapezius is working on scapula control. The pronator teres, forearm flexors, or supinators control forearm momentum.	The posterior capsule and posterior deltoid are under stress. Possible subluxation of glenohumeral joint. The long head of the biceps may be stressed with certain pitches (curveball).
Follow-through: The body moves forward, and the ipsilateral foot is planted ahead of the body.	The posterior deltoid and posterior rotator cuff contract eccentrically to slow the arm.	No significant shoulder injuries.

Lower Extremity

The aim of Part IV is to provide detailed information to the clinician on the major joints of the lower extremity along with the objective sequence. Part IV contains four chapters related to the lower extremity. Chapter 12 covers the hip, chapter 13 discusses the knee, and chapter 14 deals with the foot and ankle. As in part III, each chapter contains a description of joint articulation, type of joint, degrees of freedom, arthrokinematics, joint open- and close-packed positions, end feel, and capsular pattern. The remainder of each chapter describes stability of the joints, special tests, neurological assessment, surface palpation, muscle origins and insertions, and actions and innervations. Finally, a clinical syndrome table is included in each chapter to help the clinician perform musculoskeletal differential diagnoses. The last chapter of part IV is a synopsis of functional tests for the lower extremity.

Hip Joint

The hip joint is similar to the shoulder joint in anatomy and biomechanics, but the hip is much more stable because of its strong ligament support and deeper articulating fossa. The hip articulation is primarily weight bearing and can withstand great compressive loads. The function of the hip joint is closely associated with the function of the sacroiliac joint and lumbar spine. Therefore, any client that presents with persistent hip pain should also have the SI joint and lumbar spine examined. This chapter covers osteology, arthrokinematics, range of motion, muscle origin and insertion, muscle action, neurology, and special tests for the hip joint. Clinical syndromes are presented in a table at the end of the chapter. A recommended sequence for the subjective and objective exam is also included.

CHAPTER 12

Joint Basics

Articulation Convex head of the femur and concave acetabulum of the pelvis.

Type of Joint Diarthrodial spheroidal joint.

Degrees of Freedom

- Flexion and extension in sagittal plane about a coronal axis through the femoral head
- Abduction and adduction in coronal plane about a sagittal axis through the femoral head
- Internal rotation and external rotation in transverse plane about a longitudinal axis through the femoral head

Active Range of Motion (AAOS)

Hip flexion: 0–120°

Hip extension: 0–30°

Hip abduction: 0–45°

Hip adduction: 0–30°

Hip internal rotation: 0–45°

Hip external rotation: 0–45°

Caudal Glide

Assessment: Joint mobility.

Patient position: Supine with the hip in 30° flexion and abduction and slight external rotation.

Clinician position: Standing in a walk-stance position at the end of the examination table and facing the patient. The clinician cradles the limb at level of malleolus with both hands.

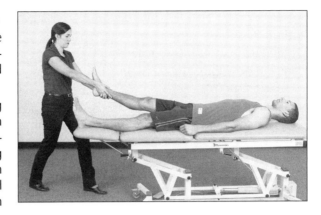

Method: While leaning back, the clinician applies a caudal mobilizing force on the lower limb. Apply first pressures gently; increase amplitude and depth of the movement if no pain response occurs. Assess quality of movement through the range and end feel; compare with the other side.

Inferior Glide at 90° Hip Flexion

Patient position: Supine with the hip and knee flexed to 90° and supported by the clinician's shoulder.

Clinician position: Standing in a walk-stance position at the side of the examination table and facing the patient. The clinician wraps the ulnar borders of his or her hands around the proximal thigh of the patient.

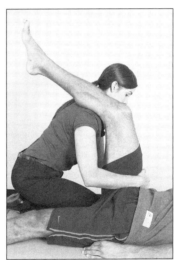

Method: While leaning back, the clinician applies a caudal mobilizing force on the proximal femur. Apply first pressures gently; increase amplitude and depth of the movement if no pain response occurs. Assess quality of movement through the range and end feel; compare with the other side.

Biomechanics: The inferior glide at 90° hip flexion increases hip joint space by separation of articulating surfaces and loosens adhesions in the anterior direction.

Posterior Glide

Assessment: Flexion and internal rotation of the hip.

Patient position: Supine with the hip in the resting position (30° flexion, 30° abduction, slight external rotation).

Clinician position: The mobilizing hand contacts the anterior aspect of the proximal femur (*a*).

Method: Apply the mobilizing force straight down in a posterior direction (*b*). Posterior glide is necessary for flexion and internal rotation.

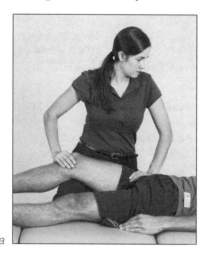

a

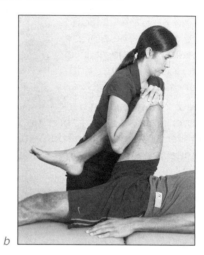

b

Anterior Glide (Right)

Assessment: Extension and external rotation.

Patient position: Left side lying with a pillow between the legs and with the hips comfortably flexed.

Clinician position: Standing in a walk-stance position perpendicular to the side of the examination table. The clinician's palm is butted against the posterior lateral trochanter, and the other hand stabilizes the pelvis.

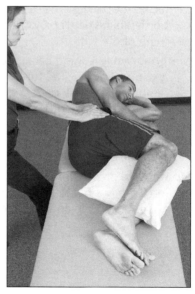

Method: The clinician applies an anterior force parallel to the joint surfaces with the distal hand. Apply first pressures gently; increase amplitude and depth of the movement if no pain response occurs. Assess quality of movement through the range and end feel; compare with the other side.

Biomechanics: According to the convex–concave rule, the femoral head glides anterior on the acetabulum during hip extension and external rotation.

Lateral Glide

Assessment: Lateral mobility of the hip.

Patient position: Supine with the leg extended (can be flexed to 90°) (see *a*).

Clinician position: One hand stabilizes the lateral aspect of the distal femur, and the other hand contacts the medial aspect of the proximal femur (*b*).

Method: The proximal hand applies a lateral force.

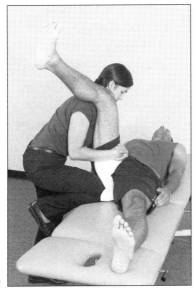
a

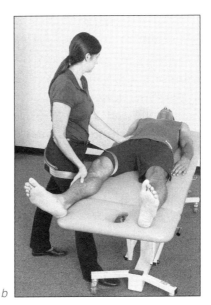
b

End Feel

Flexion: Soft (tissue approximation) due to muscle bulk of the anterior thigh and lower abdominal muscles or stretch of the hip extensors.

Extension: Firm due to tissue stretch of the anterior capsule; iliofemoral, ischiofemoral, and pubofemoral ligaments; and hip flexor muscles.

Abduction: Firm due to tissue stretch of the inferior capsule, pubofemoral and ischiofemoral ligaments, inferior band of iliofemoral ligament, and adductor muscles.

Abduction: Hard (femoral neck approximates the acetabulum).

Adduction: Soft (tissue approximation of the thighs).

Adduction: Firm due to stretch of the abductor muscles.

Internal rotation: Firm due to tissue stretch of the posterior joint capsule, ischiofemoral ligament, and external rotators of the hip.

External rotation: Firm due to tissue stretch of the anterior joint capsule, iliofemoral and pubofemoral ligaments, and internal rotator muscles.

Capsular Pattern

Equal limitation in flexion, abduction, and internal rotation with slight loss in extension, little or no loss in external rotation.

Close-Packed Position

Maximum extension, internal rotation, slight abduction.

Loose-Packed Position

30° of flexion, 30° of abduction, slight external rotation.

Stability

Iliofemoral Ligament (Y-Ligament)   From the anterior inferior iliac spine down to the upper and lower parts of the intertrochanteric line of the femur; blends with the anterior capsule, prevents overextension during standing and external rotation; during adduction the medial inferior band is under mild tension.

Ischiofemoral Ligament   From the body of the ischium near the acetabular margin upward and laterally to the greater trochanter; limits extension, internal rotation, and abduction.

Pubofemoral Ligament   From the superior ramus of the pubis down to the lower part of the intertrochanteric line; limits extension, abduction, and external rotation.

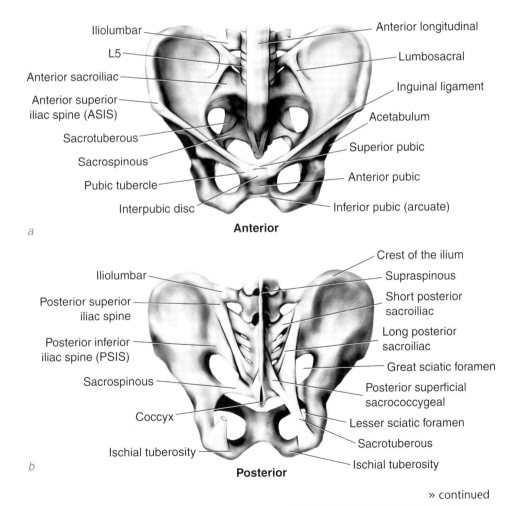

Pelvis ligaments: (*a*) anterior view; (*b*) posterior view; (*c*) the iliolumbar ligaments; hip ligaments: (*d*) anterior view; (*e*) posterior view.

» continued

Reprinted from R. Behnke, *Kinetic anatomy*, 2nd ed. (Champaign, IL: Human Kinetics), 139, 127, and 177.

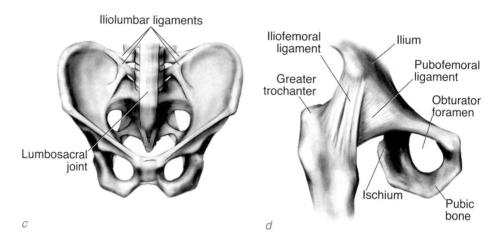

c

d

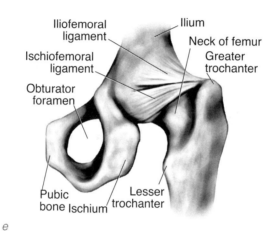

e

» continued

Patrick's or Faber Test

Assessment: Range of motion of hip and pain.

Patient position: Supine with the leg placed so that the foot is resting on top of the knee of the opposite leg. Hip in flexion, abduction, and external rotation.

Clinician position: Standing on the side of the table facing the

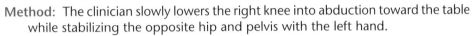

side of the patient. The clinician places the left hand on the patient's left ASIS and the right hand grasps the right knee.

Method: The clinician slowly lowers the right knee into abduction toward the table while stabilizing the opposite hip and pelvis with the left hand.

Positive response: The leg does not reach the table or pain is present in this position.

Biomechanics: The full excursion of the joint range of motion in this position normally permits the test leg to reach the table. A soft-tissue shortening or articular surface pathology will limit this ROM.

Craig's Test

Assessment: Measure femoral anteversion.

Patient position: Prone, lying with the knee flexed to 90°.

Clinician position: Standing on the side of the table facing the side of the patient. The clinician holds on to the patient's left ankle with the right hand while palpating the greater trochanter with the left index finger.

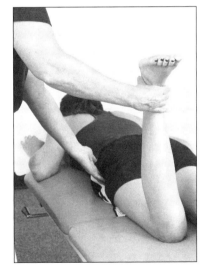

Method: The clinician passively moves the patient's leg from internal to external rotation of the hip while palpating the greater trochanter. When the trochanter reaches its most lateral position, the clinician measures the angle between the lower leg and the vertical.

Normal response: In an adult, the mean angle is 8 to 15°.

Biomechanics: Excessive anteversion presents with excessive medial rotation and decreased lateral rotation. Retroversion presents with excessive lateral rotation.

Hip Flexion and Adduction

Examination: Pathology in the articulating surface of the hip joint as with OA.

Patient position: Supine, hip in flexion with the knee bent

Clinician position: Standing on the side of the table facing the side of the patient. The clinician grasps the patient's right knee with both hands and places the right knee on the table supporting the patient's pelvis on his or her proximal thigh.

Method: The clinician gently oscillates the patient's hip into hip flexion and adduction at different points of the arc of motion where the femoral head contacts the acetabulum.

Alternative method: Hip quadrant (scour test)—the clinician applies slight resistance while the hip is taken into an arc of motion.

Positive response: Irregularity in movement, pain, and patient apprehension.

Biomechanics: Maximal compression of articulating surfaces to provoke articular cartilage pathology.

Hip Flexor Length

Assessment: Length of the hip flexors (right leg).

Patient position: Sitting at the end of the table with the distal legs supported on the table.

Clinician position: The clinician helps lower the patient to supine position while the patient holds both knees to the chest. The clinician then holds the patient's posterior right leg with the right hand and palpates the ASIS and PSIS with the left hand, while the patient holds the left knee to the chest.

Method: Step 1: The clinician lowers the right leg to the table while monitoring the low back with the left hand (*a*). Step 2: If the leg does not lower to the table with the knee flexed, the clinician extends the knee and then attempts to lower the leg to the table (*b*). Step 3: If the leg does not lower to the table with the knee extended, the clinician flexes the knee, abducts the hip, and attempts to lower the leg to the table (*c*).

Normal response: The leg lowers to the table with the knee flexed.

Positive response: If the leg does not lower to the table with the knee in extension—tightness of iliopsoas. If the leg lowers to the table with the knee in extension—tightness in rectus femoris. If the leg lowers to the table with the knee in flexion and hip in abduction—tightness in the tensor fascia latae.

Biomechanics: The hip flexors under examination are the iliopsoas, rectus femoris, and tensor fascia latae. The hip should be able to reach neutral position with the spine flat if all hip flexors are of normal length. To bias the rectus femoris, the knee can be straightened. To bias the tensor fascia latae, the hip can be abducted.

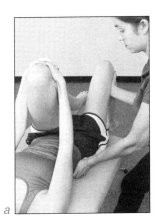
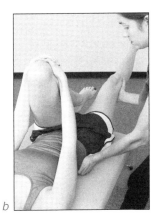
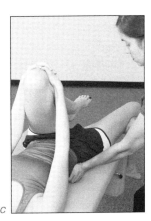

a *b* *c*

Modified Ober Test

Assessment: Length of the iliotibial band.

Patient position: Left side lying with the right knee and hip flexed.

Clinician position: Standing on the side of the table, behind the patient. The clinician stabilizes the patient's right pelvis with the left hand to prevent the lateral tilt and holds the patient's leg with the right hand.

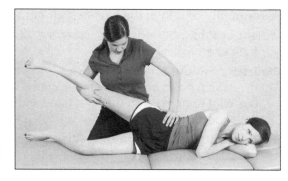

Method: The clinician brings the leg into extension, keeping the femur from rotating internally. The clinician then allows the leg to drop into adduction.

Positive response: The leg does not drop into adduction or drops less than 10° from horizontal.

Biomechanics: A tight iliotibial band (tensor fascia latae) will cause hip abduction and internal rotation of the femur.

Ely's Test

Assessment: Length of the rectus femoris.

Patient position: Prone, arms at the side, legs together.

Clinician position: Standing on the side of the patient. The clinician places one hand or forearm on the patient's pelvis and grasps the ankle with the other hand.

Method: The clinician passively flexes the patient's knee with one hand while other hand stabilizes the pelvis.

Positive response: Anterior pelvic tilt or limited knee flexion indicates tightness of the rectus femoris.

Biomechanics: The rectus femoris attaches to the anterior inferior iliac spine and the patellar tendon. Neutral pelvis with increasing knee flexion increases tension in the rectus femoris.

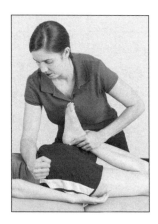

Hamstring Length (Straight-Leg Raise)

Assessment: Length of the hamstring muscle.

Patient position: Supine.

Test position: Back neutral, knee extended, hip extended.

Method: The clinician passively brings the leg up into increasing hip flexion.

Positive response: Less than 80° of hip flexion indicates tightness in the connective tissue of the posterior thigh.

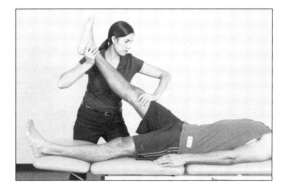

Piriformis

Assessment: Piriformis involvement.

Patient position: Left side lying. Flex the test hip to 60° with the knee flexed.

Clinician position: Standing on the side of the patient facing the front side of the patient. The clinician stabilizes the patient's pelvis with the right hand and holds the patient's medial aspect of the knee with the left hand.

Method: The clinician applies a downward force to the flexed knee and monitors the onset of resistance.

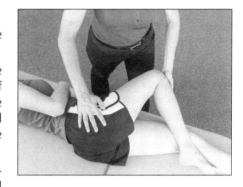

Positive response: Sciatica pain or tightness of the piriformis muscle.

Biomechanics: The piriformis attaches from the lateral sacrum to the superior border of the greater trochanter. About 15% of people have their sciatic nerve passing through the piriformis muscle rather than below it. Sciatica pain is elicited as the piriformis impinges on the nerve.

Ortolani's Test

Assessment: Congenital hip dysplasia.

Patient position: Supine.

Test position: Hip in flexion and adduction.

Method: The clinician presses the hips into a posterior direction and relocates the hip by abducting the hips and pressing anteriorly.

Positive response: Click, relocation.

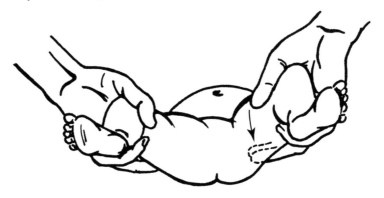

Trendelenburg's Sign

Examination: Integrity of the gluteus medius or an unstable hip.

Patient position: Standing on one limb, the affected side (*a*).

Clinician position: Standing behind the patient.

Method: The clinician observes the alignment of the contralateral limb with the pelvis.

Positive response: The pelvis on the opposite side drops when the patient stands on the affected limb (*b*).

Biomechanics: The gluteus medius (prime mover) and other hip abductors stabilize the pelvis on the femur.

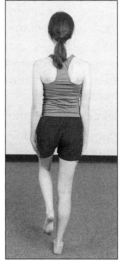

a

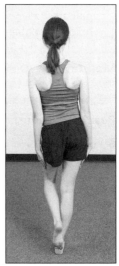

b

Arthrokinematics

Flexion

Nonweight bearing (NWB): The head spins and slightly glides posteriorly and inferiorly.

Weight bearing (WB): The pelvis glides anteriorly on the fixed femur.

Extension

NWB: The head spins and slightly glides anteriorly in extension.

WB: The pelvis glides posteriorly on the fixed femur.

Abduction

NWB: Inferior glide of the convex femoral head. With the hip flexed to 90° the femoral head glides anteriorly in abduction.

WB: In a weight-bearing state, the concave acetabulum glides toward the opposite pelvis.

Adduction

NWB: Superior glide. With the hip flexed to 90° the femoral head glides posteriorly in adduction.

Internal Rotation

NWB: Internal rotation is accomplished by posterior glide of the femoral head. With the hip flexed to 90° the femoral head glides inferiorly.

WB: The acetabulum spins about the femoral head toward the side of rotation. For right lower-extremity internal rotation, the pelvis will rotate to the right.

External Rotation

NWB: External rotation is accomplished by anterior glide of the femoral head. With the hip flexed to 90° the femoral head glides superiorly.

WB: The acetabulum spins about the femoral head opposite the side of rotation. For right lower-extremity external rotation, the pelvis will rotate to the left.

Neurology

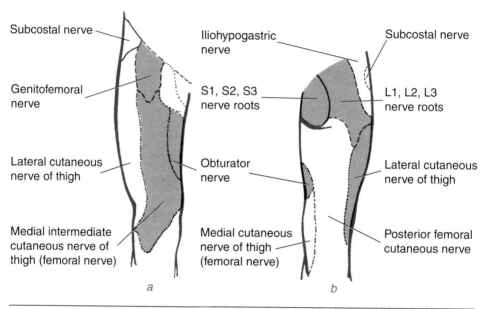

Sensory distribution around the hip: (*a*) anterior view; (*b*) posterior view.

Neurology

Nerve root	Reflex	Motor	Sensory
L2	—	Hip flexion	Anterior proximal thigh
L3	Patellar tendon	Quadriceps	Lateral thigh
L4	Anterior tibialis	Anterior tibialis	Lateral thigh to lateral knee
L5	Proximal hamstring	Extensor hallucis longus	Posterior thigh, dorsum of the foot
S1	Achilles tendon	Peroneus longus	Posterior thigh and lateral foot

Peripheral Nerves

Nerve	Motor	Sensory
Obturator	Hip adduction and external rotation	Medial inner thigh
Femoral	Hip flexion	Medial thigh (anterior femoral cutaneous)
Tibial	Plantar flex, adduct, or invert the foot	Heel
Superficial peroneal	Eversion of the foot	Lateral calf
Deep peroneal	Dorsiflexion of the foot	Cleft between first and second toe

Surface Palpation

Greater trochanter

Anterior superior iliac spine

Ischial tuberosity

Inguinal ligament

Femoral triangle

Pubic symphysis

Posterior superior iliac spine

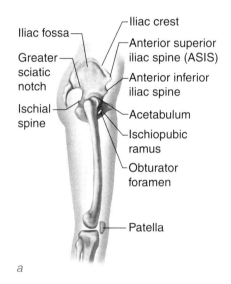

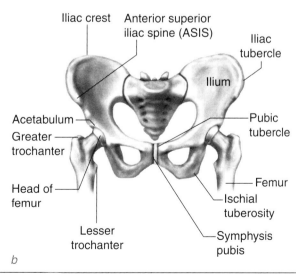

Bony structures of the hip: (*a*) lateral view; (*b*) anterior view.

Reprinted from R. Behnke, *Kinetic anatomy*, 2nd ed. (Champaign, IL: Human Kinetics), 177.

Muscle Origin and Insertion

Muscle	Origin and insertion
Psoas	Transverse processes, body L1–L5 and T12 to lesser trochanter
Iliacus	Inner surface of ilium and sacrum to lesser trochanter
Rectus femoris	Anterior inferior iliac spine to patella and tibial tuberosity
Sartorius	Anterior superior iliac spine to medial tibia (pes anserine)
Pectineus	Pectineal line on pubis to below lesser trochanter
Adductor longus	Inferior rami of pubis to middle third of posterior femur
Adductor brevis	Inferior rami of pubis to upper half of posterior femur
Gracilis	Inferior rami of pubis to medial tibia (pes anserine)
Biceps femoris	Ischial tuberosity to lateral condyle of tibia and head of fibula
Semimembranosus	Ischial tuberosity to medial condyle of tibia
Semitendinosus	Ischial tuberosity to medial tibia (pes anserine)
Gluteus maximus	Posterior ilium, sacrum, coccyx to gluteal tuberosity, iliotibial band
Gluteus medius	Anterior lateral ilium to lateral surface of greater trochanter
Adductor magnus	Anterior pubis and ischial tuberosity to linea aspera on posterior femur, adductor tubercle
Tensor fasciae latae	Anterior superior iliac spine to iliotibial tract
Obturator internus	Sciatic notch and margin of obturator foramen to greater trochanter
Obturator externus	Pubis, ischium, and margin of obturator foramen to upper, posterior femur
Quadratus femoris	Ischial tuberosity to greater trochanter
Piriformis	Anterior, lateral sacrum to superior greater trochanter
Superior gemellus	Ischial spine to greater trochanter
Inferior gemellus	Ischial tuberosity to greater trochanter

Adapted from J. Hamill and K. Knudzen, 1995, Biomechanical basis of human movement (Baltimore, MD: Lippincott, Williams, and Wilkins), 504.

Muscle Action and Innervation

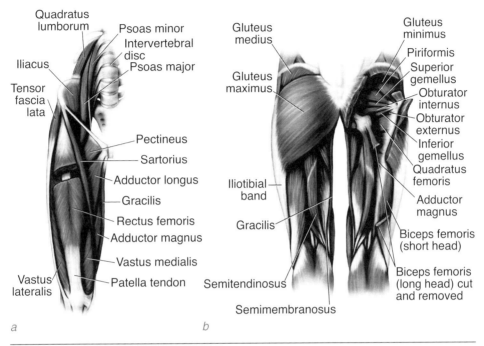

Muscles acting on the hip and pelvis: (*a*) anterior view; (*b*) posterior view.

Reprinted, by permission, from R. Behnke, *Kinetic anatomy*, 2nd ed. (Champaign, IL: Human Kinetics), 178 and 180.

Action	Muscle involved	Nerve supply	Nerve root
Hip flexion	Psoas	L1–L3	L1–L3
	Iliacus	Femoral	L2–L3
	Rectus femoris	Femoral	L2–L4
	Sartorius	Femoral	L2–L4
	Pectineus	Femoral	L2–L3
	Adductor longus	Obturator	L2–L4
	Adductor brevis	Obturator	L2–L3, L5
	Gracilis	Obturator	L2–L3
Hip extension	Biceps femoris	Sciatic	L5, S1–S2
	Semimembranosus	Sciatic	L5, S1–S2
	Semitendinosus	Sciatic	L5, S1–S2
	Gluteus maximus	Inferior gluteal	L5, S1–S2
	Gluteus medius (posterior fibers)	Superior gluteal	L5, S1
	Adductor magnus	Sciatic	L2–L4
Hip abduction	Tensor fasciae latae	Superior gluteal	L4–L5
	Gluteus minimus	Superior gluteal	L5, S1
	Gluteus medius	Superior gluteal	L5, S1
	Gluteus maximus	Inferior gluteal	L5, S1–S2
	Sartorius	Femoral	L2–L3
Hip adduction	Adductor longus	Obturator	L2–L4
	Adductor brevis	Obturator	L2–L4
	Adductor magnus	Obturator	L2–L4
	Gracilis	Obturator	L2–L3
	Pectineus	Femoral	L2–L3
Hip internal rotation	Adductor longus	Obturator	L2–L4
	Adductor brevis	Obturator	L2–L4
	Gluteus minimus (anterior portion)	Superior gluteal	L5, S1
	Gluteus medius (anterior portion)	Superior gluteal	L5, S1
	Tensor fasciae latae	Superior gluteal	L4–L5
	Gracilis	Obturator	L2–L3
	Pectineus	Femoral	L2–L3
Hip external rotation	Gluteus maximus	Inferior gluteal	L5, S1–S2
	Obturator internus	Sacral plexus	L5, S1
	Obturator externus	Obturator	L3–L4
	Quadratus femoris	Sacral plexus	L4–L5, S1
	Piriformis	L5, S1–S2	L5, S1–S2
	Superior gemellus	Sacral plexus	L5, S1
	Inferior gemellus	Sacral plexus	L4–L5, S1
	Sartorius	Femoral	L2–L3
	Gluteus medius	Superior gluteal	L5, S1

Adapted from *Orthopedic Physical Assessment,* 2nd ed., D.J. Magee, pg. 338. Copyright 1992, with permission from W.B. Saunders.

EXAMINATION SEQUENCE

HISTORY

Profile

Occupation and recreational activities—consider effect of hip pain on level of function or disability (walking, repetitive squatting, sporting activities, overuse, or abuse)

Location of Symptoms

Common patterns of referral from the L-spine nerve root: L1–L5.

May need to question stiffness, snapping, popping, grinding if not offered spontaneously.

Check symptom-free areas—LS, SI joint, knee.

Groin pain: consider OA, femoral anterior glide syndrome.

Lateral hip pain: consider greater trochanteric bursitis, OA.

Deep joint pain: consider OA, stress fracture.

Posterior hip pain: consider proximal hamstring strain, piriformis syndrome, SI joint.

Behavior of Symptoms

Aggravating Factors

Crossing legs

Sitting for long periods

Sitting to standing

Squatting

Twisting

Walking phase of gait, pivoting, inclines

Lying on side

Putting on socks

Getting in or out of vehicle

Going up or down stairs, weakness, giving way or pain

Running, jumping, performing sport-related moves

TESTS AND MEASURES

Standing

Observation

Gait (various speeds, forward, backward)

Posture (leg length: ASIS, PSIS, femur position)

Implicate or Clear the Lumbar Spine

Neurological Examination—S1 Myotome

Functional Tests: Hopping, Skipping, One-Legged Stance, Squatting, Heel Rotation, Crossing Legs

Special Test: Trendelenburg's Test

Supine

Palpation

ASIS

Iliac crest

Pubic tubercle

Greater trochanter

Soft tissue

Implicate or Clear the Knee

Neurological Examination (Segmental, Peripheral, or Central as Indicated)

AROM

Hip flexion (0–120°)

Hip ER or IR

Hip abduction (0–45°)

Hip adduction (0–30°)

PROM With OP, as Indicated

Muscle Length Test

Hamstring length

PAMs

Inferior glide at 90° hip flexion

Inferior glide at 30° hip flexion

Lateral traction

Posterior glide

Compression

Special Tests

Hip flexion and adduction or quadrant test (scour)

Faber test

Leg length

Neurodynamic Testing

Side Lying

Muscle Length Test

Iliotibial band (modified Ober test)

Piriformis test

MMT

Hip abduction (test both supine if less than fair)

Hip adduction (test both supine if less than fair)

ITB (test in long sitting if less than fair)

PAMs

Anterior glide (or can be done in prone position)

Prone

Palpation

PSIS

Iliac crest

Ischial tuberosity

Sciatic notch

SI joint

Soft tissue

Lumbar spine for clearing

Neurological Examination if Indicated

AROM With OP

Hip IR or ER

Hip extension (0–20°)

MMT

Hip extension (test in side lying if less than fair)

Knee flexion (test in side lying if less than fair)

Special Tests

Craig's test

Ely's test

Neurodynamic Testing—Prone Knee Bend (PKB)

Sitting

AROM

Hip ER (0–45°)

Hip IR (0–45°)

MMT

Hip flexion (test in side lying if less than fair)

Sartorius (test in supine if less than fair)

Hip ER or IR (test in supine if less than fair)

Special Tests

Hip Flexor Length

Clinical Syndromes

Description	Location and behavior of symptoms	History	Tests and measures, diagnostics	Intervention
BURSITIS				
Inflammation of the bursa around the hip, commonly the ischial, iliopsoas, and trochanteric.	Local pain and tenderness over area of bursa, symptoms increase with activity, snapping sensation.	Gradual or may be acute from a fall or direct blow. Profile: middle-aged.	Pain with passive and active movements, pain with reciprocal flexion or extension, tenderness to palpation. Iliopsoas: Hip ER, hip flex. Trochanteric: tight ITB, LLD, hip IR. Ischial: tight hamstrings. Special tests: + FAB,+ Ober. X ray: normal, MRI to rule out.	Acute: PRICEM. Subacute: education. Manual therapy: joint mobility for hypo. Therapeutic exercise: flexibility, biomechanical analysis. Cortisone injection usually helpful.
OSTEOARTHRITIS				
Degenerative changes in femoral head or acetabulum.	Groin or greater trochanter pain, anterior thigh, medial knee, lateral thigh. Stiffness, especially after prolonged positions or activity. May wake at night.	Insidious onset, gradual wear and tear of the hip joint.	Limited ROM in capsular pattern; stiffness after activity, increased symptoms when hip in close-packed position and weight bearing. Special tests: + scour, Faber. X ray: decreased joint space, osteophytes.	Pain control: NSAIDS, modalities. Assistive equipment: cane to unload. Education: joint stress, weight loss. Manual therapy: AROM, joint mob. Therapeutic exercise: flexibility, aerobic exercise, strengthen hip ER and abductors. Surgery: joint replacement.

Description	Location and behavior of symptoms	History	Tests and measures, diagnostics	Intervention
FEMORAL NECK STRESS FRACTURE; PELVIC STRESS FRACTURE				
	Local tenderness at GT, may radiate to inner thigh or groin. Night pain, no relief with cortisone injection. Groin pain.	Insidious onset, increased in training, aggravated by activity. Insidious onset, history of overuse.	Positive percussion test, limited IR. Antalgic gait, tenderness to palpation. X rays: may be negative, scan.	Pain control: relative rest, electrical stimulation. Assistive equipment: neoprene sleeve, crutches. Education: biomechanical training. Manual therapy: hip mobility. Therapeutic exercise: aerobic exercise like swimming, cycling.
MUSCLE STRAIN				
Microtearing of the muscle or connective tissue about the hip: adductors, hamstrings, quadriceps.	Discomfort locally at site of strain.	Acute trauma or overuse.	Local tenderness, decreased muscle power, tissue hiatus; pain with stretch and muscle contraction.	Acute: PRICEM. Subacute: flexibility, muscle balance, biomechanics: imbalance in sagittal plan.
MUSCLE IMBALANCES				
Femoral anterior glide. Decreased posterior glide of femoral head (pinch anterior joint capsule).	Pain in groin with knee or hip flexion, may progress to posterior hip.	Younger runners, females.	Sway back posture, hand and knee: decreased hip flexion; increased use of thigh muscles versus hip girdle muscles.	Joint mobilization of hip (posterior glides), passive hip or knee flexion, hip flexion, gluteus maximus, medius strengthening.
Hip adduction syndrome. Increased hip adduction.	Buttock or lat thigh pain with standing, walking, stairs.	Sleeps on side.	Weak hip abductors, hip drop with gait, increased add in stance, LLD, short adductor muscles (<35° of hip abduction).	Strengthen hip abductors, educate on standing posture.
Lateral glide (snapping hip, iliotibial band syndrome). Friction between ITB and femur.	Deep hip pain, popping, active subluxation.	Dancers, hyperflexibility.	Prominent GT, stands in hip adductors, weak hip abductors and ER (long), short TFL.	Strengthen hip abductors or ER, educate on standing and sitting posture, stabilization.

» continued

» continued

Description	Location and behavior of symptoms	History	Tests and measures, diagnostics	Intervention
PIRIFORMIS SYNDROME				
Spasm of the piriformis muscle (hip lateral rotation syndrome).	Buttock pain, may refer down LE; may be aggravated by sitting or walking.	Insidious; overuse.	Local tenderness; limited internal rotation of the hip, pain with hip IR stretch or ER MMT. Piriformis stretch test; + SLR.	Soft-tissue massage; core strengthening; hip strengthening; lumbar spine or SI joint mobilization.
DEVELOPMENTAL HIP DYSPLASIA				
Hip dislocation in newborn.		Congenital deformity.	Hip weakness, balance problems. Limb shortening. Ortolani's test, X ray.	Hip spica. Splint in flex, abduction: 5–6 months. Surgery: release hip adductors, iliopsoas. Osteotomy (>2 year-olds), created acetabulum.
LEGG-CALVÉ PERTHES DISEASE				
Osteonecrosis of epiphyseal center of proximal femur.	Groin and anterior thigh pain, medial knee pain (without knee injury). No history of trauma.	3- to 10-year-old males; 12% bilaterally; family history; insidious. Short in stature.	Limp, limited ROM in abduction, IR, flex. X ray: I. Bone death, X rays normal (1–6 weeks). II. Revascularization, X ray: increased density (up to 1 year). III. Distortion and remodeling, X ray: widening of joint, flattened ossification center (1–3 years).	Refer to orthopedic surgeon. Splinting: 30° abduction or IR (6–8 weeks). Maintain ROM as appropriate. After immobilization: stationary cycling, swimming, rowing.
SLIPPED CAPITAL FEMORAL EPIPHYSIS				
Slippage of the head of the femur at the epiphyseal.	Hip pain and tenderness, anterior thigh pain.	11- to 13-year-old females; 13- to 16-year-old males; obese. 30% bilaterally. Acute or chronic, may occur following fall.	Antalgic gait, ER of hip with hip flexion. Limited: hip abdution, IR, flex. X ray. Leg-length discrepancy.	Refer to orthopedic surgeon. Surgical reduction and pinning (NWB 6 weeks). PT: ROM, strengthening, flexibility.

Description	Location and behavior of symptoms	History	Tests and measures, diagnostics	Intervention
AVASCULAR NECROSIS				
Deterioration of femoral head secondary to occlusion of the medial or lateral circumflex artery.	Ache, stiffness, pain: worse in groin, may radiate to medial thigh, knee worse with standing, walking, crossing legs.	Occurs following severe trauma to the hip such as fracture or dislocation; may be congenital. Idiopathic: 30- to 60-year-old males, bilateral 40–80%).	Limited ROM, decreased strength. X ray.	Refer to orthopedic surgeon. Postsurgery: restore strength and flexibility.
PELVIC APOPHYSITIS				
Secondary center of ossification ASIS, AIIS.	Pain at origin of immature pelvis, rest improves symptoms.	Running and kicking sports.	Antalgic gait. Pain with active or resisted hip flexion, adduction. Palpation: tender over tendon insertion.	Pain control: ice, electric stimulation. Education: training errors. Manual therapy: soft-tissue, joint mobility. Therapeutic exercise: correct muscle imbalances, strengthen weak muscles, check biomechanics.
LABRAL TEAR				
Tear to fibrocartilage ring of acetabulum.	Anterior hip pain; possibly groin; click with hip movement.	Trauma, repetitive stress to hip; hip dysplasia; long duration of symptoms.	(+) hip quadrant. Faber could be positive. Radiograph or MRI (+).	Limited WB. PT: posture, hip strengthening; flexibility; modification of functional activities.
SPINE REFERRAL				
	Lateral hip: L4. Groin: L1, SI joint, L4. Posterior hip: DDD.	Refer to lumbar spine clinical syndromes table.	Comparable sign with palpation to specific spinal level.	Refer to lumbar spine clinical syndromes table.

Adapted, by permission, from C. Wadsworth, 1988, *Manual examination and treatment of the spine and extremities* (Baltimore, MD: Lippincott, Williams, and Wilkins), 173.

Knee

The knee joint is composed of the tibiofemoral joint, the superior tibiofibular joint, and the patellofemoral joint. The tibiofemoral joint is not a pure hinge joint, but a bicondylar joint that has movement in all three planes (sagittal, transverse, frontal). The knee joint is susceptible to injury because ligamentous support provides its main stability. This chapter covers osteology, arthrokinematics, range of motion, muscle origin and insertion, muscle action, neurology, and special tests for the three joints. A table at the end of the chapter provides clinical syndromes. Also presented is a recommended sequence for the subjective and objective exam.

TIBIOFEMORAL JOINT

Articulation   A convex medial and lateral condyle of the distal femur and the two concave medial and lateral condyles of the proximal tibia.

Type of Joint   Diarthrodial ginglymus joint.

Degrees of Freedom

- Flexion and extension in the sagittal plane about a coronal axis through the femoral condyles
- Internal and external rotation in transverse plane about a longitudinal axis through the medial intercondylar eminence
- Abduction and adduction in coronal plane about a sagittal axis throughout the center of the knee

Active Range of Motion

Flexion: 0–135°

Extension: 0–10° hyperextension

Tibial internal rotation: 0–30°

Tibial external rotation: 0–40°

Knee Flexion

Patient position: Supine.

Clinician position: Standing on the right side of the table facing the side of the patient. After the patient has achieved the available range of motion (without deviations), the clinician places the left hand over the patient's right knee and grasps the patient's right ankle with the right hand.

Method: Gently apply overpressure into flexion oscillating into the end range.

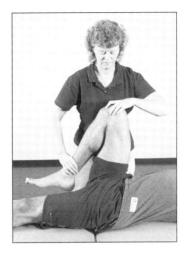

Knee Extension

Patient position: Supine.

Clinician position: Standing on the right side of the table facing the side of the patient. After the patient has achieved the available range of motion (without deviations), the clinician places the left cupped hand over the patient's right tibial tubercle with fingers pointing caudad and cups the patient's right ankle with the right hand.

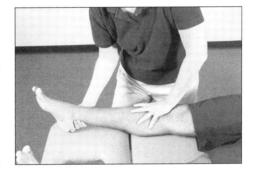

Method: Gently apply overpressure into extension oscillating into the end range.

Distraction

Patient position: Sitting with the knee flexed and femur fully supported.

Clinician position: Sitting in front of the patient. The clinician takes up the soft tissue of the posterior lower leg with the fingers of both hands and places the thenar eminences of both hands on the tibial plateaus of the knee.

Method: Apply a distraction force to the tibia (*a*). Apply first pressures gently; increase amplitude and depth of the movement if no pain response occurs. Assess quality of movement through the range and end feel; compare with the other side.

Alternative method: Apply a distraction force with both hands around the distal tibia with fingers pointing down along the distal tibia (*b*).

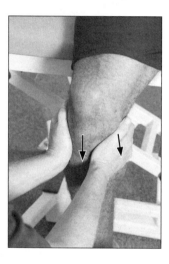
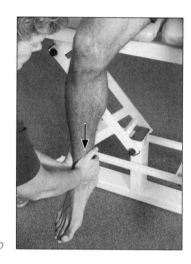

a

b

Anterior Glide

Assessment: Anterior glide of the tibia on the femur; to facilitate extension.

Patient position: Sitting with the knee flexed and femur fully supported.

Clinician position: Sitting in front of the patient. The clinician takes up the soft tissue of the posterior lower leg with the fingers of both hands and places the thumbs (or thenar eminences) of both hands on the tibial plateaus of the knee.

Method: Apply an anterior force to the tibia through the thumbs (or thenar eminences). Apply first pressures gently; increase amplitude and depth of the movement if no pain response occurs. Assess quality of movement through the range and end feel; compare with the other side.

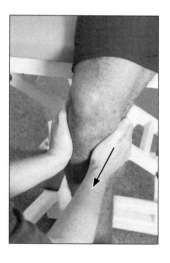

Alternative method: Hook lying position with the foot supported.

Posterior Glide

Assessment: Posterior glide of the tibia on the femur; to facilitate flexion.

Patient position: Sitting with the knee flexed and femur fully supported.

Clinician position: Sitting in front of the patient. The clinician takes up the soft tissue of the posterior lower leg with the fingers of both hands and places the thumbs (or thenar eminences) of both hands on the tibial plateaus of the knee.

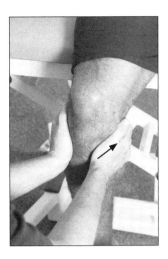

Method: Apply a posterior force to the tibia through the thenar eminences. Apply first pressures gently; increase amplitude and depth of the movement if no pain response occurs. Assess quality of movement through the range and end feel; compare with the other side.

Alternative method: Hook lying position with the foot supported.

Intervention: Use appropriate grade of movement (I–IV) to treat pain or resistance. Posterior glide increases knee flexion.

Biomechanics: According to the convex–concave rule, the concave tibia guides posteriorly on the convex femur during flexion.

Medial Glide

Assessment: Medial glide of the tibia on the femur.

Patient position: Side lying with a slightly flexed knee and leg extending over the edge of the table.

Clinician position: One hand placed on the proximal tibia and the other hand supporting the leg at the ankle.

Method: Apply a medial force to the tibia with the proximal hand.

Lateral Rotation

Assessment: Lateral rotation of the tibia on the femur.

Patient position: Sitting with the leg unsupported and the knee at 90°.

Clinician position: Grasp both hands around the proximal tibia.

Method: Apply a lateral rotation force on the tibia.

End Feel

Flexion: Soft due to contact between muscle bulk of the posterior calf and thigh; firm due to tension in the quadriceps muscle or anterior joint capsule

Extension: Firm due to posterior capsule, arcuate complex

Capsular Pattern

Greater limitation of flexion than extension; no rotary restriction.

Close-Packed Position

Maximal extension.

Loose-Packed Position

Midflexion.

Stability

Figure 13.1 displays ligaments stabilizing the knee.

Medial   Medial collateral ligament (MCL), anterior cruciate ligament (ACL), medial capsule, posterior cruciate ligament (PCL), meniscofemoral, meniscotibial.

Lateral   Lateral collateral ligament (LCL), lateral meniscus, arcuate ligament, ACL, PCL.

Anterior   ACL, MCL, LCL, quadriceps tendon.

Posterior   PCL, posterior oblique ligament, arcuate complex.

Rotation   MCL, posterior oblique ligament, ACL.

   MCL   medial condyle of the femur to anteromedial surface of the tibial condyle; controls valgus force at the knee; may limit extension, external rotation of the tibia on the femur.

   LCL   lateral condyle of the femur to inferior posterior portion of the head of the fibula; controls varus force.

   ACL   anterior intercondylar area of the tibia, passing superior, posterior, and laterally to be attached to posterior surface of medial surface of the lateral femoral condyle; two bands that are taut throughout range of motion; greatest resistance with extreme hyperextension, limits tibial internal rotation.

   PCL   posterior intercondylar area of the tibia, passes superiorly or anteriorly and medially to attach to anterior part of the medial femoral condyle; two bands—anteromedial, which is taut in flexion, and posterolateral, which is taut in extension; limits tibial internal rotation.

Menisci

    a. Medial: attached to articulating surface of the tibial plateau, deep surface of the knee joint capsule, and anterior or posterior intercondylar fossa; more C-shaped; thicker posteriorly than anteriorly.

    b. Lateral: attached to articulating surface of tibial plateau, deep surface of knee joint capsule, and anterior or posterior intercondylar fossa; more O-shaped; equal thickness anterior and posterior; thicker along periphery.

Quadriceps and patella tendon   Extension of quadriceps muscle that courses over the patella and inserts on the tibial tubercle. The patella improves the efficiency of extension because it holds the quadriceps tendon away from the axis of movement.

Arcuate ligament   Fibular head to posterolateral femoral condyle.

Arcuate complex   Arcuate ligament, LCL, popliteus, lateral head of the gastrocnemius.

Oblique popliteal ligament   Bridges the posterior femoral condyles, blends with the semimembranosus, runs with the popliteus muscle, provides reinforcement to the lateral capsule, and limits anterior medial rotation of the tibia.

Posterior oblique ligament   Posterior to MCL at the posteromedial corner of the capsule.

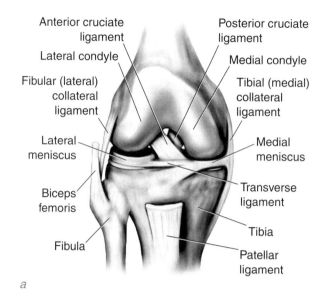

Anterior cruciate ligament

Posterior cruciate ligament

Lateral condyle

Medial condyle

Fibular (lateral) collateral ligament

Tibial (medial) collateral ligament

Lateral meniscus

Medial meniscus

Biceps femoris

Transverse ligament

Fibula

Tibia

Patellar ligament

a

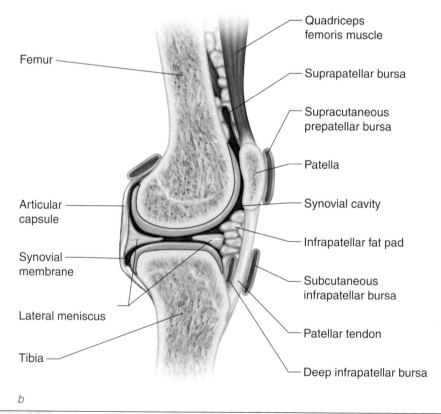

Quadriceps femoris muscle

Femur

Suprapatellar bursa

Supracutaneous prepatellar bursa

Patella

Articular capsule

Synovial cavity

Infrapatellar fat pad

Synovial membrane

Lateral meniscus

Subcutaneous infrapatellar bursa

Tibia

Patellar tendon

Deep infrapatellar bursa

b

Figure 13.1 Ligaments stabilizing the knee: (*a*) anterior view; (*b*) lateral view.

Reprinted from R. Behnke, *Kinetic anatomy*, 2nd ed. (Champaign, IL: Human Kinetics), 197 and 201.

Q-Angle

Patient position: Supine with the knee extended and relaxed. Both lower limbs must be at right angles to the line joining the two ASISs. The foot and hip should be in a neutral position.

Clinician position: Standing and facing the side of the patient.

Method: The clinician draws a line from the ASIS to the midpoint of the patella. The clinician then draws a line from the midpoint of the patella to the tibial tubercle. The angle formed by the crossings of the two lines is the Q-angle.

Normal response: Males 13°, females 18°.

Positive response: If the angle is less than 13°—chondromalacia patella or patella alta. If the angle is greater than 18°—chondromalacia patella, patella alta, subluxating patella, increase femoral anteversion, genu valgum, lateral displacement of the tibial tubercle, or increase lateral tibial torsion.

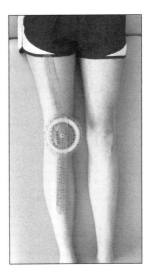

Anterior Instability: Lachman Test

Assessment: ACL integrity.

Patient position: Supine with the knee flexed to 15–30°.

Clinician position: Standing on the right side of the table facing the patient. The clinician grasps the lateral femur with the left hand and the medial tibia with the right hand.

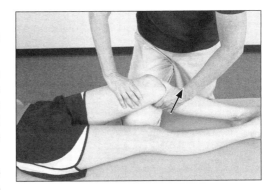

Method: Stabilize the femur while exerting an anterior force to the tibia.

Alternative method: Modified Lachman test, prone Lachman test.

Positive response: Excessive anterior translation of the tibia on the femur as compared with the opposite side.

Sensitivity: .63, specificity: .90 (Boeree and Ackroyd, 1991).

Anterior Instability: Anterior Drawer Sign

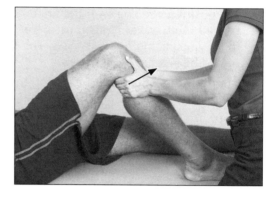

Assessment: ACL integrity.

Patient position: Supine with the knee flexed to 90° and the foot flat on the table.

Clinician position: Sit on the patient's foot and grasp the proximal tibia with both hands.

Method: Attempt to pull the tibia forward.

Positive response: Excessive anterior translation of tibia as compared with the opposite side.

Sensitivity: .76., specificity: .86 (Rubinstein et al., 1994).

Anterior Instability: Pivot Shift Test

Assessment: Anterolateral rotary instability of the knee.

Patient position: Supine with the leg relaxed, hip flexed to 30°, and slight internal rotation.

Clinician position: Hold the patient's foot with one hand while placing the other at the level of the fibular head. Place the heel of that hand behind the fibula. The knee is extended (this position actually subluxes the tibia anteriorly).

Method: Apply a valgus force to the knee while maintaining an internal rotation torque on the tibia. The leg is flexed.

Positive response: At approximately 30–40° the tibia will reduce with a clunk.

Sensitivity: .93, specificity: .89 (Rubinstein et al., 1994).

Anterior Instability: Flexion Rotation Drawer

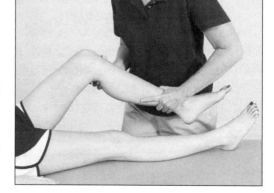

Assessment: Anterolateral instability of the knee.

Patient position: Supine.

Clinician position: The clinician holds the patient's ankle between the arms with the hands around the tibia. (The weight of the thigh causes the femur to drop posteriorly and rotate externally, producing an anterior subluxation of the lateral tibial plateau.)

Method: Flex the patient's knee to 20–30° while maintaining a neutral tibia. Then push the tibia posteriorly.

Positive response: Reduction of subluxed tibia.

Posterior Instability: Poster Drawer Sign

Posterior Instability: Posterior Drawer Sign

Assessment: PCL integrity.

Patient position: Supine, knee flexed to 90°, and foot flat on the table.

Clinician position: Sit on the patient's foot and grasp the proximal tibia with both hands. Attempt to push the tibia backward.

Positive response: Excessive posterior translation of tibia as compared to the opposite side.

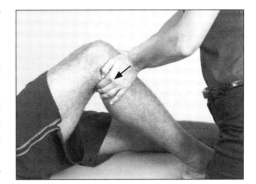

Sensitivity: .90, specificity: .99 (Rubinstein et al. 1994).

Posterior Instability: Posterior Sag

Examination: Posterior cruciate ligament integrity.

Patient position: Supine with the hip flexed to 90°, knee flexed to 90°, and foot supported by one of clinician's hands.

Clinician position: Standing and facing the side of patient. One hand supports the patient's feet, and the other hand is placed over the patient's thighs.

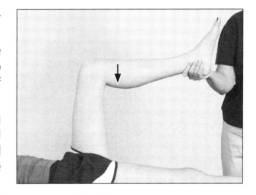

Method: The clinician looks at the tibial plateaus of both knees.

Normal response: The medial tibial plateau is 1 cm anterior to the femoral condyle.

Positive response: The tibia drops back or sags back.

Biomechanics: The PCL prevents posterior translation of the tibia on the femur.

Medial Instability: Valgus Stress Test

Assessment: MCL integrity.

Patient position: Supine with the knee flexed at 0–5° and 20–30°, right lower leg off the table (supported by clinician), and thigh resting on the table.

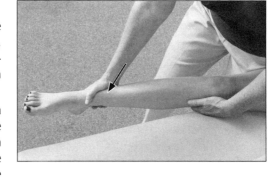

Clinician position: Standing in a walk-stance position facing the head of the table. The clinician places the left hand on the lateral knee to stabilize the thigh on the table. The clinician grasps the patient's medial ankle with right hand.

Method: Apply a valgus force to the knee.

Positive response: Excessive gapping of the medial joint line with or without pain.

Lateral Instability: Varus Stress Test

Assessment: LCL integrity.

Patient position: Supine with the knee flexed at 0–5° and 20–30°, right lower leg off the table (supported by clinician), and thigh resting on the table.

Clinician position: Standing in a walk-stance position facing the end of the table. The clinician places the right hand on the medial knee to stabilize the thigh on the table. The clinician grasps the patient's lateral ankle with the left hand.

Method: Apply a varus force to the knee.

Positive response: Excessive gapping of the lateral joint with or without pain.

Meniscal Instability: McMurray's Test

Patient position: Supine with the knee in full flexion.

Clinician position: Standing and facing the patient's right side. The clinician grasps the patient's right knee with the left hand while palpating the medial or lateral joint line and cups the patient's right heel with the right hand.

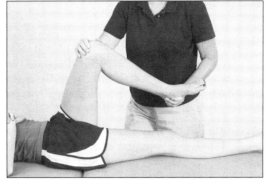

Method: The clinician applies medial rotation and a varus force through the tibia while extending the knee (lateral meniscus). The clinician then applies lateral rotation and a valgus force through the tibia while extending the knee (medial meniscus).

Sensitivity: .16, specificity: .98 (Evans et al. 1993).

Sensitivity: .25–.29, specificity: .25–.90 (Boeree and Ackroyd 1991).

Meniscal Instability: Grind Test

Assessment: Meniscus.

Patient position: Supine with the knee flexed in varying degrees of flexion.

Method: The clinician applies compressive and rotation force through the tibia.

Positive response: Click or pain.

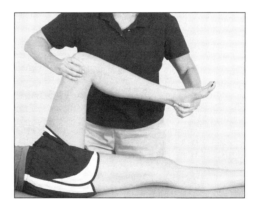

Meniscal Instability: Apley's Compression and Distraction Test (Right)

Assessment: Meniscal integrity.

Patient position: Prone with the knee flexed to 90°.

Clinician position: Standing and facing the side of the patient with the right knee stabilizing the patient's right thigh on the table. For compression, the clinician cups the plantar aspect of the patient's heel and midfoot with both hands (*a*). For distraction, the clinician cups the patient's heel and dorsal aspect of the midfoot with both hands (*b*).

Method: Rotate the tibia while applying a compressive force through the tibia. Rotate the tibia while applying a distractive force through the tibia.

Positive response: Pain or clicking, pain or reproduction of symptom.

Sensitivity: .16, specificity: .80 (Fowler and Lubliner 1989).

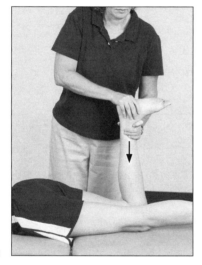

a

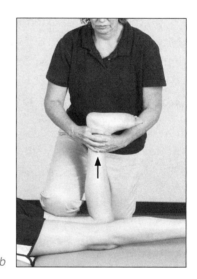

b

PROXIMAL TIBIOFIBULAR JOINT

Articulation   Concave facet on the head of the fibula and the convex facet on the lateral condyle of the tibia.

Type of Joint   Synovial plane gliding joint.

Degrees of Freedom

None; only accessory movement occurs.

Active Range of Motion

None.

Superior Glide

Assessment: Superior glide of the fibula.

Patient position: Supine with the knee flexed to 90° with the foot flat.

Test position: Have the patient actively dorsiflex the foot.

Clinician position: Assess superior motion of the fibular head.

Method: For this assessment, no force applied.

Anterior and Posterior Glide

Assessment: Joint play at the tibiofibular joint. The fibular head must move posteriorly on knee flexion and anteriorly on knee extension.

Patient position: Supine with the knee flexed to 90° and the foot flat.

Clinician position: Stabilize the knee with the medial hand. Grasp the head and neck of the proximal fibula with the lateral hand. The thumb contacts anteriorly, and the index and long finger pads contact posteriorly. (Be cautious of the peroneal nerve.)

Method: The lateral hand may glide the proximal fibula posteriorly or anteriorly.

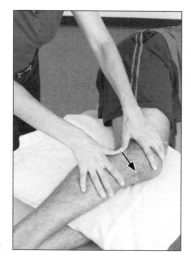
a

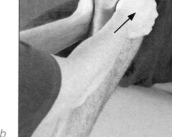
b

End Feel

None.

Capsular Pattern

Pain when joint stressed.

Close-Packed Position

Not applicable.

Loose-Packed Position

Not applicable.

Stability

Anterior Tibiofibular Ligament   From the fibula to anterior tibia, provides anterior stability.

Posterior Tibiofibular Ligament   From the fibula to posterior tibia, provides posterior stability.

Special Tests

None.

PATELLOFEMORAL JOINT

Articulation   Patella articulates with femoral condyles in the trochlear groove.

Type of Joint   Diarthrodial plane joint.

Degrees of Freedom

- Medial and lateral glide in frontal plane
- Superior and inferior glide in frontal plane
- Internal and external rotation in frontal plane

Active Range of Motion

None.

Patellar Alignment

Patient position: Supine with the quadriceps relaxed and knees straight.

Clinician position: Standing to the side of the patient.

Method:

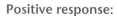

- Glide: Measure the distance from the mid-patella to the medial and lateral epicondyles of the femur. Compare static and dynamic.
- Tilt: Compare the heights of the medial and lateral borders of the patella. Compare static and dynamic.
- Rotation: Determine the position of the patella relative to the long axis of the femur.
- Anterior-posterior tilt: Determine the position of the inferior pole of the patella relative to the superior pole of the patella.

Positive response:

- Glide: medial—the distance from the medial epicondyle to the midpatella is .5 cm less than the distance from the lateral epicondyle to the midpatella; lateral—the distance from the lateral epicondyle to the midpatella is .5 cm less than the distance from the medial epicondyle to the midpatella.
- Tilt: medial—the lateral border is higher than the medial border; lateral—the medial border is higher than the lateral border.
- Rotation: external—the inferior pole is lateral to the long axis of the femur; internal—the inferior pole is medial to the long axis of the femur.
- Anterior-posterior tilt: the inferior pole of the patella is posterior to the superior pole.

Lateral Glide

Assessment: Lateral glide.

Patient position: Supine with the knee extended and relaxed.

Clinician position: Place the fingers and thumbs along the medial and lateral borders of the patella.

Method: Glide the patella in a lateral direction.

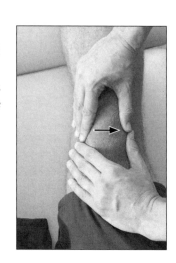

Medial Glide

Assessment: Medial glide.

Patient position: Supine with the knee extended and relaxed.

Clinician position: Place the fingers and thumbs along the medial and lateral borders of the patella.

Method: Glide the patella in a medial direction.

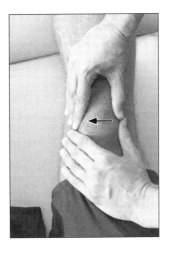

Superior Glide

Assessment: Patellar mobility for knee extension.

Patient position: Supine with the knee extended and relaxed.

Clinician position: Place the heel of one hand on the inferior aspect of the patella.

Method: Glide the patella cranially.

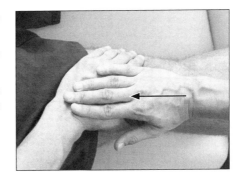

Inferior Glide

Assessment: Patellar mobility for knee flexion.

Patient position: Supine with the knee extended and relaxed.

Clinician position: Place the web space of one hand around the superior border of the patella.

Method: Glide the patella caudally.

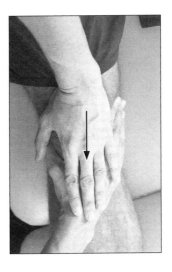

End Feel

Not applicable.

Capsular Pattern

Not applicable.

Close-Packed Position

Full flexion.

Loose-Packed Position

Full extension.

Stability

Retinaculum Distal connective tissue of quadriceps complex, reinforces patella.

Patellofemoral Ligaments Inferior pole of patella to tibial tuberosity.

Critical Test

Assessment: Patellofemoral pain.

Patient position: Sitting at the edge of the table.

Clinician position: Sitting to the side of the patient with one hand on the patient's distal anterior ankle and the other hand stabilizing the hip at the ASIS.

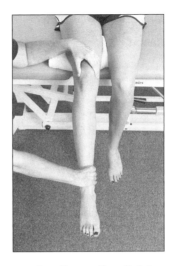

Method: The clinician applies resistance to the quadriceps muscle through the ankle while the patient performs an isometric contraction (10-second hold) at 120°, 90°, 60°, 30°, and 0°. If pain occurs at any of the angles, the clinician passively returns the knee to full extension. The patient's leg is then fully supported on the clinician's knee while the clinician applies a sustained medial glide to the patella as the knee is returned to the painful angle. The patient performs an isometric quadriceps contraction as the clinician maintains the patella medial glide at the initial painful angle.

Positive response: Pain decreases with the medial glide.

Apprehension Test

Assessment: Lateral patella subluxation or dislocation.

Patient position: Supine with the quadriceps relaxed and the knee supported with a towel roll at 30° of knee flexion.

Clinician position: Standing to the side of the patient. The clinician places the thumbs on the medial side of the patella.

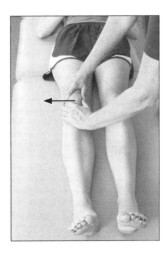

Method: The clinician carefully and slowly glides the patella laterally.

Positive response: The patient isometrically contracts the quadriceps or has an apprehensive look on his or her face.

Arthrokinematics

Weight-Bearing

Knee Extension   Femoral condyles roll anteriorly and slide posteriorly; near end extension, the femur rotates internally on the tibia, the patella slides superiorly and laterally, and the menisci follow the femur and move anteriorly.

Knee Flexion   Femoral condyles roll posteriorly and slide anteriorly; at beginning of flexion, the femur rotates externally on the tibia, the patella slides inferiorly, and the menisci follow the femur and move posteriorly.

Non-weight-bearing

Knee Extension   The tibial condyle slides and rolls anteriorly. The patella slides superiorly. During last 15–20° of extension, the tibia rotates externally on the femur. The fibular head moves posteriorly.

Knee Flexion   The tibia glides and rolls posteriorly on the femur. The patella slides inferiorly. Internal rotation of the tibia on the femur during first 15–20° of knee flexion; the fibula moves inferiorly and anteriorly.

Tibial Internal Rotation   The posterior horn of the lateral meniscus is compressed with tension on the anterior horn; the lateral meniscus moves posteriorly, and the medial meniscus moves anteriorly.

Tibial External Rotation   The posterior horn of the medial meniscus is compressed with tension on the anterior horn; the lateral meniscus moves anteriorly, and the medial meniscus moves posteriorly.

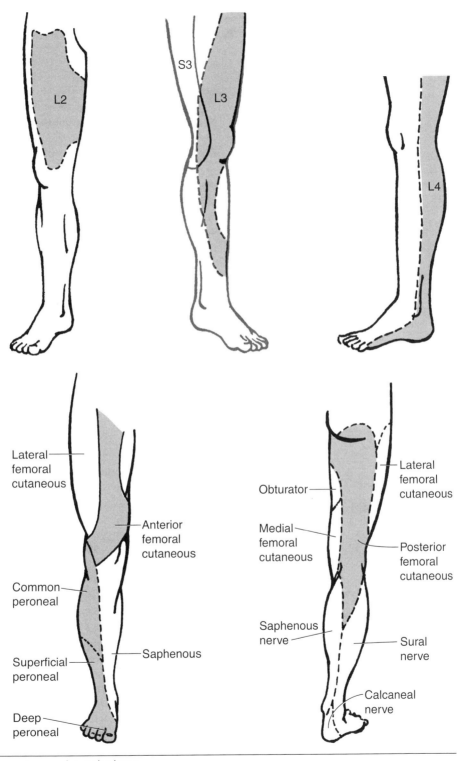

Dermatomes about the knee.

Neurology

Nerve root	Reflex	Motor	Sensory
L2	—	Hip flexion	Anterior proximal thigh
L3	Patellar tendon	Quadriceps	Lateral thigh
L4	Anterior tibialis	Anterior tibialis	Medial distal leg
L5	Proximal hamstring	Extensor hallucis longus	Dorsum of the foot
S1	Achilles tendon	Peroneus longus	Lateral foot

Peripheral Nerves

Nerve	Motor	Sensory
Obturator	Hip adduction and external rotation	Medial inner thigh
Femoral	Hip flexion	Medial thigh (anterior femoral cutaneous)
Tibial	Plantar flex, adduct, or invert the foot	Heel
Superficial peroneal	Eversion of the foot	Lateral calf
Deep peroneal	Dorsiflexion of the foot	Cleft between first and second toe

Surface Palpation

Femoral condyles
Adductor tubercle
Tibial tuberosity
MCL
Quadriceps
Joint line
LCL
Popliteal fossa
Pes anserine
Fibular head
Gastrocnemius
Gerdy's tubercle
Patella

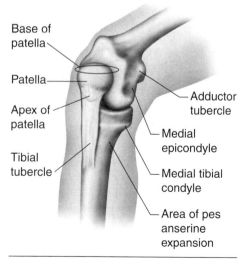

Landmarks of the knee.

Muscle Origin and Insertion

Muscle	Origin and insertion
Rectus femoris	Anterior inferior iliac spine to patella and tibial tuberosity
Gastrocnemius	Medial and lateral condyles of femur to calcaneus
Gracilis	Inferior rami of pubis to medial tibia (pes anserine)
Popliteus	Lateral condyle of femur to proximal tibia
Sartorius	Anterior superior iliac spine to medial tibia (pes anserine)
Biceps femoris	Ischial tuberosity to lateral condyle of tibia and head of fibula
Semimembranosus	Ischial tuberosity to medial condyle of tibia
Semitendinosus	Ischial tuberosity to medial tibia (pes anserine)
Vastus intermedius	Anterior, lateral femur to patella and tibial tuberosity
Vastus lateralis	Intertrochanteric line, linea aspera to patella and tibial tuberosity
Vastus medialis	Linea aspera, trochanteric line to patella and tibial tuberosity

Adapted from J. Hamill and K. Knudzen, 1995, *Biomechanical basis of human movement* (Baltimore, MD: Lippincott, Williams, and Wilkins).

Muscle Action and Innervation

Action	Muscle involved	Nerve supply	Nerve root
Knee flexion	Biceps femoris	Sciatic	L5, S1–S2
	Semimembranosus	Sciatic	L5, S1–S2
	Semitendinosus	Sciatic	L5, S1–S2
	Sartorius	Femoral	L2–L4
	Gracilis	Obturator	L2–L3
	Popliteus	Tibial	L4–5, S1
	Gastrocnemius	Tibial	S1–S2
	Tensor fascia latae	Superior gluteal	L4–5, S1
	Plantaris	Tibial	L4–5, S1
Knee extension	Rectus femoris	Femoral	L2–L4
	Vastus medialis		
	Vastus lateralis		
	Vastus intermedius		
	Tensor fasciae latae		
Tibial internal rot	Popliteus	Tibial	L4 – 5, S1
	Semimembranosus	Sciatic	L5, S1–S2
	Semitendinosus	Sciatic	L2–L4
	Sartorius	Femoral	L2–L3
	Gracilis	Obturator	
Tibial external rot	Biceps femoris	Sciatic	L5, S1–S2

Reprinted from *Orthopedic Physical Assessment*, 2nd ed., D.J. Magee, pg. 385. Copyright 1992, with permission from W.B. Saunders.

HISTORY

Profile

Occupation and recreational activities—consider effect of knee pain on level of function or disability (repetitive squatting, kneeling, sporting activities, overuse or abuse)

Location of Symptoms

Tibiofemoral Joint

Deep in joint compartment involved.

Ligaments and tendons usually hurt at the site.

Meniscal injuries usually have local pain or catching.

Pain may spread down shin or calf.

Posterior pain can be from L5–S2.

Patellofemoral Joint

Around patellar margins

Lateral knee

Posterior knee

Inferior patella

Retropatellar

Superior Tibia–Fibula Joint

Referred along fibula

Down front of shin

Local pain

Behavior of Symptoms

Aggravating Factors

Kneeling

Sitting for long periods of time

Sitting to standing

Squatting

Twisting

Walking phase of gait, pivoting, inclines

Running, jumping, sport-related moves

Going up or down stairs, weakness, giving way or pain

Special Aggravating Questions

» Locking: look for consistent mechanism—differentiate true locking from pain inhibition. Loose body or meniscal tear—TF, may be unable to flex—PF.

» Giving way or buckling—establish position or movement, could be due to weakness or pain inhibition, may be due to ligament instability, meniscal injury, PF tracking disorder.

» Crepitus or clicking—establish type, location, with or without pain, snapping of tendon or ITB.

» Swelling location, variability.

TESTS AND MEASURES

Standing

Observation—Hyperextension or Lack of Extension, Varus or Valgus Deformity, Q-Angle

Implicate or Clear Lumbar Spine

Neurological Examination—S1 Myotome

Functional Tests—Gait (Forward, Backward, Change Directions, Heel Walk, Toe Walk), Running, Cutting, Twisting, Squatting, Stairs, Kneeling, Balance, Rotation

Supine

Palpation
Skin (temperature, sweating, skin rolling)
Soft tissue or bony structures

- Medial: MCL, joint line, vastus medialis
- Anterior: tibial condyles, tibial plateau, tibial tuberosity, patellar tendon, fat pad, quadriceps femoris, patellar position
- Lateral: LCL, joint line, femoral condyles, ITB, fibular head, vastus lateralis

Girth Measurements and Patellar Tap Test

Implicate or Clear Hip and Ankle

Neurological Examination (Segmental, Peripheral, or Central as Indicated)

AROM of Knee With OP—Extension With OP, Flexion With OP (0–135°)

PROM of Tibiofemoral Joint if Appropriate

Muscle Length Testing—Hamstrings

MMT—Quads (Static, Through Range, Quad Lag)

PAMs—Tibiofemoral Joint
Anterior glide at 90° flexion
Posterior glide at 90° flexion

PAMs—Proximal Tibiofemoral Joint
AP or PA in hook lying or side lying

PAMs—Patellofemoral Joint
Superior and inferior glides

Medial and lateral glides

Special Tests—Tibiofemoral Joint
ACL—anterior drawer, Lachman test

PCL—posterior drawer, Godfrey test, posterior sag sign

LCL—varus stress test

MCL—valgus stress test

Meniscal tests—palpation of the joint line, McMurray's test

Special Tests—Patellofemoral Joint
Q-angle

Apprehension test

Patellar position

Patella alta

Patella baja

Medial or lateral glide

Medial or lateral tilt

External or internal rotation

Anterior or posterior tilt

Neurodynamic Testing
Passive neck flexion (PNF)

Straight-leg raise (SLR)

Slump

Reassessment purposes, subjective indicators, postsurgical patients, symptoms that do not fit a normal pain pattern, symptoms in absence of joint signs

Side Lying

Muscle Length—Ober Test

MMT—Gluteus Medius

Prone

Palpation—Lumbar Spine for Clearing, ITB Insertion at Fibular Head, Biceps Femoris, Gastrocnemius, Posterior Capsule, Semimembranosus or Tendinosis, Gracilis or Sartorius Insertion at Gerdy's Tubercle, Tibial or Peroneal Nerve

Neurological Examination, as Indicated

Muscle Length—Ely's test

MMT

Hamstrings (medial and lateral)—test in side lying if less than fair

Hip extension—test in side lying if less than fair

Special Tests—Tibiofemoral Joint—Apley's Compression or Distraction Test

Neurodynamic Testing—Prone Knee Bend (PKB)

Sitting

Muscle Length Test, Hip Flexor Length Test

MMT

Quadriceps—test in side lying if less than fair

PAMs—Tibiofemoral Joint: Distraction, Anterior Glide, Posterior Glide

Special Tests—Patellofemoral Joint: Critical Test

Clinical Syndromes: Tibiofemoral Joint

Description	Location and behavior of symptoms	History	Tests and measures, diagnostics	Intervention
DJD				
Degenerative changes in articular cartilage. Present in females more than males. >55 years old.	General knee pain, usually intermittent but can become constant. May complain of diffuse swelling or tightness to posterior knee. Deep knee ache. Aggravation: prolonged standing, sitting to standing, going up and down stairs, squatting.	Repetitive stress to knee complex. History of trauma. History of obesity.	Observation: varus or valgus deformity. Slight to moderate knee effusion may be present. Gait: decreased WB on involved limb. May lack full knee extension in mid and terminal stance. Pain at end range of active extension. Pain with flexion > 90°. Negative meniscus and stability tests. Diagnostics: X rays—AP show diminished joint space, varus or valgus deformity.	Weight reduction. Limiting stress on joint—arch support. Modify ADLs. Strengthening of whole extremity—functional and nonweight bearing. Stretching, pool exercises, aerobic exercise. Surgical management: arthroscopy, debridement, carticel, hemiarthroplasty, TKR.
MENISCAL INJURY				
Tear in fibrocartilage ring. May be a younger patient with an acute injury or an older patient with a degenerative tear.	May complain of sharp pain, locking, giving way, catching, clicking, or snapping. Aggravation: Getting up from sitting, squatting, sitting to standing, stairs, weight-bearing activities.	Peak age 20–30 years old. Traumatic injuries usually occur in patients 40 years old and younger. Mechanism of injury: flexion, compression, rotation.	Limited AROM. Limited and painful passive movement testing. Tenderness along joint line. A-P tibiofemoral increases pain. Special tests: Apley's and McMurray's may be positive. Diagnostics: arthrograms combined with CT, arthroscopy, MRI.	Rest, ice, crutches, quad sets—acute phase. Restore ROM and strength. Surgical management: arthroscopy, meniscus repair, meniscus transplant.

Description	Location and behavior of symptoms	History	Tests and measures, diagnostics	Intervention
INSTABILITY				
Increased laxity in joint secondary to ligamentous tear.	Intermittent generalized ache, deep. Complaints of unstable, undependable knee. Chronic swelling—mild or moderate with stressful activities. Aggravation: medial or lateral movements or pivoting, prolonged weight bearing.	If acute, the patient can describe the exact moment of injury with severe pain. May complain of hearing a snap or pop. Blow to knee with foot planted or a quick pivot on affected knee. Immediate swelling often occurs. Method of injury: • ACL: cutting, deceleration, hyperextension. • MCL: valgus. • LCL: varus. • PCL: hyperflexion, dashboard injury.	Observation: swelling to knee. Functional: may avoid extension in gait—look for compensation. Passive movement testing: Passive and accessory movements should be greater than normal excursion (decreased if swelling present). Palpation: may be tender over specific ligament (MCL or LCL) if partially torn. Special tests: Stability tests are positive for specific ligament torn. Diagnostics: X rays (lateral view), arthroscopy, MRI.	Acute: modalities, bracing, assistive devices, decrease activity. Chronic: LE strengthening—closed chain, balance or proprioceptive training, bracing as needed. Surgical management: ACL repair (allograft, autograft), PCL repair (allograft, autograft). MCL and LCL—treated conservatively in most cases.

Clinical Syndromes: Patellofemoral Joint

Description	Location and behavior of systems	History	Tests and measures, diagnostics	Intervention
PATELLOFEMORAL DYSFUNCTION				
May involve articular cartilage destruction; usually chronic in nature, more common in females.	Pain about the patella or on the undersurface, stiffness, complaints of giving way going up or down stairs, prolonged sitting, may get catching sensation in knee but is able to unlock it actively.	Insidious onset. Sudden change in activity.	Poor control of terminal knee extension, hesitation to flex knee during gait, tender to palpation. Functional testing: single-leg squat or double-leg squat, stepping down, jumping, sitting to standing. Special test: critical test. Muscle length (ITB, hip flexors, hamstrings). Diagnostics: X rays (AP, lateral, intercondylar notch, axial).	Treatment is based on OE findings. Stretching tight structures. Patellar taping. Muscle strengthening. Modalities. Surgical management: arthroscopy, lateral release, Carticel.
FAT PAD IRRITATION				
Inflammation of inferior patellar fat pad.	Complaints of pain in infrapatellar region and puffiness of the anterior knee. Aggravation: pain with prolonged standing, climbing stairs.	Trauma. Complication from surgery—scope.	Observation: hyperextended knees. ROM: pain with extension plus OP. Palpation: pain with palpation of inferior pole of patella and fat pad. Positive for AP tilt. Diagnostics: X rays—patellar position.	• Protect fat pad. • Ice. • US. • Interferential electrical stimulation.

Description	Location and behavior of systems	History	Tests and measures, diagnostics	Intervention
PATELLAR TENDINITIS				
Inflammation of patellar tendon; jumper's knee.	Complaints of pain infrapatellar region with jumping, mid to full squat.	Sports that involve sprinting, sudden starts and stops, repetitive jumping or kicking. Overuse.	Q-angle WNL or small, AP tilt normal, tendon is painful to palpation. Muscle tightness. Muscle weakness.	• Modify activity. • Ice. • NSAIDS. • Taping. • Eccentric loading program to quads. Surgical management: arthroscopy.
BURSITIS				
Inflammation of the bursa about the knee.	Prepatellar (housemaid's knee). Infrapatellar: pain usually in proportion to swelling.	Trauma. Overuse.	Swelling to bursa, discomfort with palpation over bursa.	• Ice, US. • Interferential electrical stimulation. • Protective pads. • NSAIDS. Surgical management: usually treated conservatively, bursectomy.

Miscellaneous Knee Syndromes

Description	Location and Behavior of Symptoms	History	Tests and measures, diagnostics	Intervention
OSGOOD- SCHLATTER'S DISEASE				
Dysfunction of apophyseal area of tibial tubercle, more common in young boys than in young girls.	Local pain with increased activity (sprinting, jumping, kicking). Pain with kneeling.	The tuberosity does not appear as a discrete structure until 12–15 weeks of fetal life. In the newborn the proximal epiphysis of the tibia consists of cartilaginous plate which remains until 11 to 13 years old. Ossification centers and eventually forms the tuberosity with closure and disappearance of the epiphyseal cartilaginous plate at 18 to 19 years old.	Enlargement of tibial tubercle. Diagnostics: X rays (lateral).	Treat with rest as needed. Stretch tightened structures, strap or tape patellar tendon to decrease stress on epiphysis. Surgical management: shave tibial tubercle and reattach the patellar tendon.
ITB SYNDROME				
Irritation of distal iliotibial band; usually due to repeated friction between ITB and lateral femoral condyle.	Complaints of crepitus or popping along lateral knee. Local ache to lateral knee.	Overuse. Training errors. Terrain. Biomechanical malalignment.	Examine using the modified Ober test. Tibia externally rotated. Gait: may walk with leg extended during foot strike to midstance.	• Treat tight ITB and other biomechanical faults. • Modalities. • Modify activity. Surgical management: lateral release.
BAKER'S CYST				
Posterior capsule effusion.	Aching in popliteal fossa.		Popliteal swelling. Frequently a palpable mass that fluctuates. Decreased knee flexion. Diagnostics: CT arthrograms.	Aspiration usually reveals a jellylike substance or clear synovial fluid. Surgical management: removal.

Description	Location and Behavior of Symptoms	History	Tests and measures, diagnostics	Intervention
PLICA SYNDROME				
Irritation of synovial tissue.	Usually asymptomatic. Symptoms most common in adolescents in the medial parapatellar area. Aggravation: running and jumping, prolonged sitting.	A plica exists when any portion of the embryonic synovial septa persist into adulthood (20–60%). May become inflamed due to repetitive stress from activity or direct trauma.	Palpation. Diagnostics: arthrography or CT arthrograms.	• Modify activity. • Ice, US. • Flexibility exercises. • Patellar mobilization. • Patellar taping. Surgical management: removal.
SPINE REFERRAL—DDD				
	Medial knee—L3. Posterior knee—L5, S1.	Refer to lumbar spine clinical syndromes table.	Comparable sign with palpation to specific spinal levels. Comparable sign with LS clearing tests.	Refer to lumbar spine clinical syndromes table.

Adapted, by permission, from C. Wadsworth, 1988, *Manual examination and treatment of the spine and extremities* (Baltimore, MD: Lippincott, Williams, and Wilkins), 194.

Foot and Ankle

The foot and ankle are the distal link to the lower extremity. As the foot strikes the ground, kinetic forces are dissipated through each joint of the foot and ankle. The joints above the foot and ankle are directly affected by the biomechanics of these structures. This chapter covers the distal tibiofibular joint; talocrural joint; subtalar joint; and transtarsal, tarsometatarsal, metatarsalphalangeal, and interphalangeal joints in the toes as well as the midfoot in which no active motion occurs. This chapter covers osteology, arthrokinematics, range of motion, muscle origin and insertion, muscle action, neurology, and special tests for all these joints. Clinical syndromes are presented in a table at the end of the chapter. The chapter also includes a recommended sequence for the subjective and objective exam.

DISTAL TIBIOFIBULAR JOINT (DTF)

Articulation   The convex lower end of the fibula and the concave fibular notch at the distal end of the tibia.

Type of Joint   Synarthrosis syndesmosis.

Degrees of Freedom

None.

Active Range of Motion

No active motion.

Posterior Glide

Assessment: Accessory motion of dorsiflexion.

Patient position: Supine with the knee in extension.

Clinician position: Place the fingers of the medial hand under the tibia and the thumb over the tibia to stabilize it. Place the lateral hand using the thenar eminence over the lateral malleolus, with the fingers underneath.

Method: Glide the lateral malleolus posteriorly, directing force through the left thenar eminence.

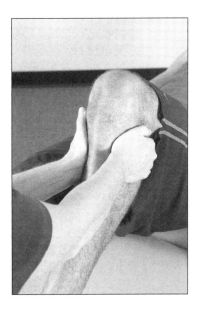

End Feel

Not applicable.

Capsular Pattern

Pain when joint stressed.

Close-Packed Position

Not applicable.

Loose-Packed Position

Not applicable.

Stability

Anterior and Posterior Tibiofibular Ligaments   Connect the tibia and fibula together anterior and posterior to the interosseous ligament.

Crural Interosseous Tibiofibular Ligament   Connects the tibia and fibula and is continuous with the interosseous membrane.

Special Tests

None.

TALOCRURAL JOINT (TC)

Articulation   The tibia, fibula, and talus; the superior convex dome of the talus fits into the concave surface formed by the medial malleolus, distal tibial, and lateral malleolus.

Type of Joint   Diarthrodial hinge joint.

Degrees of Freedom

Dorsiflexion and plantarflexion in sagittal plane about a coronal axis that passes approximately through fibular malleolus and the body of the talus; forms an 80° angle from vertical; lateral malleolus slightly posterior and inferior to medial malleolus.

Active Range of Motion

Dorsiflexion: 0–20°
Plantarflexion: 0–50°

Distraction

Assessment: To increase joint play at the ankle mortise. Oscillations may also be used for pain control.

Patient position: Sitting with the knee flexed and the femur fully supported.

Clinician position: Sitting in front of the patient. The clinician takes up the soft tissue of the posterior lower leg with the fingers of both hands and places the thenar eminences of both hands on the tibial plateaus of the knee.

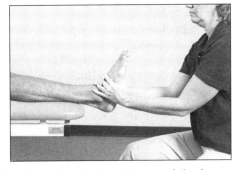

Method: Apply a distraction force to the tibia. Apply first pressures gently; increase amplitude and depth of the movement if no pain response occurs. Assess quality of movement through the range and end feel; compare with the other side.

Alternative method: Apply a distraction force with both hands around the distal tibia with the fingers pointing down along the distal tibia.

Intervention: Use appropriate grade of movement (I–IV) to treat pain or resistance. Inferior glide increases the range of motion of the hip and decreases the joint pain.

Biomechanics: Distraction of the tibia from the femur may increase motion and decrease pain.

Talocrural Anterior Glide

Assessment: Plantarflexion.

Patient position: Supine with the leg supported on table, the ankle in a resting position, and the foot off the edge of the plinth.

Clinician position: Standing at the end of the table facing the side of the patient in a walk-stance position. The clinician stabilizes the distal tibia against the plinth with the left hand, wrapping the fingers around posteriorly. The clinician grasps the neck of the talus just distal to malleoli with the web space of the right hand.

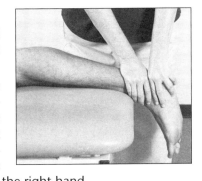

Method: The clinician applies an anterior force on the talus in the mobilization plane. Apply first pressures gently; increase amplitude and depth of the movement if no pain response occurs. Assess quality of movement through the range and end feel; compare with the other side.

Intervention: Use appropriate grade of movement (I–IV) to treat pain or resistance. To increase plantarflexion of the talocrural joint.

Biomechanics: According to the convex–concave rule, the convex talar head glides anteriorly on the concave distal tibiofibular mortise during talocrural plantarflexion.

Posterior Glide

Assessment: Dorsiflexion

Patient position: Supine with the knee relaxed and the foot off the edge of the end of the table.

Clinician position: Standing at the end of the table facing the side of the patient in a walk-stance position. The clinician grasps the anterior or distal surface of the tibia and fibula with the web space of the left hand and grasps the anterior talus with the web space of the right hand.

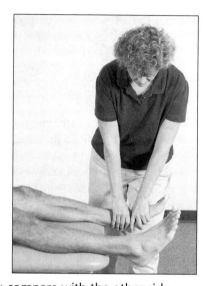

Method: The clinician applies a posterior force on the calcaneus and talus in the mobilizing plane. Apply first pressures gently; increase amplitude and depth of the movement if no pain response occurs. Assess quality of movement through the range and end feel; compare with the other side.

Intervention: Use appropriate grade of movement (I–IV) to treat pain or resistance. To increase dorsiflexion of the talocrural joint.

Biomechanics: According to the convex–concave rule, the convex talar head glides posteriorly on the concave distal tibiofibular mortise during talocrural dorsiflexion.

End Feel

Dorsiflexion: Firm due to tension in the posterior capsule, Achilles tendon, posterior portion of deltoid and calcaneofibular ligament, and posterior talofibular ligament

Plantarflexion: Firm due to tension in the anterior capsule, anterior portion of deltoid and anterior talofibular ligament, anterior tibial muscle, and long extensors of the toes

Plantarflexion: Hard due to the posterior tubercle of the talus contacting posterior tibia

Capsular Pattern

Dorsiflexion limited more than plantarflexion.

Close-Packed Position

Maximum dorsiflexion.

Loose-Packed Position

10° of plantarflexion midway between inversion and eversion.

Stability

Figure 14.1 illustrates the ligaments that stabilize the talocrural joint.

Medial Ligaments

Deltoid   Consists of the posterior tibiotalar, tibiocalcaneal, tibionavicular, and anterior tibiotalar ligaments.

Posterior tibiotalar   From the medial malleolus to the posterior talus process.

Tibiocalcaneal   From the medial malleolus to the sustentaculum tali.

Tibionavicular   From the medial malleolus to the navicular bone and spring ligament.

Anterior tibiotalar   From the medial malleolus to the navicular bone; stabilizes the medial ankle.

Lateral Ligaments

Anterior talofibular ligament   From the lateral malleolus to the lateral talus.

Calcaneofibular ligament   From the tip of the lateral malleolus downward and backward to the lateral surface of calcaneus.

Posterior talofibular ligament   From the lateral malleolus to the posterior tubercle of the talus; stabilizes the lateral ankle.

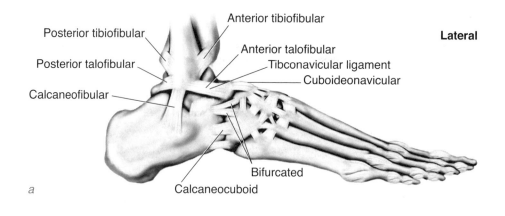

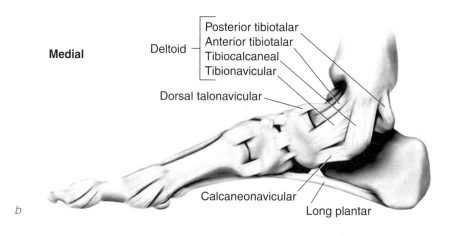

Figure 14.1 Ligaments supporting the foot and ankle: (*a*) medial aspect; (*b*) lateral aspect.

Reprinted from R. Behnke, *Kinetic anatomy*, 2nd ed. (Champaign, IL: Human Kinetics), 213.

Lateral Instability (Talar Tilt)

Assessment: Integrity of the calcaneofibular ligament.

Patient position: Sitting with the leg supported on the table, the lower leg hanging off the edge of the table, and the foot relaxed.

Clinician position: Sitting in front of the patient. The clinician stabilizes the distal tibiofibular joint with the web space of the right hand and grasps the lateral talus and calcaneus with the left hand.

Method: The clinician applies an inversion force to the talocrural and subtalar joint.

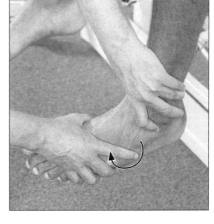

Alternative method: The technique can be performed with the patient in the supine position.

Positive response: Lateral gapping or pain as compared with the opposite side.

Biomechanics: The calcaneofibular ligament stabilizes the lateral ankle.

Anterior Instability (Anterior Drawer)

Assessment: Integrity of the anterior talofibular ligament.

Patient position: Sitting with the leg supported on the table, the lower leg hanging off the edge of the table, and the foot relaxed.

Clinician position: Sitting in front of the patient. The clinician stabilizes the distal tibiofibular joint with the web space of the left hand and grasps the calcaneus with the right hand.

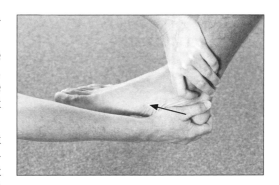

Method: The clinician applies an anterior force with the right hand.

Alternative method: The technique can be performed with the patient in the supine position.

Positive response: Excessive movement of the talus forward as compared with the opposite side.

Biomechanics: The anterior talofibular ligament checks the talus from excessive anterior movement. The calcaneofibular ligament is a secondary stabilizer in this test.

Sensitivity: .96, specificity: .84 (van Dijk et al. 1996).

Medial Instability

Assessment: Integrity of the deltoid ligament.

Patient position: Supine with the foot in slight plantarflexion.

Method: The clinician grasps the foot and applies an eversion force to the TC and subtalar joint.

Positive response: Medial gapping or pain as compared with the opposite leg.

Achilles Tendon: Thompson's Test

Assessment: Integrity of the Achilles tendon.

Patient position: Prone with the feet over the edge of a table.

Method: The clinician squeezes the calf at the middle of the muscle belly.

Positive response: A normal response would be plantarflexion of the foot. If the tendon is ruptured, this movement is markedly decreased or absent.

Biomechanics: The Achilles tendon is the common tendon insertion of the gastrocnemius, soleus, and plantaris (triceps surae). Squeezing of this muscle bundle should produce passive plantarflexion of the ankle.

Sensitivity: .96 (Maffulli, 2004).

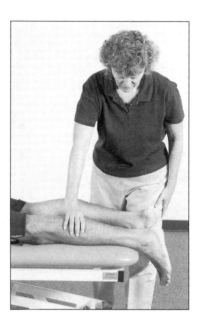

Homans' Sign

Patient position: Supine with the leg supported on the table, the ankle in a resting position, and the foot off the edge of the plinth.

Clinician position: Standing at the end of the table facing the side of the patient. The clinician grasps the patient's plantar aspect of the right foot with the right hand.

Method: The clinician passively dorsiflexes the patient's right foot with the knee extended.

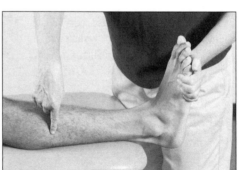

Positive response: Pain in the calf.

Biomechanics: Forced dorsiflexion creates increased pressure within the posterior compartment of the calf, including the vascular structures.

SUBTALAR JOINT (STJ; TALOCALCANEAL JOINT)

Articulation   The superior talus and inferior calcaneus; posteriorly, the concave facet on the inferior surface of the talus and convex facet on the body of the calcaneus. The anterior and middle articulations are formed by two convex facets on the talus with two concave facets on the calcaneus.

Type of Joint   Diarthrodial bicondylar joint with triplane motion: motion consisting of inversion and eversion (frontal plane), abduction and adduction (transverse plane), plantarflexion and dorsiflexion (sagittal plane).

Degrees of Freedom

Pronation and supination in three planes

Axis of motion—oblique axis from posterolateral plantar aspect to anteromedial dorsal aspect

Active Range of Motion

Inversion: 0–30°

Eversion: 0–15°

Calcaneal Inversion (Right)

Patient position: Prone with the lower extremity extended and the ankle in a resting position.

Clinician position: Standing or sitting at the end of the table. The clinician wraps one hand around the distal calcaneus and stabilizes the distal tibiofibular joint with the other hand.

Method: Apply an inversion force to assess maximum calcaneal inversion. This can be measured with a goniometer. Compare bilaterally.

Biomechanics: Normal STJ inversion is 30°.

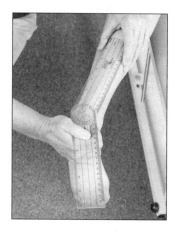

Calcaneal Eversion (Right)

Patient position: Prone with the lower extremity extended and the ankle in a resting position.

Clinician position: Standing or sitting at the end of the table. The clinician wraps one hand around the distal calcaneus and stabilizes the distal tibiofibular joint with the other hand.

Method: Apply eversion force to assess maximum calcaneal eversion. This can be measured with a goniometer. Compare bilaterally.

Biomechanics: Normal STJ eversion is 10–15°.

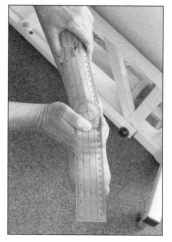

Distraction

Assessment: General mobility, pain control.

Patient position: Supine with the leg supported on the table, the ankle in a resting position, and the foot off the edge of the plinth.

Clinician position: Standing or sitting at the end of the table facing the side of the patient. The clinician cups the calcaneus from the posterior aspect of the foot with the right hand and fixates the talus with the web space of the left hand.

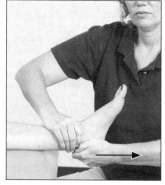

Method: The clinician pulls the calcaneus distally with respect to the long axis of the leg. Apply first pressures gently; increase amplitude and depth of the movement if no pain response occurs. Assess quality of movement through the range and end feel; compare with the other side.

Intervention: Use appropriate grade of movement (I–IV) to treat pain or resistance. To increase general mobility and decrease pain.

Biomechanics: This technique will distract the calcaneus from the talus.

Medial Glide

Assessment: Inversion.

Patient position: Left side lying with the leg supported on the table with pillows.

Clinician position: Standing at the end of the table facing the side of the patient in a walk-stance position. The clinician stabilizes the talus with the web space of the left hand and places the base of the right hand on the side of the calcaneus laterally while wrapping the fingers around the plantar surface of the patient's left foot.

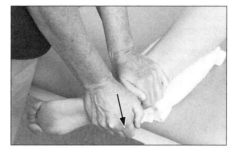

Method: The clinician applies a medial glide. Apply first pressures gently; increase amplitude and depth of the movement if no pain response occurs. Assess quality of movement through the range and end feel; compare with the other side.

Alternative method: The technique can be performed with the patient in the prone or supine position.

Intervention: Use appropriate grade of movement (I–V) to treat pain or resistance and increase inversion of the subtalar joint.

Biomechanics: The posterior facet of the calcaneus is concave. Therefore, to increase inversion, according to the convex–concave rule, the calcaneus must glide medially.

Lateral Glide

Assessment: Eversion.

Patient position: Right side lying with the leg supported on the table with pillows.

Clinician position: Standing at the end of the table facing the side of the patient in a walk-stance position. The clinician stabilizes the talus with the left hand and places the base of the right hand on the side of the calcaneus medially while wrapping the fingers around the plantar surface of the patient's right foot.

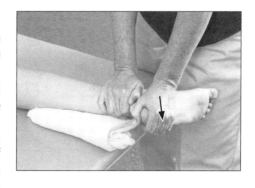

Method: The clinician applies a lateral glide. Apply first pressures gently; increase amplitude and depth of the movement if no pain response occurs. Assess quality of movement through the range and end feel; compare with the other side.

Intervention: Use appropriate grade of movement (I–IV) to treat pain or resistance and increase eversion of the subtalar joint.

Biomechanics: The posterior facet of the calcaneus is concave. Therefore, to increase eversion, according to the convex–concave rule, the calcaneus must glide laterally.

End Feel

Inversion: Firm (lateral joint capsule and lateral ligaments)

Eversion: Firm (joint capsule, deltoid ligament, and posterior tibialis muscle)

Eversion: Hard (calcaneus and sinus tarsi)

Capsular Pattern

Supination limited more than pronation; inversion limited more than eversion.

Close-Packed Position

Supination.

Loose-Packed Position

Pronation.

Stability

Cervical Talocalcaneal Ligament From inferolateral aspect of talar neck downward and lateral to dorsum of calcaneus; restricts inversion.

Interosseous Talocalcaneal Ligament From the underside of the talus at sustentaculi tali downward and lateral to the dorsum of the calcaneus; restricts eversion.

Subtalar Joint Neutral (Right)

Assessment: STJ neutral.

Patient position: Prone with the leg supported on the table, the ankle in a resting position, and the foot off the edge of the plinth.

Clinician position: Sitting or standing at the end of the table facing the head of the table. The clinician grasps the patient's foot over the fourth and fifth metatarsal heads with the index finger and thumb of the right hand while palpating both sides of the talus on the dorsum of the foot using the thumb and index finger of the left hand *(a)*.

Method: The clinician supinates and pronates the foot until the talar head does not bulge laterally or medially and then passively dorsiflexes the foot to resistance. This can be measured with a goniometer *(b)*.

Alternative method for forefoot to rear foot relationship: In the subtalar joint neutral position, the clinician can assess the neutral rear foot position and also assess the forefoot to rear foot relationship. The operator is looking for rear foot varus or forefoot varus or valgus. Both rear foot and forefoot measures can be assessed with a goniometer *(c)*.

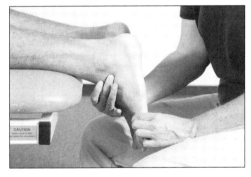

a

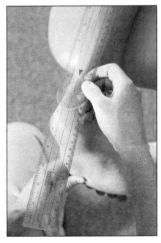

b

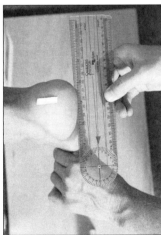

c

Navicular Drop Test

Assessment: Excessive STJ pronation.

Patient position: Standing.

Clinician position: Kneeling on the floor facing the patient.

Method: Use a pen to place a horizontal mark on the navicular tubercle. Guide the patient to place his or her subtalar joint in neutral *(a)*. Measure the vertical distance from the floor to the marked tubercle *(b)*. Record this amount. Now ask the subject to march in place for five steps to maintain relaxed foot position. Remeasure the marked tubercle *(c)*.

Positive response: A difference greater than 10 mm between the two measures is indicative of overpronation.

Biomechanics: Normal pronation of the subtalar joint during gait is 4°, and this occurs following initial contact until midstance.

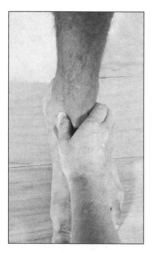 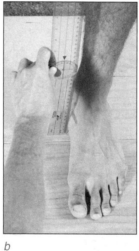 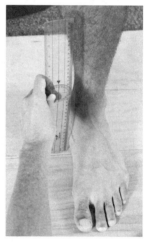

a   b   c

TRANSTARSAL JOINT
(JOINT OF CHOPART, MIDTARSAL JOINT)

Articulation   The calcaneus and cuboid and the talus and navicular. The talonavicular joint is composed of the large convex head of the talus and the concave posterior portion of the navicular bone. The calcaneocuboid joint is composed of the shallow convex (proximal, distal)–concave (medial, lateral) surfaces on the anterior calcaneus and the convex (medial, lateral)–concave (proximal, distal) surfaces on the posterior cuboid (figure 14.2).

Type of Joint   The calcaneocuboid joint is a sellar-shaped joint; the talonavicular joint is a condyloid joint.

Degrees of Freedom

Pronation and supination consisting of

inversion and eversion in the frontal plane,

abduction and adduction in the transverse plane, and

plantarflexion and dorsiflexion in the sagittal plane.

Active Range of Motion

Longitudinal (8° of motion): 15° upward from transverse plane, 16° medially from longitudinal reference

Oblique (22° of motion): 52° upward from transverse plane and 64° medially from longitudinal foot reference

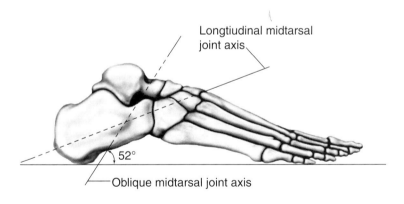

Longtiudinal midtarsal joint axis

52°

Oblique midtarsal joint axis

Figure 14.2   Lateral view of the oblique and longitudinal transtarsal joint axes.
Reprinted from R. Behnke, *Kinetic anatomy*, 2nd ed. (Champaign, IL: Human Kinetics), 210.

Plantar Glide

Assessment: To increase the arch.

Patient position: Supine with the knee relaxed.

Clinician position: The clinician fixates the more proximal bone with the finger by grasping dorsally at the level of the talar neck; the thumb wraps around laterally, and the rest of the fingers wrap around medially. The other hand grasps the mobilizing bone, the thumb contacts dorsally, and the hand and fingers wrap around the foot medially and plantarly.

Method: Move the distal bones plantarly.

Dorsal Glide

Assessment: To decrease the arch.

Patient position: Prone with the hip and knee flexed.

Clinician position: The clinician fixates the calcaneus with one hand. The fingers of the other hand wrap around the lateral side of the foot.

Method: Move the distal bones in a dorsal direction.

End Feel

Supination: Firm (lateral joint capsule and lateral ligaments)

Pronation: Firm (joint capsule, deltoid ligament, and posterior tibialis muscle)

Pronation: Hard (calcaneus and sinus tarsi)

Capsular Pattern

Dorsiflexion more limited than plantarflexion.

Close-Packed Position

Dorsiflexion.

Loose-Packed Position

Plantarflexion.

Stability

Plantar Calcaneonavicular (Spring Ligament)   Attached from the anterior margin of the sustentaculum tali to the inferior surface and tuberosity of the navicular bone; reinforces the medial arch.

Bifurcated (Y-Ligament of the Foot)   Stem attached to the upper surface of the anterior portion of the calcaneus, lateral limb attached to the upper surface of the cuboid, and medial limb attached to the upper navicular bone; reinforces laterally.

Long Plantar   Attached from the undersurface of the calcaneus behind and to the undersurface of the cuboid and the bases of the third, fourth, and fifth metatarsal bones in front.

Short Plantar   Attached from the anterior tubercle on the undersurface of the calcaneus and to the adjoining part of the cuboid bone.

Special Tests

None.

MIDFOOT

Articulation   Naviculocuboid, naviculocuneiform, intercuneiform joint.

Type of Joint   Plane synovial joints; cuneonavicular—plane synovial joints; cuboideonavicular and cuneocuboid—fibrous joint.

Degrees of Freedom

No active motion occurs.

Active Range of Motion

None.

End Feel

Not applicable.

Capsular Pattern
Not applicable.

Close-Packed Position
Supination.

Loose-Packed Position
Pronation.

Stability

Plantar Calcaneonavicular (Spring Ligament) Attached from the anterior margin of the sustentaculum tali to the inferior surface and tuberosity of the navicular bone; reinforces the medial arch.

Bifurcated (Y-Ligament of the Foot) Stem attached to the upper surface of the anterior portion of the calcaneus; lateral limb attached to the upper surface of the cuboid, and medial limb attached to the upper navicular bone; reinforces laterally.

Long Plantar Attached from the undersurface of the calcaneus behind and to the undersurface of the cuboid and the bases of the third, fourth, and fifth metatarsal bones in front.

Short Plantar Attached from the anterior tubercle on the undersurface of the calcaneus and to the adjoining part of the cuboid bone.

Special Tests
None.

FOREFOOT (TARSOMETATARSAL JOINTS)

Articulation Five tarsometatarsal joints. The concave base of the first metatarsal articulates with the convex surface of the medial cuneiform. The bases of the second and third metatarsals articulate with the mortise formed by the intermedial cuneiform and the sides of the medial and lateral cuneiforms. The base of the third metatarsal articulates with the lateral cuneiform, and the bases of the fourth and fifth metatarsals articulate with the cuboid.

Type of Joint Tarsometatarsal and intermetatarsal joint (first ray): diarthrodial plane joint.

Degrees of Freedom

Flexion and extension in sagittal plane about a coronal axis

Abduction and adduction in the frontal plane about a sagittal axis

Active Range of Motion
Each ray has its own oblique axis.

Distraction

Assessment: Mobility.

Patient position: Sitting with the leg supported.

Clinician position: The clinician stabilizes the tarsal with one hand, grasping with the thumb dorsally and the index finger plantarly. The other hand grasps around the proximal portion of the metatarsal.

Method: Apply long-axis distraction to the metatarsal to separate the joint.

Plantar/Dorsal Glide

Assessment: Plantar or dorsal glide of tarso-metatarsal joint (TMT joint) for flexion and extension.

Patient: Lying prone with the knee bent to 90°.

Clinician position: The clinician stabilizes the tarsal with one hand, grasping with the thumb dorsally and index finger volarly. The other hand grasps around the proximal portion of the metatarsal.

Method: The thumb on the dorsum of the metatarsal glides the proximal portion of the bone in a volar or dorsal direction.

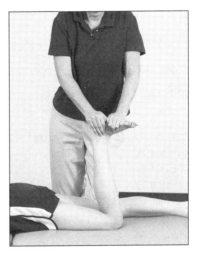

End Feel

Firm end feel in all planes due to ligamentous constraints.

Capsular Pattern

Equal limitation in all directions.

Close-Packed Position

Not defined.

Loose-Packed Position

Not defined.

Stability

Dorsal Ligaments   From the tarsals to the metatarsals; support the arch.

Plantar Ligaments   From anterior margin of calcaneus to the inferior surface of the navicular; support the arch.

Interosseous Ligaments   From the undersurface of the talus to the superior surface of the calcaneus; reinforce the foot and limit pronation, supination, and abduction.

Special Tests

None.

METATARSALPHALANGEAL JOINTS (MTP)

Articulation   Formed proximally by the convex heads of the five metatarsals and distally by the concave bases of the proximal phalanges.

Type of Joint   Diarthrodial condyloid joint.

Degrees of Freedom

Flexion and extension about an oblique axis
Abduction and adduction not defined

Active Range of Motion

Flexion: 0–20°
Extension: 0–70°
Abduction: 0–10°

End Feel

Flexion: Firm due to tension in the dorsal joint capsule, collateral ligaments, and short toe extensors

Extension: Firm due to tension in the plantar joint capsule, short toe flexors, and plantar fascia

Abduction: Firm due to tension in the joint capsule, collateral ligaments, plantar interosseous, and adductor muscle fascia

Capsular Pattern

Greater limitation in extension than flexion 2–5 MTP joints: variable.

Close-Packed Position

Full extension.

Loose-Packed Position

10° of extension.

Stability

Plantar Aponeurosis   From inferior calcaneus, blends with the metatarsal heads, reinforces the arch of the foot; responsible for windlass effect.

Fibrous Capsule   Surrounds the joint and is strengthened by plantar and collateral ligaments.

Deep Transverse Metatarsal Ligament   Blends with the plantar ligament, connects the MTP.

Squeeze Test or Morton's Test

Examination: Morton's neuroma.

Patient position: Supine with the leg supported on the table, the ankle in a resting position, and the foot off the edge of the plinth.

Clinician position: Standing or sitting at the end of the table facing the head of the table. The clinician grasps the foot around the metatarsal heads.

Method: Squeeze the metatarsal heads together.

Positive response: Excruciating pain on the outer border of the forefoot.

INTERPHALANGEAL JOINTS (IP)

Articulation   Concave base of the distal phalanx and convex head of the proximal phalanx.

Type of Joint   Diarthrodial hinge joint.

Degrees of Freedom

Flexion and extension in the sagittal plane about a coronal axis.

Active Range of Motion

PIP flexion: 0–90°
DIP flexion: 0–40°

Distraction

Assessment: Mobility of the joint.

Patient position: Leg and foot resting on the treatment table.

Clinician position: The clinician fixates the proximal bone with the fingers of one hand and wraps the fingers and thumb of the other hand around the distal bone close to the joint.

Method: Apply long-axis traction to separate the joint surfaces.

Glides

Volar Glide

Assessment: Flexion.

Dorsal Glide

Assessment: Extension.

Patient position: Sitting with the leg supported.

Clinician position: The clinician fixates the proximal bone with the fingers of one hand and wraps the fingers and thumb of the other hand around the distal bone close to the joint.

Method: Apply the glide force by the thumb against the proximal end of the bone.

End Feel

PIP flexion: Soft due to soft tissues of plantar surfaces contacting each other

PIP flexion: Firm due to tension in the dorsal joint capsule and collateral ligaments

PIP extension: Firm due to tension in the plantar joint capsule and plantar fascia

DIP flexion: Firm due to tension in the dorsal joint capsule, collateral ligaments, and oblique retinacular ligament

DIP extension: Firm due to tension in the plantar joint capsule and plantar fascia

Capsular Pattern

Flexion more limited than extension.

Close-Packed Position

Full flexion.

Loose-Packed Position

Slight flexion.

Stability

Same as with MTP.

Special Tests

None.

Range of Motion (Talocrural Joint, Subtalar Joint, Great Toe)

Motion	Range of motion (AAOS)
Plantarflexion	0–50°
Dorsiflexion	0–20°
Inversion	0–35°
Eversion	0–15°
Subtalar joint inversion	0–30°
Subtalar joint eversion	0–10°
Great toe extension	0–70°

Arthrokinematics

Non-weight-bearing

Dorsiflexion

DTF: The fibula rotates laterally and glides proximally to accommodate the wider portion of the talus engaging the mortise.

TC: The talus slides posteriorly and abducts on the tibia wedging into the mortise.

STJ: Pronation.

Plantarflexion

DTF: The fibula rotates medially, narrowing the mortise as the talus disengages from the mortise.

TC: The talus slides anteriorly on the tibia and disengages from the mortise.

STJ: Supination.

Inversion

STJ: The calcaneus slides medially on fixed talus.

TMT: The navicular slides medially and dorsally on the talus.

Eversion

STJ: The calcaneus slides laterally on fixed talus.

TMT: The navicular slides laterally and toward the plantar surface on the talus.

Pronation   Occurs at the STJ and involves calcaneal dorsiflexion, abduction, and eversion.

Supination   Occurs at the STJ and involves calcaneal plantarflexion (coronal axis), adduction (vertical axis), and inversion (longitudinal axis through the foot).

First MTP flexion: Plantar glide of the base of phalanges on the heads of the metatarsal

First MTP extension: Dorsal glide

2–5 MTP flexion: Plantar glide

2–5 MTP extension: Dorsal glide

Abduction   The concave base of phalanges slide on convex heads of metatarsals in lateral direction away from the second toe.

IP Flexion   The concave base of distal phalanx slides on the convex head of the proximal phalanx in the same direction as the shaft of the distal bone; the concave base slides toward plantar surface of the foot IP extension: concave base slides toward dorsum of the foot during extension.

Weight-Bearing

Dorsiflexion

DTF: The fibula glides anteriorly to a greater extent than the tibia on the talus; results in internal rotation of the tibia.

TC: The talus glides posteriorly and medially.

STJ: Pronation.

Plantarflexion

DTF: The fibula glides posteriorly to a greater extent than the tibia on the talus; results in external rotation of the tibia.

TC: The talus glides anteriorly and laterally.

STJ: Supination.

Pronation   Occurs at the STJ and involves adduction and plantarflexion of the talus and eversion of the calcaneus; when the talocalcaneal joint is pronated, two sets of axes at the midtarsal joint are parallel and allow maximal amount of motion.

Supination   Occurs at the STJ and involves abduction and dorsiflexion of the talus and inversion of the calcaneus; when the talocalcaneal joint is supinated, two sets of axes at the midtarsal joint are divergent and allow little motion.

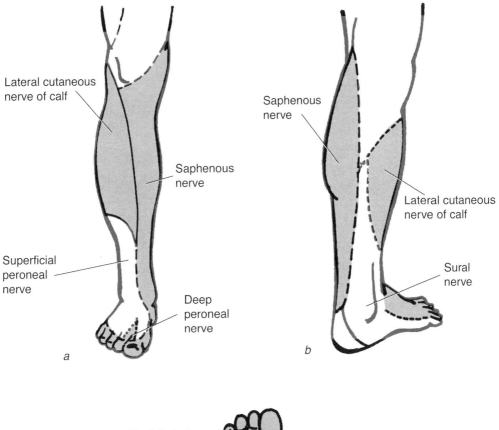

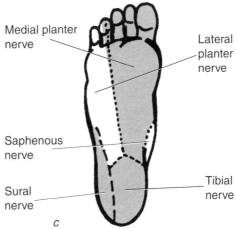

Peripheral nerve distribution in the lower leg, ankle, and foot: (*a*) anterior view; (*b*) posterior view; (*c*) in the foot.

Neurology

Nerve root	Reflex	Motor	Sensory
L3	Patellar tendon	Quadriceps	Lateral thigh
L4	Anterior tibialis	Anterior tibialis	Medial distal leg
L5	Proximal hamstring	Extensor hallucis longus	Dorsum of the foot
S1	Achilles tendon	Peroneus longus	Lateral foot

Peripheral Nerves

Nerve	Motor	Sensory
Obturator	Hip adduction and external rotation	Medial inner thigh
Femoral	Hip flexion	Medial thigh (anterior femoral cutaneous)
Tibial	Plantarflex, adduct, or invert the foot	Heel
Superficial peroneal	Eversion of the foot	Lateral calf
Deep peroneal	Dorsiflexion of the foot	Cleft between first and second toe

Surface Palpation

Navicular tubercle

Extensor digitorum longus

Cuboid

Extensor hallucis longus

Peroneal tubercle

Extensor digitorum brevis

Peroneus longus

Dorsal pedal pulse

Peroneus brevis

Anterior tibialis tendon

Peroneus tertius tendon

Muscle Origin and Insertion

Muscle	Origin and insertion
Abductor digiti minimi	Lateral calcaneus to base of proximal phalanx of fifth toe
Abductor hallucis	Medial calcaneus to medial base of proximal phalanx of first toe
Adductor hallucis	Second, third, and fourth metatarsal to lateral side of proximal phalanx of big toe
Dorsal interossei	Sides of metatarsals to lateral side of proximal phalanx
Extensor digitorum brevis	Lateral calcaneus to proximal phalanx of first, second, and third toes
Extensor digitorum longus	Lateral condyle of tibia, fibula, interossei membrane to dorsal expansion of toes 2–5
Extensor hallucis longus	Anterior fibula, interosseous membrane to distal phalanx of big toe
Flexor digiti minimi brevis	Fifth metatarsal to proximal phalanx of little toe
Flexor digitorum brevis	Medial calcaneus to middle phalanx of toes 2–5
Flexor digitorum longus	Posterior tibia to distal phalanx of toes 2–5
Flexor hallucis brevis	Cuboid to medial side of proximal phalanx of big toe
Flexor hallucis longus	Lower two-thirds of posterior fibula and interosseous membrane to the plantar aspect of the base of the distal phalanx of the great toe
Gastrocnemius	Medial and lateral condyles of femur to posterior calcaneus
Lumbricales	Tendon of FDL to base of proximal phalanx of toes 2–5
Peroneus brevis	Lower lateral fibula to fifth metatarsal
Peroneus longus	Lateral condyle of tibia and upper, lateral fibula to first cuneiform, lateral first metatarsal
Peroneus tertius	Lower, anterior fibula, interosseous membrane to base of fifth metatarsal
Plantar interossei	Medial side of third to fifth metatarsal to medial side of proximal phalanx of toes 3–5
Plantaris	Linea aspera of femur to calcaneus
Quadratus plantae	Medial, lateral inferior calcaneus to flexor digitorum tendon
Soleus	Upper posterior tibial fibula interosseous membrane to posterior calcaneus
Tibialis anterior	Upper lateral tibia, interosseous membrane to medial, plantar surface of 1st cuneiform
Tibialis posterior	Upper posterior tibia, fibula, interosseous membrane to inferior navicular

Adapted from J. Hamill and K. Knudzen, 1995, *Biomechanical basis of human movement* (Baltimore, MD: Lippincott, Williams, and Wilkins), 506.

Muscle Action and Innervation

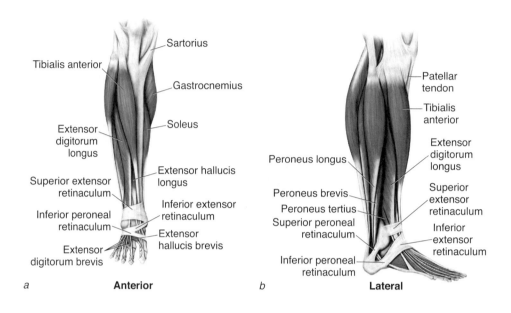

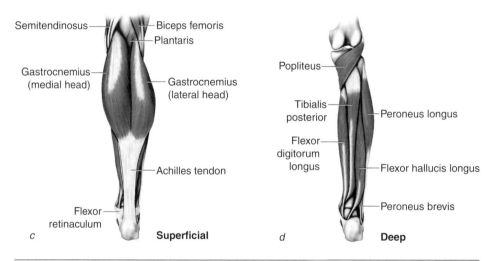

Lower leg muscles: (*a*) anterior view; (*b*) lateral view; (*c*) posterior view of superficial aspect; (*d*) posterior view of deep aspect.

Reprinted from R. Behnke, *Kinetic anatomy*, 2nd ed. (Champaign, IL: Human Kinetics), 217.

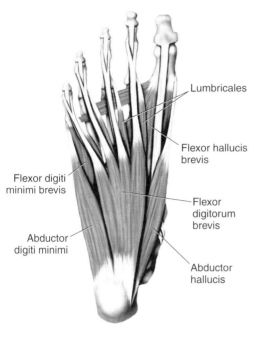

Lumbricales

Flexor hallucis brevis

Flexor digiti minimi brevis

Flexor digitorum brevis

Abductor digiti minimi

Abductor hallucis

a   **First plantar layer**

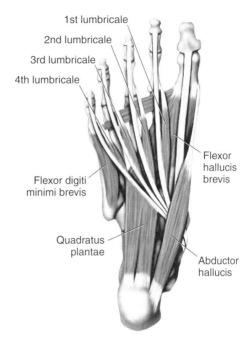

1st lumbricale

2nd lumbricale

3rd lumbricale

4th lumbricale

Flexor hallucis brevis

Flexor digiti minimi brevis

Quadratus plantae

Abductor hallucis

b   **Second plantar layer**

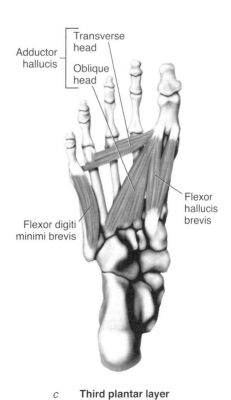

Adductor hallucis

Transverse head

Oblique head

Flexor hallucis brevis

Flexor digiti minimi brevis

c   **Third plantar layer**

Ligaments and tendons of the plantar aspect of the foot.

Reprinted from R. Behnke, *Kinetic anatomy*, 2nd ed. (Champaign, IL: Human Kinetics), 225, 226.

Muscle Action and Innervation

Action	Muscle involved	Nerve supply	Nerve root
Plantarflexion	Gastrocnemius	Tibial	S1–S2
	Soleus	Tibial	S1–S2
	Plantaris	Tibial	S1–S2
	Flexor digitorum longus	Tibial	S2–S3
	Peroneus longus	Superficial peroneal	L5, S1–S2
	Peroneus brevis	Superficial peroneal	L5, S1–S2
	Flexor hallucis longus	Tibial	S2–S3
	Tibialis posterior	Tibial	L4–L5
Dorsiflexion	Tibialis anterior	Deep peroneal	L4–L5
	Extensor digitorum longus	Deep peroneal	L5, S1
	Extensor hallucis longus	Deep peroneal	L5, S1
	Peroneus tertius	Deep peroneal	L5, S1
Inversion	Tibialis posterior	Tibial	L4–L5
	Flexor digitorum longus	Tibial	S2–S3
	Flexor hallucis longus	Tibial	S2–S3
	Tibialis anterior	Deep peroneal	L4–L5
	Extensor hallucis longus	Deep peroneal	L5, S1
Eversion	Peroneus longus	Superficial peroneal	L5, S1–S2
	Peroneus brevis	Superficial peroneal	L5, S1–S2
	Peroneus tertius	Deep peroneal	L5, S1
	Extensor digitorum longus	Deep peroneal	L5, S1
Flexion of the toes	Flexor digitorum longus	Tibial	S2–S3
	Flexor hallucis longus	Tibial	S2–S3
	Flexor digitorum brevis	Tibial	S2–S3
	Flexor hallucis brevis	Tibial	S2–S3
	Interossei	Tibial	S2–S3
	Flexor digiti minimi brevis	Tibial	S2–S3
	Lumbricals (MCP)	Tibial	S2–S3
Extension of the toes	Extensor digitorum longus	Deep peroneal	L5, S1
	Extensor hallucis longus	Deep peroneal	L5, S1
	Extensor digitorum brevis	Deep peroneal	S1–S2
	Lumbricals	Tibial	S2–S3
Abduction of the toes	Abductor hallucis	Tibial	S2–S3
	Abductor digiti minimi	Tibial	S2–S3
	Dorsal interossei	Tibial	S2–S3
Adduction of the toes	Adductor hallucis	Tibial	S2–S3
	Plantar interossei	Tibial	S2–S3

Adapted from *Orthopedic Physical Assessment,* 2nd ed., D.J. Magee, pg. 475. Copyright 1992, with permission from W.B. Saunders.

EXAMINATION SEQUENCE

HISTORY

Profile

Occupation and recreational activities—consider effect of foot and ankle pain on level of function and disability (walking, repetitive squatting and kneeling, sporting activities, overuse and abuse)

Location of Symptoms:

Common patterns of referral from the L-spine nerve root: L4, L5, S1, S2.

May need to question stiffness, snapping, popping, laxity if not offered spontaneously.

Check symptom-free areas—LS, SI joint, hip, knee.

Lateral ankle: consider lateral ankle sprain, peroneal tendon strain.

Medial ankle: consider medial ankle sprain, posterior tibia strain.

Posterior ankle: consider Achilles tendon injury, bursitis.

Plantar surface of foot: consider plantar fasciitis, Morton's neuroma.

Anterior shin: shinsplints.

Behavior of Symptoms

Aggravating Factors

Walking phase of gait, pivoting, inclines

Prolonged standing

Heel raises

Running, jumping, sport-related moves

Going up or down stairs, weakness, giving way or pain

TESTS AND MEASURES

Standing

Observation—Posture, Tibial Position, Pes Planus, Pes Cavus, Calluses, Swelling, Position of Toes, Position and Symmetry of Calcaneus, Muscle Bulk

MMT: Gastrocnemius or Soleus (Test in Prone if Less Than Poor)

Implicate or Clear Lumbar Spine

Neurological Examination: S1 Myotome

Functional Tests: Hopping, Skipping, One-Legged Stance, Squatting, Stairs, Twisting, Walking on Outside of Feet, Gait

Special Test: Navicular Drop Test

Supine

Palpation: Skin Temperature, Soft Tissue, Bony Structures, Dorsal Pedal Pulse

Girth Measurements: Figure 8

Implicate or Clear Knee

Neurological Examination (Central, Peripheral, or Segmental as Indicated)

AROM: TCJ
DF (0–20°)

PF (0–50°)

AROM: Tarsal Joints
Inversion (0–35°)

Eversion (0–15°)

AROM: Great Toe Extension (0–70°)

PROM

PAM: TCJ
Distraction

Posterior glide

PAM: STJ
Distraction of the calcaneus

Special Tests
Homan's sign: DVT

Squeeze test for Morton's neuroma versus stress fracture

Neurodynamic Testing
Passive neck flexion (PNF): Indicated for all LQ dysfunctions.

Straight-leg raise (SLR): Indicated in lower limb and lumbar symptoms.

SLR or DF: lateral calf, heel or foot symptoms, S1 nerve root, plantar fasciitis.

SLR, DF, or inversion: lateral calf, heel or foot symptoms, S1 nerve root, Achilles tendinitis.

SLR or PF: L5 nerve root dysfunction, chronic ankle sprains, anterior compartment syndrome, shinsplints, and common peroneal nerve dysfunction.

Prone

Palpation: Lumbar Spine for Clearing, Callus Formation, Achilles Tendon, Arches

Neurological Examination: Myotomes—Knee Flexion, Hip Extension (S1–2)

AROM (Muscle Length of Gastrocnemius and Soleus Complex)
TCJ (knee straight, knee bent): DF

PROM
STJ: inversion (0–30°)

STJ: eversion (0–15°)

PAM: Talocrural Joint
  Anterior glide

PAM: Subtalar Joint
  Medial glide

  Lateral glide

Special Tests
  Thompson's test

  Subtalar joint neutral

-   Forefoot–rear foot relationship

-   First ray position

Sitting

AROM: TCJ
  DF (0–20°)

  PF (0–50°)

AROM: Tarsal Joints
  Inversion (0–35°)

  Eversion (0–15°)

AROM: Great Toe Extension (0–70°)

PROM

MMT: Tibialis Anterior, Tibialis Posterior, Ankle Eversion, EHL, EDL, FHL, FDL

Special Tests
  Anterior drawer

  Talar tilt

Clinical Syndromes

Description	Location and behavior of symptoms	History	Tests and measures, diagnosis	Intervention
ACHILLES TENDINITIS				
Inflammation of Achilles tendon.	Dull aching pain in Achilles tendon, walking, heel raise, and jumping.	Gradual onset, overuse, recent change in activity.	May be observable, palpable edema and thickening of the tendon; crepitus may be felt with active PF and DF; check TC and ST joint motion. Diagnostics: MRI.	Eccentric exercise program, soft-tissue work, biomechanical correction, taping or heel lift.
ACHILLES TENDON RUPTURE				
Tear of the Achilles tendon.	Sudden pain in Achilles; complaints of someone kicking them.	Sudden explosive push-off; males 30–40 years old.	Inability to walk or perform single heel raise, balling up of triceps surae, Thompson's test (+), palpable defect. Diagnostics: MRI.	Medical management: surgery is usually required.
BURSITIS				
Inflammation of Achilles bursa.	Pain in posterior aspect of heel between tendon and skin.	Irritated by poorly fitted shoes, overuse from repetitive DF.	Pain with pinching of Achilles bursa, pain with walking and AROM, swelling near Achilles insertion, poor talar motion. Diagnostics: MRI.	Rest from activity causing irritation, modalities, heel cushion, orthotics.
ANKLE SPRAIN				
Injury to lateral or medial ligaments of TC joint.	Immediate pain under lateral or medial malleolus, unable to bear weight.	Sudden turning of the ankle during weight bearing.	Increasing severity of swelling, discoloration, and inability to bear weight with grade 1, 2, 3 or anterior drawer (+), talar tilt (+). Diagnostics: MRI	Progressive functional exercise program, proprioceptive training, hip and core strengthening, support for activity.

Description	Location and behavior of symptoms	History	Tests and measures, diagnosis	Intervention
PLANTAR FASCIITIS				
Inflammation of the plantar fascia.	Heel pain with weight bearing, worse in morning, first step out of bed is the worst.	Overuse, acute from stepping on hard object, sometimes being overweight contributes.	Point tender over plantar surface of calcaneus. Diagnostics: X ray may show bone spur.	Orthotics, stretching, soft-tissue massage, iontophoresis, check neurodynamics, night splint.
HYPOMOBILE ANKLE				
Postimmobiliza-tion, postop.	Deep ache in the joint and sharp with end range movement, increased stiffness in morning.	Occurs after a period of immobi-lization.	Glides stiff often painful, pain with OP and usually hard end feel, gait with foot more abducted. Diagnostics: X ray.	Glides, active range, stretching short-ened musculature.
HALLUX RIGIDUS				
OA of the first MT joint.	Pain at base of the great toe, aggra-vated with walk-ing.	Chronic instability of the great toe.	Decreased mobility of first MT, exces-sive supination with toe-off. Diagnostics: X ray.	Joint mobilization if not inflamed, NSAIDS; orthotics (rocker bottom).
HALLUX ABDUCTO VALGUS (HAV)				
Lateral deviation of the first metatarsal.	Asymptomatic, may have pain in the great toe.	Chronic: predis-posing factors include abnormal foot mechanics, improper foot-wear.	Lateral deviation of the big toe. Diagnostics: X ray.	Biomechanical correction, joint mobilization.
MORTON'S NEUROMA				
Inflammation of the heads of the third and fourth metatarsals.	Burning, aching, or numbness and tingling in third and fourth metatarsals.	Unilateral, common in 25- to 50-year-old women, chronic pronator.	Tissue thickening at the area of the MT heads, tenderness, paresthesia and pain increased by weight bearing, squeeze test (+).	Metatarsal pad, wide toe box, biomechanical correction, steroid injection.

» continued

» continued

Description	Location and behavior of symptoms	History	Tests and measures, diagnosis	Intervention
SHINSPLINTS				
Medial tibial stress syndrome; posterior tibialis, soleus, FDL.	Diffuse shin pain most commonly located at the distal medial two-third of the tibia, pain with weight-bearing activities, usually eases rapidly with rest.	Overuse: increased pronation, incorrect footwear, hard running surface, recent increase in activity.	Swelling lower leg, inflammation, check footwear, biomechanics, pain with MMT and passive stretch.	Medical management: May require fasciotomy in extreme cases. Biomechanical correction, adjust training errors, eccentric endurance training, orthotics.
Stress fracture.	Pain is more local and less diffuse. Usually distal or middle third of tibia. Early: pain with activity Late: pain even at rest.	Overuse: muscle fatigue leading to increased bone loading, pronation, incorrect footwear, hard running surface, recent increase in activity.	Local swelling, percussion, tuning fork, no pain with passive stretch. Diagnostics: bone scan, X ray.	Rest, biomechanical correction.
Chronic compartment syndrome.	Diffuse posteromedial pain, tingling and numbness possible, pain only during activity, time of onset during activity is the same.	Overtraining, sudden increase in exercise intensity, etiology uncertain.	Muscle weakness, visible hypertrophy of specific compartment, diminished pulses. Diagnostics: EMG, Doppler flow study	Nonoperative treatment is usually unsuccessful; first look at training errors, poor techniques, shoes, and biomechanics.
NERVE ENTRAPMENT				
Sural, saphenous, superficial peroneal.	Pain, tingling, numbness, burning, night pain.	Acute: sharp blow, unrelieved pressure; chronic: postures, tumor, aneurysm, enclosed compartment.	Limited ROM, weakness, sensory changes, neurodynamic. Diagnostics: nerve conduction velocity, EMG.	Check biomechanics, soft tissue, neurodynamics.
SPINE REFERRAL: DDD				
	Posteromedial lower leg or foot—L4; anterolateral lower leg and dorsum of foot with MT 1, 2, 3—L5; plantar surface and last two MT—S1; posterior lower leg and Achilles—S2.	Refer to lumbar spine clinical syndrome table.	Comparable sign with palpation to specific spinal levels. Comparable sign with LS clearing tests.	Refer to lumbar spine clinical syndrome table.

Adapted, by permission, from C. Wadsworth, 1988, *Manual examination and treatment of the spine and extremities* (Baltimore, MD: Lippincott, Williams, and Wilkins), 219.

Functional Assessment of the Lower Extremity

This chapter begins by describing muscle imbalances associated with the lower extremity. Next, functional ranges of motion needed for most activities of daily living involving the hip, knee, foot, and ankle are listed. The remainder of the chapter is a list of common functional tests used by clinicians to assess the hip, knee, and ankle.

Muscle Imbalances

- Tight hip extensors cause increased lumbar flexion when the thigh is flexed.

- Tight hip flexors cause increased lumbar extension and anterior tilt as the thigh extends.

- Tight adductors cause lateral pelvic tilt opposite the side of tightness and side bending toward the side of tightness during weight bearing.

- Tight abductors cause lateral pelvic tilt toward the side of tightness and side bending away from the side of tightness during weight bearing.

- Short leg results in abduction of the hip on the short side, adduction of the hip on the long side, convexity of the lumbar spine toward the short side, iliotibial band (ITB) tightness on the short side, and gluteus medius weakness on the long side.

- Overuse of two-joint hip flexor muscles rather than iliopsoas may cause faulty hip mechanics or knee pain.

- Overuse of hamstring muscles rather than gluteus maximus may cause overuse problems of the hamstrings.

- Anterior pelvic tilt results in hip flexion and lumbar extension caused by combined shortness of hip flexors and back extensors. Abdominals, glutei, and hamstrings are lengthened.

- Posterior pelvic tilt results in hip extension and lumbar flexion caused by shortness of hip extensors and trunk flexors. Hip flexors and erector spinae are lengthened.

- In forward bending as the head and upper trunk begin flexion, the pelvis moves posteriorly no more than 2 in. (5 cm) to maintain the center of gravity. Continued forward bending is accompanied by hip flexion until approximately 45°. Hip flexion at end-range forward bending should be between 70° and 95°. The return to upright position begins with posterior translation of the pelvis and then back extension.

- Pelvic rotation in transverse plane: Rotation occurs around one lower extremity that is fixed on the ground. With weight bearing, forward rotation of the pelvis results in internal rotation of the hip on the stance side. Backward rotation of the pelvis results in external rotation of the hip on the stance side. On forward rotation the adductors, obliques, and sartorius become tight while the gluteus medius and tensor fascia lata become lengthened. On backward rotation, the gluteus medius and tensor become short and the adductors, obliques, and sartorius become lengthened.

- Pelvic elevation in frontal plane: Asymmetry of the pelvis in the frontal plane due to a leg-length difference causes changes in muscle length for many hip muscles. On the long side, the hip is in relative adduction, resulting in shortness of the adductors and quadratus lumborum and lengthening of the gluteus medius and tensor fascia lata.

Functional Ranges of Motion Necessary for Lower Extremity

	Gait	Stair ascent	Stair descent
Hip	0–40°	0–60°	0–45°
Knee	0–60°	0–90°	0–100°
Ankle			
Dorsiflexion	0–10°	0–20°	0–20°
Plantarflexion	0–30°	0–30°	0–30°

Functional Strength Testing of the Hip

The following table and reproducible scale relate to the strength testing of the hip.

Functional Tests

Starting position	Action	Functional test
Standing	Lift foot onto 20 cm step and return (hip flexion and extension)	5 to 6 reps: functional 3 to 4 reps: functionally fair 1 to 2 reps: functionally poor 0 reps: nonfunctional
Standing	Sit in chair and return to standing (hip flexion and extension)	5 to 6 reps: functional 3 to 4 reps: functionally fair 1 to 2 reps: functionally poor 0 reps: nonfunctional
Standing	Lift leg to balance on one leg, keeping pelvis straight (hip abduction)	Hold 60 to 90 s: functional Hold 30 to 59 s: functionally fair Hold 1 to 29 s: functionally poor Cannot hold: nonfunctional
Standing	Walk sideways 6 m (hip adduction)	6 to 8 m one way: functional 3 to 6 m one way: functionally fair 1 to 3 m one way: functionally poor 0 m: nonfunctional
Standing	Test leg off floor (patient may hold on to something for balance), medially rotate	10 to 12 reps: functional 5 to 9 reps: functionally fair 1 to 4 reps: functionally poor 0 reps: nonfunctional
Standing	Test leg off floor (patient may hold on to something for balance), laterally rotate	10 to 12 repetitions: functional 5 to 9 repetitions: functional fair 1 to 4 repetitions: functional poor 0 repetitions: nonfunctional

Adapted, by permission, from M.L. Palmer and M. Epler, 1990, *Clinical assessment procedures in physical therapy* (Baltimore, MD: Lippincott, Williams, and Wilkins).

Harris Hip Function Scale

(Circle one in each group)

Pain (44 points)		Range of motion (5 points max)
None or ignores	44	*Instructions*: Record 10° of fixed adduction as "−10° abduction"
Slight, occasional, no compromise in activity	40	Record 10° of fixed external rotation as "−10° internal rotation"
Mild, no effect on ordinary activity, pain after unusual activity, uses aspirin	30	Record 10° of fixed external rotation with 10° further external rotation as "−10° internal rotation"
Moderate, tolerable, makes concessions, strong meds	20	
Marked, serious limitation	10	
Totally disabled	0	

Function (47 points)			Range	Index factor	Index value*
Gait (walking max distance; 33 points max)		Permanent flexion (1)_____	_____°		
1. *Limp*		A. Flexion to			
None	11	(0–45°)		1.0	
Slight	8	(45–90°)		0.6	
Moderate	5	(90–120°)		0.3	
Unable to walk	0	(120–140°)		0.0	
2. *Support*					
None	11	B. Adduction to			
Cane, long walks	7	(0–15°)		0.8	
Cane, full time	5	(15–30°)		0.3	
Crutch	4	(30–60°)		0.0	
Two canes	2				
Two crutches	02	C. Adduction to			
Unable to walk	0	(0–15°)		0.2	
		(15–60°)		0.0	
3. Distance walked					
Unlimited	11	D. External rotation in extension to			
Six blocks	8	(0–30°)		0.4	
Two or three blocks	5	(30–60°)		0.0	
Indoors only	2				
Bed and chair	0				

Functional activities (14 points max)

1. *Stairs*		E. Internal rotation in extension to	
Normally	4	(0–60°)	0.0
Normally with banister	2		
Any method	1		
Not able	0		
2. Socks and tie shoes		*Index value = range × index factor	
With ease	4		
With difficulty	2	Total index value = (A + B + C + D + E) _____	
Unable	0		
3. *Sitting*		Total range of motion points _____	
Any chair, 1 hour	5	(multiply total index value × 0.05)	
High chair, 1/2 hour	3		
Unable to sit 1/2 hour any chair	0	Pain points _____	
4. Enter public transport		Function points _____	
Able to use public transport	1	Absence of deformity points _____	
Not able to use public transport	0	Range of motion points _____	
		Total points (100 points max) _____	

Absence of deformity (requires all four; 4 points max)

1. Fixed adduction <10°	4	Comments:
2. Fixed internal rotation in extension <10°	0	
3. Leg-length discrepancy <1 1/4 in. (3.2 m)		
4. Pelvic flexion contracture <30°		

From J. Loudon, M. Swift, and S. Bell, 2008, *The clinical orthopedic assessment guide, 2nd ed.* (Champaign, IL: Human Kinetics). Reprinted, by permission, from W.H. Harris, 1969, "Traumatic arthritis of the hip after dislocation and acetabular fracture: Treatment by mold arthroplasty," *Journal of Bone and Joint Surgery* 51: 737-755.

Functional Strength Testing of the Knee

The following two reproducible scales relate to the strength testing of the knee.

Cincinnati Rating Scale

Left	Right	Points	Symptoms (50 points)
			1. Pain
		20	No pain, normal knee, performs 100%.
		16	Occasional pain with strenuous sports or heavy work, knee not entirely normal, some limitations but minor and tolerable.
		12	Occasional pain with light recreational sports or moderate work activities, often brought on by vigorous activities, running, heavy labor, strenuous sports.
		8	Pain, usually brought on by sports, light recreational activities, or moderate work. Occasionally occurs with walking, standing, or light work.
		4	Pain is a significant problem with activities as simple as walking. Relieved by rest. Unable to do sports.
		0	Pain present all the time, occurs with walking, standing, and at nighttime. Not relieved with rest. I don't know what my pain level is. I have not tested my knee.

Intensity of pain

❏ Mild   ❏ Moderate   ❏ Severe

Frequency of pain

❏ Intermittent   ❏ Constant

Location of pain

❏ Medial   ❏ Anterior patella   ❏ Posterior diffuse

Pain occurs on

❏ Stairs   ❏ Sitting   ❏ Kneeling   ❏ Standing

Type of pain

❏ Sharp   ❏ Aching   ❏ Throbbing   ❏ Burning

Left	Right	Points	Symptoms
			2. Swelling
		10	No swelling, normal knee, 100% activity.
		8	Occasional swelling with strenuous sports or heavy work. Some limitations but minor and tolerable.
		6	Occasional swelling with light recreational sports or moderate work activities, frequently brought on by vigorous activities, running, heavy labor, strenuous sports.
		4	Swelling limits sports and moderate work. Occurs infrequently with simple walking activities or light work (about three times per year).

Left	Right	Points	Symptoms (50 points)
		2	Swelling brought on by simple walking activities and light work. Relieved with rest.
		0	Severe problem all the time with simple walking activities. I don't know what my swelling level is. I have not tested my knee.

If swelling occurs it is (check one box on each line)

Intensity

❏ Mild ❏ Moderate ❏ Severe

Frequency

❏ Intermittent ❏ Constant

Left	Right	Points	Symptoms (50 points)
			3. Giving way
		20	No giving way.
		16	Occasional giving way with strenuous sports or heavy work. Can participate in all sports but some guarding or limitations are still present.
		12	Occasional giving way with light recreational activities or moderate work. Able to compensate; limits vigorous activities, sports, or heavy work; not able to cut or twist suddenly.
		8	Giving way limits sports and moderate work; occurs infrequently with walking or light work (about three times per year).
		4	Giving way with simple walking activities and light work. Occurs once a moth. Requires guarding.
		0	Severe problem with simple walking activities; cannot turn or twist while walking without giving way. I do not know my level of giving way. I have not tested my knee.

4. Other symptoms (unscored)

Knee stiffness	Kneecap grinding	Knee locking
❏ None	❏ None	❏ None
❏ Occasional	❏ Mild	❏ Occasional
❏ Frequent	❏ Moderate	❏ Frequent
❏ Severe		

Function (50 points)

Left	Right	Points	
			5. Overall activity level
		20	No limitation, normal knee, able to do everything, including strenuous sports or heavy labor.

» continued

» continued

Left	Right	Points	Symptoms (50 points)
		16	Perform sports, including vigorous activities, but at a lower performance level; involves guarding or some limits to heavy labor.
		12	Light recreational activities possible with rare symptoms; more strenuous activities cause problems.
		8	No sports or recreational activities possible. Walking activities possible with rare symptoms; limited to light work.
		4	Walking, activities of daily living cause moderate symptoms, frequent limitations.
		0	Walking, activities of daily living cause severe problems, persistent symptoms. I do not know what my real activity level is, I have not tested my knee, or I have given up strenuous sports.
			6. Walking
		10	Normal, unlimited.
		8	Slight or mild problem.
		6	Moderate problem; smooth surface possible up to 800 m.
		4	Severe problem: only two or three blocks possible.
		2	Severe problem: requires cane, crutches.
			7. Stairs
		10	Normal, unlimited.
		8	Slight or mild problem.
		6	Moderate problem: only 10–15 steps possible.
		4	Severe problem: requires banister support.
		2	Severe problem: 1–5 steps possible.
			8. Running activity
		5	Normal, unlimited: fully competitive, strenuous.
		4	Slight or mild problem: run half speed.
		3	Moderate problem: only 2–4 km possible.
		2	Severe problem: only one or two blocks possible.
		1	Severe problem: only a few steps possible.
			9. Jumping or twisting activities
		5	Normal, unlimited: fully competitive, strenuous.
		4	Slight or mild problem: some guarding, but sports possible.
		3	Moderate problem: gave up strenuous sports, recreational sports possible.
		2	Severe problem: affects all sports; must constantly guard.
		1	Severe problem: only light activity possible (golf, swimming).

Total: Left _____ Right _____ (Maximum: 100 points)

From J. Loudon, M. Swift, and S. Bell, 2008, *The clinical orthopedic assessment guide, 2nd ed.* (Champaign, IL: Human Kinetics). Adapted, by permission, from F.R. Noyes, G.H. McGinniss, and G.H. Mooar, 1984, "Functional disability in the anterior cruciate insufficient knee syndrome," *Sports Medicine* 1: 3287-3288.

Lysholm Knee Scale

Limp *(5 points)*
None	5 _____
Slight or periodic	3 _____
Severe and constant	0 _____

Support *(5 points)*
Full support	5 _____
Cane or crutch	3 _____
Weight bearing impossible	0 _____

Stair climbing *(10 points)*
No problems	5 _____
Slightly impaired	3 _____
One step at a time	2 _____
Unable	0 _____

Squatting *(5 points)*
No problems	5 _____
Slightly impaired	3 _____
Not past 90°	2 _____
Unable	0 _____

Total _____

Walking, Running, Jumping

Instability
Never gives way	30 _____
Rarely gives way except for athletic or other severe exertion	25 _____
Gives way frequently during athletic events or other severe exertion	0 _____
Occasionally in daily activities	10 _____
Often in daily activities	5 _____
Every step	0 _____

Swelling
None	10 _____
With giving way	7 _____
On severe exertion	5 _____
On ordinary exertion	2 _____
Constant	0 _____

Pain
None	30 _____
Inconstant and slight during severe exertion	25 _____
Marked on giving way	20 _____
Marked during severe exertion	15 _____
Marked on or after walking more than 1 1/4 miles (2 km)	10 _____
Marked on or after walking less than 1 1/4 miles (2 km)	5 _____
Constant and severe	0 _____

Atrophy of thigh *(5 points)*
None	5 _____
1–2 cm	3 _____
>2 cm	0 _____

Total (total score = 100 points) _____

From J. Loudon, M. Swift, and S. Bell, 2008, *The clinical orthopedic assessment guide, 2nd ed.* (Champaign, IL: Human Kinetics). Adapted, by permission, from J. Lysholm and J. Gillquist, 1982, "Evaluation of the knee ligament surgery results with special emphasis on use of a scoring scale," *American Journal of Sports Medicine 10:* 1150-154.

Functional Strength Testing of the Foot and Ankle

The following table and reproducible scale relate to the strength testing of the foot and ankle.

Functional Tests

Starting position	Action	Functional test
Standing on one leg	Lift toes and forefeet off ground	10 to 15 reps: functional 5 to 9 reps: functionally fair 1 to 4 reps: functionally poor 0 reps: nonfunctional
Standing on one leg	Lift heels off ground	10 to 15 reps: functional 5 to 9 reps: functionally fair 1 to 4 reps: functionally poor 0 reps: nonfunctional
Standing on one leg	Lift lateral aspect of foot off ground	10 to 15 reps: functional 5 to 9 reps: functionally fair 1 to 4 reps: functionally poor 0 reps: nonfunctional
Standing on one leg	Lift medial aspect of foot off ground	10 to 15 reps: functional 5 to 9 reps: functionally fair 1 to 4 reps: functionally poor 0 reps: nonfunctional
Seated	Pick up and release marbles	10 to 15 reps: functional 5 to 9 reps: functionally fair 1 to 4 reps: functionally poor 0 reps: nonfunctional
Seated	Lift toes off ground	10 to 15 reps: functional 5 to 9 reps: functionally fair 1 to 4 reps: functionally poor 0 reps: nonfunctional

Adapted, by permission, from M.L. Paler and M. Epler, 1990, *Clinical assessment procedures in physical therapy* (Baltimore, MD: Lippincott, Williams, and Wilkins).

Functional Rating Scale for Ankles

Condition	Score
Pain	
Never hurts	5 _____
Hurts with strenuous sports	4 _____
Hurts with light sports	3 _____
Hurts with walking more than 5km	2 _____
Hurts walking less than 5 km	1 _____
Hurts at rest or at night	0 _____
Stability	
Never turns (no support)	5 _____
Never turns (with support)	4 _____
Turns occasionally (no support)	3 _____
Turns frequently during daily living activities	0 _____
Stiffness	
Never stiff	2 _____
Stiff untill warmed up	1 _____
Stiff at all times	0 _____

Condition	Score
Swelling	
Never swells	2 _____
End of day or after activity	1 _____
Swells most of time	0 _____
Activity	
Able to hop	2 _____
Not as good as normal side	1 _____
Cannot hop	0 _____
Range of motion	
Full range of motion	4 _____
Full plantarflexion, limited dorsiflexion	2 _____
Limited dorsi- and plantarflexion	0 _____
Total	_____

From J. Loudon, M. Swift, and S. Bell, 2008, *The Clinical Orthopedic Assessment Guide, 2nd ed.* (Champaign, IL: Human Kinetics). Adapted, by permission, from D. Seligson, J. Sassman, and M. Pope, 1980, "Ankle instability: Evaluation of lateral ligaments," *American Journal of Sports Medicine* 8: 39.

Other Foot and Ankle Tests

The following three reproducible scales and tests contribute to the overall functional assessment.

Physical Scales of the AIM 2

Please check (X) the most appropriate answer for each question.	All days (1)	Most days (2)	Some days (3)	Few days (4)	No days (5)
These questions refer to mobility level.					

During the past month

1. How often were you physically able to drive a car or use public transportation? _____ _____ _____ _____ _____
2. How often were you out of the house for at least part of the day? _____ _____ _____ _____ _____
3. How often were you able to do errands in the neighborhood? _____ _____ _____ _____ _____
4. How often did someone have to assist you to get around outside your home? _____ _____ _____ _____ _____
5. How often were you in a bed or chair for most or all of the day? _____ _____ _____ _____ _____

These questions refer to walking and bending.

During the past month

6. Did you have trouble doing vigorous activities such as running, lifting heavy objects, or participating in strenuous sports? _____ _____ _____ _____ _____
7. Did you have trouble either walking several blocks or climbing a flight of stairs? _____ _____ _____ _____ _____
8. Did you have trouble bending, lifting, or stooping? _____ _____ _____ _____ _____
9. Did you have trouble either walking one block or climbing a flight of stairs? _____ _____ _____ _____ _____
10. Were you unable to walk unless assisted by another person or by a cane, crutches, or walker? _____ _____ _____ _____ _____

These questions refer to hand and finger function.

During the past month

11. Could you easily write with a pen or pencil? _____ _____ _____ _____ _____
12. Could you easily button a shirt or blouse? _____ _____ _____ _____ _____
13. Could you easily turn a key in a lock? _____ _____ _____ _____ _____
14. Could you easily tie a knot or a bow? _____ _____ _____ _____ _____
15. Could you easily open a new jar of food? _____ _____ _____ _____ _____

These questions refer to mobility level.

During the past month

16. Could you easily wipe your mouth with a napkin? _____ _____ _____ _____ _____
17. Could you easily put on a pullover sweater? _____ _____ _____ _____ _____
18. Could you easily comb or brush your hair? _____ _____ _____ _____ _____
19. Could you easily scratch your lower back with your hand? _____ _____ _____ _____ _____
20. Could you easily reach shelves that were above your head? _____ _____ _____ _____ _____

These questions refer to self-care tasks.

During the past month

21. Did you need help to take a bath or shower? _____ _____ _____ _____ _____
22. Did you need help to get dressed? _____ _____ _____ _____ _____
23. Did you need help to use the toilet? _____ _____ _____ _____ _____
24. Did you need help to get in or out of bed? _____ _____ _____ _____ _____

These questions refer to household tasks.

During the past month

25. If you had the necessary transportation, could you go shopping for groceries without help? _____ _____ _____ _____ _____
26. If you had kitchen facilities, could you prepare your own meals without help? _____ _____ _____ _____ _____
27. If you had household tools and appliances, could you do your own housework without help? _____ _____ _____ _____ _____
28. If you had laundry facilities, could you do your laundry without help? _____ _____ _____ _____ _____

From J. Loudon, M. Swift, and S. Bell, 2008, *The Clinical Orthopedic Assessment Guide,* 2nd ed. (Champaign, IL: Human Kinetics). Reprinted, by permission, from Boston University School of Public Health, 1990.

Tinetti Balance Test

Subject is seated in hard, armless chair. The following maneuvers are tested.

1. **Sitting balance**
   Leans or slides in chair = 0
   Steady, safe = 1 _____

2. **Arises**
   Unable without help = 0
   Able, uses arms to help = 1
   Able, without using arms = 2 _____

3. **Attempts to arise**
   Unable without help = 0
   Able, requires more than one attempt = 1
   Able to arise, one attempt = 2 _____

4. **Immediate standing balance** (first 5 seconds)
   Unsteady (swaggers, moves feet, trunk sways) = 0
   Steady but uses cane or other support = 1
   Steady without walker or other support = 2 _____

5. **Standing balance**
   Unsteady = 0
   Steady but wide stance (medial heels > 4 in. [10 cm] apart) and uses = 1
    cane or other support
   Narrow stance without support = 2 _____

6. **Nudged** (subject at maximum position with feet as close together as possible; examiner pushes lightly on subject's sternum with palm of hand three times)
   Begins to fall = 0
   Staggers, grabs, catches self = 1
   Steady = 2 _____

7. **Eyes closed** (at maximum position no. 6)
   Unsteady = 0
   Steady = 1 _____

8. **Turning 360°**
   Discontinuous steps = 0
   Continuous = 1 _____
   Unsteady (grabs, staggers) = 0
   Steady = 1 _____

9. **Sitting down**
   Unsafe (misjudged distance, falls into chair) = 0
   Uses arms or not a smooth motion = 1
   Safe, smooth motion = 2 _____

   Balance score: _____/16

Tinetti Gait Test

Subject stands with examiner, walks down hallway or across room, first at "usual" pace, then back at "rapid" pace using usual walking aids.

10.Initiation of gait (immediately after told to go)
    Any hesitancy or multiple attempts to start   = 0
    No hesitancy   = 1 _____

11.Step length and height

    a. Right swing foot
        Does not pass left stance foot with step   = 0
        Passes left stance foot   = 1
        Right foot does not clear floor completely with step   = 0
        Right foot completely clears floor   = 1 _____

    b. Left swing foot
        Does not pass right stance foot with step   = 0
        Passes right stance foot   = 1
        Left foot does not clear floor completely with step   = 0
        Left foot completely clears floor   = 1 _____

12.Step symmetry
    Right and left step length not equal (estimate)   = 0
    Right and left step appear equal   = 1 _____

13.Step continuity
    Stopping or discontinuity between steps   = 0
    Steps appear continuous   = 1 _____

14.Path (estimated in relation to floor tiles, 12 in. [30 cm] diameter; observe excursion of one foot over about 10 ft [3 m] of the course)
    Marked deviation   = 0
    Mild or moderate deviation or uses walking aid   = 1
    Straight without walking aid   = 2 _____

15.Trunk
    Marked sway or uses walking aid   = 0
    No sway but flexion of knees or back or spreads arms out while walking   = 1
    No sway, no flexion, no use of arms, and no use of walking aid   = 2 _____

16.Walking time
    Heels apart   = 0
    Heels almost touching while walking   = 1 _____

                Gait score: _____/12
        Balance + gait score: _____/28

From J. Loudon, M. Swift, and S. Bell, 2008, *The clinical orthopedic assessment guide, 2nd ed.* (Champaign, IL: Human Kinetics). Reprinted, by permission, from M. Tinetti, 1986, "Performance oriented assessment of mobility problems in elderly patients," *Journal of the American Geriatrics Society 39*: 119-126. Copyright 1990, American Geriatrics Society.

Posture and Gait

The fifth part of the text is designed to familiarize the clinician with normal and abnormal posture and gait. Part V of the text contains three chapters that focus on posture and gait. The chapter on posture contains numerous tables that describe normal and abnormal posture, based on the work of Florence Kendall. The chapter on gait is taken from the descriptions of Rancho Los Amigos Medical Center in Los Angeles. A table condenses the information for each phase of gait and includes joint arthrokinematics, muscle action, and joint movements. The final chapter of part V describes other types of gait that pertain to stair climbing and running.

Posture

This chapter reviews normal and abnormal standing posture in the sagittal and frontal views. Normal posture is probably a misnomer because most people do not have "normal" posture. But by identifying normal or ideal posture, the clinician has a standard posture by which to make comparisons. A standard posture also helps identify asymmetries that may potentially lead to musculoskeletal dysfunction. This chapter describes faulty anatomy for each major joint. Accompanying these descriptions are the associated muscle imbalances.

Terminology

Lordosis   Anterior curve of the spine.

Kyphosis   Posterior curve of the spine.

Scoliosis   Lateral curvature of the spine.

Cervical curvature   Convex anteriorly.

Thoracic curvature   Convex posteriorly.

Lumbar curvature   Convex anteriorly.

Sacral curvature   Convex posteriorly.

Ideal Posture

Below are some standards of "normal" posture against which to compare imbalances (see figure 16.1). Plumb-line alignment, distribution of weight, and electromyography (EMG) activity are three means of assessing posture.

Plumb-Line Alignment

1. Slightly anterior to the lateral malleolus; through the calcaneocuboid joint
2. Just in front of the center of the knee joint
3. Through the greater trochanter of the femur; slightly posterior to the center of the hip joint
4. Midway through the trunk; through bodies of lumbar vertebrae
5. Through the shoulder joint
6. Through bodies of cervical vertebrae
7. Through the odontoid process
8. Through the lobe of the ear; through external auditory meatus

Pressure Distribution of Weight

45–65% of body weight should be carried over the heels.

30–47% of body weight should be carried on the forefoot.

1–8% of body weight should be carried over the midfoot.

EMG Activity in Quiet Standing

1. The muscles of the feet are quiet.
2. The soleus is active to maintain upright position.
3. The quadriceps and hamstrings for the most part are quiescent, although they may show slight activity from time to time.
4. The iliopsoas remains constantly active.
5. The gluteus maximus is quiescent.
6. The gluteus medius and tensor fascia lata are active to control lateral pelvic tilt.
7. The erector spinae is active to counterac anterior moment.
8. The abdominal muscles remain quiescent.
9. Minimal activity occurs in the upper trapezius, serratus anterior, supraspinatus, and posterior deltoid.

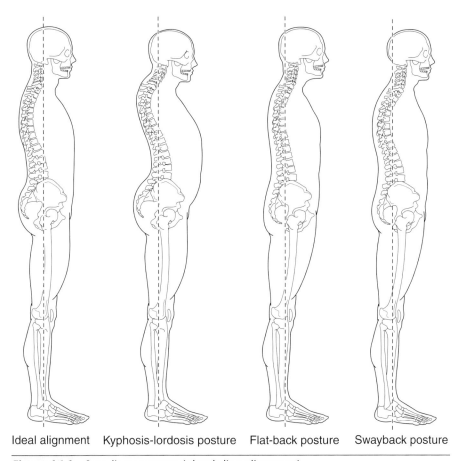

Ideal alignment   Kyphosis-lordosis posture   Flat-back posture   Swayback posture

Figure 16.1   Standing postures (plumb-line alignment).

Body Posture

Good posture	Part	Faulty posture
In standing, the longitudinal arch has the shape of a half dome. The feet toe out slightly.	Foot	Low longitudinal arch or flat feet. Low metatarsal arch, usually indicated by calluses under the foot. Weight borne on the inner or outer border of the foot. Toeing out or toeing in.
The toes should be straight without curling downward or bending upward. They should extend forward in line with the foot.	Toes	Hallux valgus, or curling of the toes as in hammertoes.
The legs are straight in frontal and sagittal planes. Patellae face straight ahead.	Knee and legs	Genu valgus, genu varum, genu recurvatum, flexed knee. Patellae ride high, low, inward, or outward.
Body weight is distributed evenly; hips are symmetrical. The spine does not curve (slight deviation to the left for a right-handed person and vice versa for a left-handed person is common).	Hips, pelvis, spine (back view)	One hip is higher than the other. Hips are rotated so that one is anteriorly rotated.
The front of the pelvis and thighs are in a straight line. ASIS and pubic symphysis are aligned. Four natural curves are present; in the neck and low back the curve is forward; in the upper back and sacral region it is backward.	Hips and pelvis (side view)	Increased lordosis, anterior pelvic tilt. The low back is flat; the pelvis is in posterior tilt. Kyphosis is present in the thoracic spine. Forward-head posture.
In adults the abdomen should be flat.	Abdomen	The abdomen protrudes.
The chest is slightly up and slightly forward.	Chest	Hollow chest; lifted and held too high by arching in the back; ribs are not symmetrical.
The arms hang relaxed and equidistant from sides with palms of the hands facing toward the body. The shoulders are level in all planes. Scapulae lie flat against the rib cage. There is about a 4 in. (10 cm) separation between them.	Arms and shoulders	The shoulders are forward and are asymmetrical. One arm hangs lower than the other. Scapulae are abducted, winged, or excessively rotated.
The head is held erect in a position of good balance.	Head	The chin is up too high. The head protrudes forward and is tilted or rotated.
The mouth remains closed.	Jaw	The mouth hangs open.

Adapted, by permission, from C. Norkin, Gait analysis. In *Physical Rehabilitation: Assessment and treatment* (Philadelphia, PA: F.A. Davis), 117-179.

Postural Musculature

Postural fault	Anatomic position	Muscles (short)	Muscles (long)
Lordosis	Lumbar spine hyperextension Anterior tilt pelvis Hip joint flexion	Lower back erector spinae Hip flexors	Abdominals External obliques Hip extensors
Flat back	Lumbar spine flexion Posterior tilt pelvis Hip joint extension	Anterior abdominals Hip extensors	Erector spinae Hip flexors
Swayback	Lumbar spine flexion Posterior tilt Hip joint extension	Rectus abdominis Internal obliques Hip extensors	External obliques One joint Hip flexors
Forward head	Cervical spine hyperextension	Cervical spine extensors Upper trapezius, levator	Cervical spine flexors
Kyphosis	Thoracic spine flexion Decrease in intercostal space	Internal obliques (upper lateral) Shoulder adductors Pectoralis minor intercostals	Thoracic spine extensors Midtrapezius Low trapezius
Forward shoulders	Scapulae abductors Scapulae elevated	Serratus anterior Pectoralis minor and upper trapezius	Midtrapezius Low trapezius
Scoliosis Slight left C-curve Thoracolumbar scoliosis (Opposite for right C-curve) (Opposite for right C-curve)	Thoracolumbar spine lateral flexion Convex toward left	Right latissimus dorsi Trunk muscles Left psoas	Latissimus dorsi Trunk muscles Right psoas
High right hip (Opposite for posture with right C-curve and high left hip)	Pelvis, lateral tilt high on right Right hip adduction Left hip abduction	Right lateral trunk Left hip abduction, TFL Right hip adduction	Left lateral trunk Right hip abduction, gluteus medius Left hip adduction
Hyperextended knee	Knee hyperextension Ankle plantarflexion	Quadriceps Soleus	Popliteus Hamstrings
Flexed knee	Knee flexion	Popliteus Hamstrings	Quadriceps Soleus
Medial rotation of femur	Hip joint medial rotation	Hip medial rotators	Hip lateral rotators
Genu valgum	Hip joint adduction Knee joint abduction	Fascia lata Lateral knee joint structures	Medial knee joint structures
Pronation	Calcaneal eversion	Peroneals Toe extensor	Post tibialis Long toe flexor
Supination	Calcaneal inversion	Tibials	Peroneals
Hammertoes Low MT arch	MTP extension	Toe extensors PIP flexion	Lumbricales

Adapted, by permission, from F.P. Kendall, 1993, *Muscles: Testing and function* (Philadelphia, PA: Lippincott, Williams, and Wilkins), 106-108.

Gait

Gait assessment should be a component of every musculoskeletal examination. This chapter facilitates gait examination by offering information in an accessible manner. The chapter lists common terminology used with gait examination, describes the gait sequence (Rancho Los Amigos terminology; figure 17.1), and includes a table that lists joint range of motion and muscle activity associated with each phase of gait for all major joints (table 17.1 on page 405). Additionally, this chapter identifies faulty gait characteristics for each major joint and where it occurs in the gait cycle. Gait examination is a technical skill that requires precision. The breakdown of each gait phase should help the clinician identify gait faults.

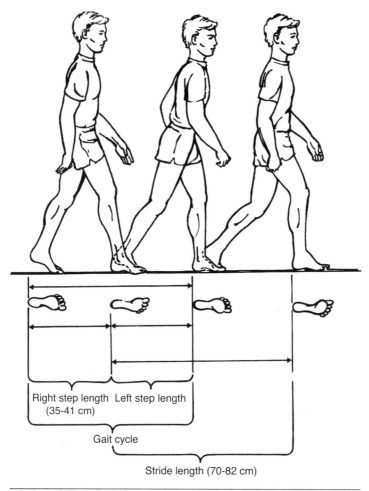

Figure 17.1 Gait sequence.

Adapted from *Orthopedic Physical Assessment*, 2nd ed., D.J. Magee, pg. 564. Copyright 1992, with permission from W.B. Saunders.

Terminology

Gait cycle   From heel strike to heel strike of the same foot.

Stance phase   Phase of the gait in which one foot contacts the ground and remains in contact with it; includes initial contact, loading response, mid-stance, terminal stance, and preswing.

Swing phase   Phase of the gait that is determined when one foot leaves the ground until that same foot returns to the ground; includes initial swing, midswing, and terminal swing.

Stance time   Amount of time spent in stance; includes single support and double support.

Swing time   Amount of time spent in swing.

Double support   Phase of the gait during which both lower extremities are in contact with the ground.

Single support   Phase of the gait during which only one lower extremity is in contact with the ground.

Ground reaction force   Force created as a result of foot contact with the supporting surface.

Stride length   Distance between two successive events accomplished by the same lower extremity.

Stride duration   Amount of time spent in stride.

Step length   Distance between the heel strike of one leg and the heel strike of the contralateral leg.

Step duration   Time between the heel strike of one leg and the heel strike of the contralateral leg.

Cadence   Number of steps per unit of time.

Step width   Linear distance between the midpoint of the heel on one foot and same point on the other foot.

Gait Sequence

Stance (60% of Gait Cycle)   Rancho Los Amigos terminology is used; traditional terms are in parentheses (Perry, J. *Gait analysis: Normal and pathological function.* Thorofare, New Jersey: Slack, 1992).

1. 1% initial contact (heel strike): Contact of the foot with the ground
2. 2–10% loading response (foot flat): From initial contact until the point at which the contralateral leg leaves the ground (figure 17.2)
3. 10–30% midstance: From loading response until the body is directly over the supporting limb
4. 30–50% terminal stance (heel-off): From midstance to a point just before initial contact of the contralateral extremity
5. 50–60% pre-swing (toe-off): From terminal stance to just before the liftoff of the reference extremity

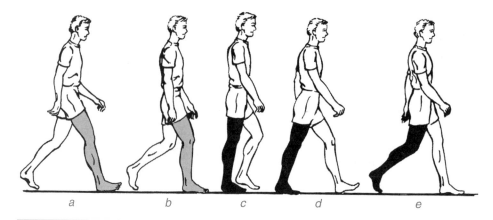

Figure 17.2 Stance phase of gait: (*a*) initial contact, (*b*) loading response, (*c*) midstance (single-leg stance), (*d*) terminal stance, and (*e*) preswing.

Swing (40% of Gait Cycle)

1. 60–73% initial swing (acceleration): Point of lift to maximum knee flexion

2. 73–87% midswing: From maximum knee flexion to the point at which the tibia is in a vertical position (figure 17.3)

3 87–100% terminal swing (deceleration): From midswing to initial contact

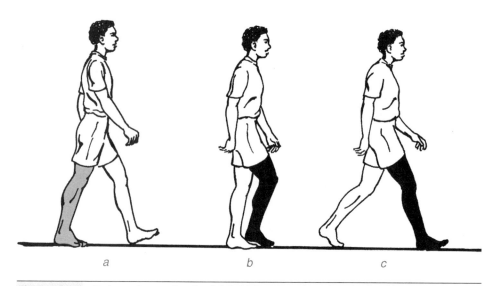

Figure 17.3 Swing phase of gait: (*a*) initial swing (acceleration), (*b*) midswing, and (*c*) terminal swing (deceleration).

Gait Sequence With Joint Position and Muscle Activity

Gait phase	Joint and muscle	Pelvis	Hip	Knee	Ankle	Foot
Initial contact	Joint position	Level in sagittal and coronal planes; forward in transverse plane on stance leg	30° hip flexion, slight external rotation	Knee extension (0–5°)	Neutral	2° inverted
	Muscle activity	Gluteus medius, adductors eccentric	Hamstrings, gluteus maximus eccentric	Vasti, ITB eccentric hamstrings concentric	Pre-tibialis eccentric	Post-tibialis eccentric
Loading response	Joint position	Contralateral pelvis drops	20° flexion, internal rotation	15° flexion	Neutral to10° plantarflexion	Pronated 5°
	Muscle activity	Gluteus medius, minimus, TFL eccentric	Gluteus maximus, adductor magnus concentric	Quadriceps eccentric, slight hamstring	Pre-tibialis eccentric	Post-tibialis eccentric
Midstance	Joint position	Level	Neutral, external rotation	0–5° flexion	8° plantarflexion to 5° dorsiflexion	Supinating
	Muscle activity	Gluteus medius, TFL concentric	Gluteus medius concentric	Early: quadriceps concentric	Soleus, gastrocnemius eccentric	Post-tibialis concentric
Terminal stance	Joint position	Anterior tilt, pelvis rotates 5° backward	Extension 20°, external rotation, abduction	Extension	5° to 10° dorsiflexion	Supinated (maximal) MTP extends to 30°
	Muscle activity	Rectus abdominis	TFL eccentric	Hamstrings eccentric, gastrocnemius	Soleus eccentric	Peroneals eccentric
Preswing	Joint position	Lateral tilt ipsilateral side	Neutral to flex, external rotation	40° flexion	20° plantarflexion	Supinated MTP to 60°

» continued

» continued

Gait phase	Joint and muscle	Pelvis	Hip	Knee	Ankle	Foot
	Muscle activity	Hip adduction eccentric	Add longus eccentric, iliopsoas concentric; late: hamstrings eccentric	Popliteus concentric, rectus femoris eccentric	Plantarflexion concentric; pre-tibialis late	Peroneals, FDL, EHL concentric
Initial swing	Joint position	Posterior tilt, lateral tilt	Flexion, neutral transverse rotation	60° flexion	5° plantarflexion to dorsiflexion	Supinated
	Muscle activity	Gluteus medius	Iliopsoas concentric	Biceps femoris concentric	Pre-tibialis concentric	Pre-tibialis concentric
Midswing	Joint position	Posterior tilt	30° flexion, adduction, neutral transverse rotation	Flexion to extension	Dorsiflexion	Neutral
	Muscle activity	Gluteus medius	Adductors concentric	Sartorius concentric	Anterior tibialis EHL	
Terminal swing	Joint position	Anterior tilt, rotated forward	30° flexion, external rotation	Extension	Neutral	Supinated
	Muscle activity	Adductors	Gluteus maximus, hamstrings eccentric	Quadriceps concentric	Anterior tibialis isometric, concentric	

Adapted from C. Norkin, 1994, Gait analysis. In *Physical rehabilitation: Assessment and treatment*, 3rd ed. edited by S.B. O'Sullivan and T.J. Schmitz (Philadephia: F.A. Davis), 482.

Range of Motion Needed During Gait

Stance Phase

Hip flexion: 0–30°

Hip extension: 0–20°

Knee flexion: 0–40°

Knee extension: 0°

Plantarflexion: 0–20°

Dorsiflexion: 0–10°

Subtalar joint inversion: 35°

Subtalar joint eversion: 15°

Swing Phase

Hip flexion: 0–30°

Hip extension: 0–20°

Knee flexion: 0–60°

Knee extension: 0°

Plantarflexion: 0–10°

Dorsiflexion: 0°

Gait Disturbances and Mechanical Faults

Initial Contact

Pelvis: Pelvic drop.

Hip: Excessive hip flexion (greater than 30°); tightness in iliopsoas; limited hip flexion—weakness of hip flexors, weakness of gluteus maximus.

Knee: Excessive knee flexion—knee remains in flexion during initial contact; possible causes—weak quadriceps, short leg on contralateral side, joint pain.

Ankle and foot: Foot slap—at heel strike, forefoot slaps to the ground; possible causes include weak dorsiflexors.

Toes first: Toes contact ground instead of heel; possible causes—leg-length discrepancy, contracted heel cord, plantarflexion contracture, painful heel, flaccidity of dorsiflexors.

Flat footed: Entire foot contacts ground at heel strike—capsular restriction at ankle.

Loading Response

Hip

a. Limited hip extension (does not return to neutral): tight hip flexors

b. Internal rotation: weak external rotators, anteversion of the femur

c. External rotation: retroversion of the femur

Knee: knee hyperextension—weak quadriceps, gastrocnemius

Ankle: limited plantarflexion—joint restriction, decreased muscle strength

Midstance

Pelvis

a. Lateral trunk lean: weak gluteus medius

b. Backward trunk lean: weak gluteus maximus

c. Forward trunk lean: weak quadriceps

Hip

a. Excessive lordosis: tight hip flexors

b. Contralateral hip drop: weakness of the gluteus medius

c. Increased knee flexion: decreased hip extension, decreased back extension

Knee

a. Knee hyperextension: weak quadriceps, gastrocnemius

b. Patella facing outward: retroversion

c. Knee flexion: capsular restriction of the knee

Ankle and foot

a. Early heel lift: heel lifting early in midstance; tightness in dorsiflexion (soft tissue or joint)

b. Toe clawing: toes grabbing floor; tightness in intrinsic musculature, poor stability of first metatarsal

c. Valgus deviation: femoral anteversion, overpronation, late pronation

Terminal Swing

Pelvis

a. Medial heel whip: weakness in hip external rotators

b. Hip flexion: hip extension restriction

Knee: excessive knee flexion—more than 40° of knee flexion during pushoff

Ankle and foot: medial heel whip—tight gastrocnemius–soleus complex

Preswing

Hip: lack of pushoff—hip extension restricted

Ankle and foot: no pushoff—insufficient transfer of weight from lateral heel to medial forefoot, limited range of motion; pain in forefoot

Swing

Hip

a. Circumduction: weak hip flexors, long leg

b. Hip hiking: lack of knee flexion or ankle dorsiflexion, weak hip flexors

c. Excessive hip flexion: weak dorsiflexion

Knee: limited knee flexion—less than 65° of knee flexion, joint pain, limited range of motion.

Ankle and foot

a. Toe drag: insufficient dorsiflexion, weak dorsiflexors and toe extensors

b. Varus: foot excessively inverted—weak peroneals

Other Gait Sequences

Orthopedic clinicians deal with various gait sequences such as running gait and stair climbing. Additionally, they commonly recommend assistive devices for clients following surgery or during the rehabilitation process. This chapter highlights running gait, stair climbing, and assisted gait. For each gait, joint range of motion and muscle activity are described. Also included is a short section on foot type and footwear.

Running

Running is different from walking in three distinct ways. Running involves

1. a double-float period in which both lower extremities are off the ground,
2. occurrence of motions at the hips through a greater range except for hip extension, and
3. a ground reaction force that is four to seven times body weight.

The running gait sequence includes the contact and swing phases.

Contact Phase   One foot is in contact with the ground; occurs during 38% of the running cycle.

Foot strike: The runner contacts the ground with either the heel, midfoot, or forefoot.

Midsupport phase: The foot is loose, adapting to terrain and absorbing shock; it begins to supinate as the heel rises from the ground.

Takeoff: The foot leaves the ground.

Swing Phase   The leg and foot are off the ground; occurs during 62% of the running cycle.

Follow-through: End of backward momentum of leg.

Forward swing: Limb begins to drive forward.

Foot descent: Limb prepares for foot strike.

Running Gait

Gait phase	Joint and muscle	Hip	Knee	Foot
Foot strike	Joint motion	20–50° flexion	15° flexion	10° dorsiflexion
	Muscle activity	Gluteus maximus, gluteus medius, TFL eccentric	Hamstrings, gastrocnemius popliteus concentric; quadriceps co-contraction	Anterior tibialis, toes extensors eccentric
Midsupport	Joint motion	30° flexion	20° flexion	20° dorsiflexion
	Muscle activity	Gluteus medius and TFL active control pelvis; gluteus maximus, hamstring eccentrically control limb in flexion	Quadriceps eccentric to control knee flexion	Gastrocnemius Soleus, posterior tibialis eccentric
Takeoff	Joint motion	10° extension	0° flexion	25° plantarflexion
	Muscle activity	Hamstrings, gluteus maximus, gluteus medius concentric, trunk musculature eccentric	Quadriceps eccentric	Gastrocnemius Soleus, peroneals, toe flexors concentric; toe extensors eccentric
Follow-through	Joint motion	5° extension	20° flexion	10° plantarflexion
	Muscle activity	Adductors to control pelvis, hip flexors eccentric to control hip extensors	Medial hamstrings concentric	Gastrocnemius concentric
Forward swing	Joint motion	10–60° flexion	125° flexion	10° plantarflexion
	Muscle activity	Iliopsoas, rectus femoris, TFL concentric	Hamstrings and quadriceps co-contract	Pre-tibialis eccentrically control ankle
Foot descent	Joint motion	40° flexion	40–20° flexion	10° dorsiflexion
	Muscle activity	Gluteus maximus and hamstrings decelerate flexing thigh, gluteus medius, TFL concentric	Hamstrings eccentric	Pre-tibialis concentric

Footwear

Clients often ask their clinicians what type of footwear is appropriate for them. Different types of feet require different types of shoes (figure 18.1). Rigid feet need shoes with more cushioning and shock absorption, and flexible feet need a more stable shoe. Shoes must fit properly according to the various components of the shoe in the list that follows.

Shoe Shape

The bottom of the shoe (last) can be shaped either straight, curved, or semicurved (see figure 18.1). The straight last is for the person who overpronates, and the curved last is for the person who has a rigid, high-arched foot.

Midsole The cushioned layers between the foot and the ground can be made of varying densities of materials. Both the inside and outside of the shoe may have various densities. Generally the inside should be firmer than the outside.

Heel Counter The heel counter is the portion of the shoe that stabilizes the rearfoot. A firm heel counter is necessary for all shoes but is more important for people who have a flexible foot.

Inner Last The inner last refers to the inner border of the shoe. Underneath the sock liner (insole) on the inside of the shoe is either stitching (slip lasting) or a piece of fiberboard laminated to the shoe (board lasting). A slip-lasted shoe is used for the rigid foot, whereas a board last is used for the more flexible foot. Combination lasts are for combination feet.

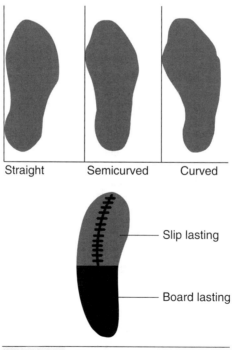

Figure 18.1 Shoe types.

Stair Climbing

Ascent (0–14%): Weight Acceptance Through 14–32% (Pull-Up)

Motion

- Hip extension from 60° to 30° of flexion

- Knee extension from 80° to 35° of flexion

- Ankle dorsiflexion from 20° to 25° (figure 18.2)

Muscles Used Gluteus maximus, semitendinosus, gluteus medius, vastus lateralis, rectus femoris, anterior tibialis, soleus, gastrocnemius; all concentric.

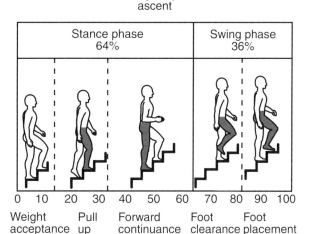

Figure 18.2 Gait cycle phases during stair climbing.

Reprinted, by permission, from C. Norkin and P. Levangie, 1992, *Joint structure and function* (Philadelphia, PA: F.A. Davis), 482.

32–64%: Forward Continuance (Pull-Up Through Forward Continuance)

Motion

- Hip extension from 30° to 50° flexion

- Hip flexion from 5° to 10° flexion

- Knee extension from 35° to 10° flexion

- Knee flexion from 5° to 10° flexion

- Ankle plantarflexion: 15° dorsiflexion to 10° plantarflexion

Muscles Used

- Gluteus maximus, gluteus medius, semitendinosus—concentric

- Gluteus maximus, gluteus medius—eccentric

- Vastus lateralis, rectus femoris—concentric

- Rectus femoris, vastus lateralis—eccentric

- Soleus—concentric

- Gastrocnemius, anterior tibialis—eccentric

64–100%: Foot Clearance Through Foot Placement

Motion

- Hip flexion from 10° to 60° flexion

- Hip extension from 40° to 50° flexion

- Knee flexion from 10° to 90° flexion
- Knee extension from 90° to 85° flexion
- Ankle dorsiflexion: 10° of plantarflexion to 20° dorsiflexion

Muscles Used
- Gluteus medius—concentric
- Semitendinosus and semimembranosus—concentric
- Vastus lateralis—concentric
- Rectus femoris, anterior tibialis—concentric
- Leg pull: iliopsoas (concentric), rectus femoris
- Foot placement: hamstrings
- Pull-up: knee extension, quadriceps
- Forward propelling: ankle
- Descent: hamstrings at toe-off
- Leg pull: hip flexors
- Weight acceptance: knee—eccentric
- Support: knee—eccentric

Assisted Gait

Three-point gait Crutches and affected limb move together, nonweight bearing, modified with toe-touch weight bearing; advance crutches with involved leg.

Four-point gait One crutch, opposite limb, other crutch, other limb.

Two-point gait Right crutch and left leg together, left crutch and right leg together.

Swing-to gait Crutches and then leg swing forward (paraplegics).

Swing-through gait Crutches and then legs swing forward through the crutches.

Stair Climbing With Assistive Device

Cane

Ascend: The uninvolved lower extremity leads up the cane and the involved leg.

Descend: The involved limb and the cane lead down; the uninvolved leg follows.

Crutches (Non-weight-bearing)

Ascend: Pushing firmly on crutches lifts the uninvolved leg to step. Crutches and the involved limb follow.

Descend: The user places crutches on step below, pushing down on crutches to lift body weight; steps down with the involved leg followed by the uninvolved leg.

Adverse Neurodynamics

Part VI contains one chapter related to neurodynamic testing. Neurodynamic tests for the spine, upper extremity, and lower extremity are described. The chapter provides detailed information on the anatomy and pathology related to neurodynamic testing as well as a detailed description of the examination sequence, including the various neurodynamic tests.

Upper-Extremity and Lower-Extremity Neurodynamics

This chapter addresses neurodynamics. Neurodynamics are important because these problems often occur together with other musculoskeletal problems. This chapter discusses historical background, anatomy, pathology, and examination sequences, including seven tests and interventions.

Historical Background

Neurodynamic testing dates back to 1978 when Geoffrey Maitland devised the slump test. In 1979 Robert Elvey developed the brachial tension test, or Elvey's test, which formed the basis for the standard upper-limb neurodynamic test 1 (ULNT1). Finally, in 1991, David Butler developed additional neurodynamic tests that are functional refinements of the standard ULNT1. Examples include tests that bias the median, radial, and ulnar nerves. The upper-limb neurodynamic test 2 (ULNT2 [Mb]) is sensitive to the median nerve. The upper-limb neurodynamic test 2 (ULNT2 [Rb]) is sensitive to the radial nerve, and the upper-limb neurodynamic test 3 (ULNT3) is sensitive to the ulnar nerve.

Anatomy

Below are explanations of the major anatomical systems involved in upper-extremity and lower-extremity neurodynamics.

Central Nervous System   The nervous system is a dynamic organ that possesses plastic and elastic properties. This continuous structure runs from the brain to the end terminals in the periphery and contains the brain and spinal cord, which are made up of a large number of nerve cells and their processes. Axoplasmic fluid within the nervous system allows movement of materials (cytoskeletal elements, neurotransmitters, and neuropeptides) along the axon between the cell body and target tissues. The materials are transported bidirectionally along the axon (antegrade and retrograde transportation). The different layers of connective tissue within the nervous system (dura mater, arachnoid mater, and pia mater) provide structural support to protect the neurons from excessive stress and help maintain the neural environment. In addition, neuroglial cells located in the plasma membrane surround the neuron and provide a metabolically balanced environment for the neuron. The dura mater is continuous with the cranial dura mater, is tough, and is innervated by the sinuvertebral nerve (enters the spinal canal segmentally and innervates four segments). The arachnoid mater is inside the dura mater, is thin, encloses the subarachnoid space, and has the same innervation as the dura mater. The pia mater surrounds the spinal cord, is thin, and is innervated by small branches from the dorsal root.

Peripheral Nervous System   The nervous system contains 12 pairs of cranial nerves and 31 pairs of spinal nerves. As the spinal nerves pass through the intervertebral foramen, the epidural tissue, dura, and arachnoid of the nerve root become continuous with the connective tissue of the peripheral nervous system. The connective tissue of the peripheral nervous system (endoneurium, perineurium, epineurium, and mesoneurium) provides structural support to protect the neural tissue from excessive stress and helps to maintain the neural environment. The endoneurium, the innermost layer, protects against tensile forces (due to collagen orientation) and contains fibroblasts, capillaries, mast cells, and Schwann cells. The perineurium protects the contents of the endoneurial tube and is more resistant to tensile forces. The epineurium is the outermost layer. The mesoneurium is made of loose areolar tissue around peripheral nerve trunks and allows gliding of peripheral nerves along adjacent tissue. The nervi nervorum (innermost layer of connective tissue) innervates the peripheral nervous system, which is why a patient may complain of pain.

Somatic and Autonomic Nervous System The somatic nervous system (SNS) controls voluntary movement. The autonomic nervous system (ANS) controls involuntary movement. Mechanical impairment of the sympathetic chain could cause nausea, vague thoracic pain, headache with straight-leg raise (SLR), deep abdominal pain, flushes, or sweating with the slump test.

Tension Points Tension points are spots where there is no movement of the nervous system in relation to the mechanical interface tissues. Tension points are located at C6, T6, L4, the posterior knee, and the anterior elbow.

Pathology

Extraneural pathology involves a movement dysfunction in relation to the mechanical interface and can be due to scar, myofascial band formation, or altered or degenerative bony changes. Examples of interface tissue are (1) soft tissue, (2) tunnels (nerve root at the intervertebral foramen, median nerve at the carpal tunnel), (3) areas where nerves branch (e.g., radial nerve at the elbow), and (4) points along the nervous system that are relatively fixed (e.g., common peroneal nerve at the fibular head).

Intraneural pathology Intraneural pathology involves a direct dysfunction of the nervous system connective tissue or neural tissue. Edema within the nerve and fibrosis within the dura are two examples of intraneural pathology that can alter axoplasmic flow.

Altered Axoplasmic Flow Pressure gradients are present within the fluids of the nervous system, tissues within the nervous system, and surrounding structures of the nervous system. An alteration in these pressure gradients can be sufficient to effect changes in blood flow and axonal transport. Decreased blood supply to the neuron can occur with a low compression force, which leads to an alteration in the axoplasmic flow. Subsequently the nerve is more susceptible to compromise, and the target tissue is more susceptible to trophic changes.

Syndromes Double crush, as described by Upton and McComas in 1973, is an injury at a proximal site along the nerve that could have an additive effect, ultimately contributing to injury to a distal site along the nerve. Reverse crush, as described by Lundborg in 2005, is an injury at a distal site along the nerve that could have an additive effect, ultimately contributing to injury to a proximal site along the nerve.

EXAMINATION SEQUENCE

HISTORY

Neurodynamic problems often occur in conjunction with other musculoskeletal problems. The following is a list of items to include within a subjective examination to help determine neurodynamic contributions to various patient presentations.

Location and Description of Symptoms

The patient will complain of symptoms at or near the vulnerable anatomical site, which can include the entire limb. A patient with extraneural pathology will complain of symptoms such as pulling like a tight string, catches of pain, and tightness. A patient with intraneural pathology will complain of symptoms such as bizarre clumps of pain, crawling, antlike, dry, woody, and dragging, and report sensations of swelling, burning, or electricity.

Aggravating and Easing Factors

Aggravating factors that would guide a clinician to perform the slump test include getting in or out of a car, taking a bath, kicking a football, and prolonged sitting, especially with the legs elevated (long sitting). Aggravating factors that would guide a clinician to perform the straight-leg raise test (SLR) include any activity in which the leg is extended, such as kicking a football. Aggravating factors that would guide a clinician to perform the prone knee bend (PKB) test include any activity in which the knee is bent toward the buttocks, such as hurdling, that results in a complaint of anterior thigh pain. Aggravating factors that would guide a clinician to perform the ULNT include reaching for a seat belt, repetitive movement combinations of the upper extremity (playing a keyboard or violin, holding a phone in the crook of the neck, hammering overhead all day, and so on). Easing factors for all aggravating movements include a position out of tension (such as standing with the knee in slight flexion if the straight-leg raise is aggravating). Symptoms may be worse at night because of constrained postures of sleep. Symptoms may be worse in the morning following strained night positions and worse at the end of the day because of a latent effect from a sustained posture or repetitive activity.

History

A patient with a neurodynamic component to his or her disorder may report a history of whiplash, postsurgical (neuromeningial invasion), history of trauma (may be a long time ago), or a predisposing occupation (one that requires repetitive activity).

TESTS AND MEASURES

Observation: Look for Postures That Fit With a Neurodynamic Dysfunction

- Knee flexed in standing
- Lateral shift
- Forward head

- Cervical spine lateral flexion
- Shoulder elevated
- Arm folded across body

Active Movements

Observe quality of movement with active movement testing. Identify any compensatory movements during active movement testing that fit with a neurodynamic dysfunction (neck side bend with shoulder movements, and so on).

Functional Tests

Have the patient perform the functional test that provokes the symptoms and then add or subtract the distal or proximal component to determine the effect on symptoms.

Tension Stress

Increase tension to active movements.

- Add neck flexion with LS flexion.
- Add shoulder shrug with CS flexion.

Nerve Palpation

Location of Nerve

Tibial: lateral to popliteal artery in posterior knee; posterior to medial malleolus

Common peroneal: posterior knee medial to biceps femoris tendon; fibular head

Superficial peroneal: anterior to lateral malleolus, lateral dorsum of foot (inversion/plantarflexion)

Sural: along side of Achilles tendon, lateral aspect of foot

Median (at elbow): just lateral to biceps tendon; at carpal tunnel

Ulnar: ulnar groove (medial elbow); wrist between pisiform and hamate (Guyon's canal)

Radial: just distal to deltoid insertion; at supinator muscle (posterior interosseous)

Method

Follow nerve. Use thumbnail, fingernail, or fingertip for small or superficial nerves, pads of thumb or finger for deep nerves. Direct palpation versus flick across nerve with thumb or finger ("twang"). May need to increase tension. May not be able to palpate or locate because of excessive soft tissue.

Normal Response

Hard (harder than tendon), round, capable of lateral movement.

Positive Response

Swollen, hard, thick; provokes symptoms, decreased mobility. Look for symptom reproduction.

General Guidelines for Performing Neurodynamic Tests

- Communicate to the patient what you are doing and why. Communicate to the patient what you want him or her to do during the test (report symptoms, sensitize neck flexion, and so on).
- Always test the asymptomatic side first.
- Know normal responses to each test before performing it.
- Establish baseline neurological status before testing and monitor frequently.
- Use the same starting position for each performance of the neurodynamic test.
- Continually monitor symptoms. Establish resting symptoms and monitor symptoms throughout the test.
- Assessment always includes (1) range of movement with each added component, (2) quality of movement with each added component (noting onset of resistance), (3) symptom response with each added component. (Subtle changes often effect change.)
- The clinician can choose to change the order of adding components depending on the working hypothesis. The neurodynamic test is more sensitive if the examiner begins with the component that is closest to the symptom complaint. For example, the clinician can take up the distal component for the patient with distal symptoms that are nonirritable.
- Document in order of components added. Document the quality of movement with each added component. Document the range of motion available with each added component. Document the symptom response with each added component.
- Contraindications and precautions to neurodynamic testing include irritable and severe dysfunctions, unstable conditions (disc prolapse with impending nerve root compression), elderly patients (caution with slump), tests that cause dizziness, tests that cause acute head pain, pathologies affecting the nervous system (MS, diabetes, Guillain-Barre syndrome, HIV+), and circulatory disturbances.
- Absolute contraindications include tethered cord syndrome, spinal cord injuries, cauda equina lesions, and recent neurological changes.

Passive Neck Flexion

Patient position: Supine, with or without a pillow, head in neutral position (*a*), and legs extended (assess).

Clinician position: Standing on the side of the patient. The clinician supports the occiput of the cervical spine with one hand and stabilizes the thorax with the other hand (*b*).

Method: Lift the patient's head in a chin-to-chest direction (assess).

Sensitization: Sensitize with SLR, SLR with DF (assess).

Normal response: Pulling in the cervicothoracic region.

Positive response: Provokes or reproduces comparable signs and symptoms (pain, resistance, restriction of movement). Range of motion or symptom response is altered in one component when there is a release of another component.

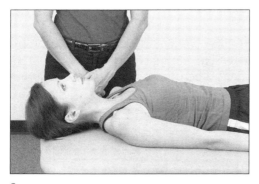

a

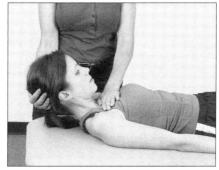

b

STRAIGHT-LEG RAISE

Patient position: Supine, legs extended, with or without a pillow (*a*).

Clinician position: Standing on the side of the patient. The clinician places one hand on the distal thigh and grasps the ankle with the other hand (*b*).

Method: The clinician passively flexes the patient's leg, maintaining neutral hip rotation and full knee extension (assess).

Sensitization: Sensitize with DF (tibial branch of sciatic nerve) (*c*), DFInv (sural branch of sciatic nerve), HMR (peroneal), PFI (common peroneal branch of sciatic nerve) (*d*), Had (sciatic nerve), CF or CE (assess).

Alternative method: Well straight-leg-raise test (cross SLR). Contralateral SLR reproduces symptoms. Diagnostically useful with patients with prolapsed discs (the irritated or adhered dural theca is brought into contact with the prolapsed or extruded disc material). Bilateral SLR, side lying SLR, prone SLR, hip flexion or knee extension—irritable symptoms.

Normal response: 50–120°, stretch in the posterior thigh, posterior knee, and posterior calf into foot.

Positive response: Provokes, reproduces comparable signs and symptoms (pain, resistance, restriction of movement). Range of motion or symptom response is altered in one component when there is a release of another component.

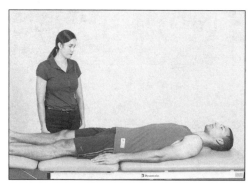

a

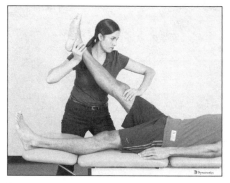

b

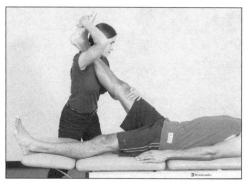

c

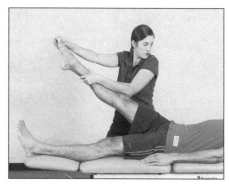

d

PRONE KNEE BEND

Patient position: Prone, arms at the side, legs together (*a*) (assess).

Clinician position: Standing on the side of the patient. The clinician places one hand on the patient's pelvis and grasps the ankle with the other hand.

Method: The clinician passively flexes the patient's knee with one hand while the other hand stabilizes the pelvis (assess) (*b*).

Sensitization: Sensitize with HE (lateral femoral cutaneous nerve) (*c*), hip IR or ER, hip extension or knee extension, hip abduction, hip ER (saphenous) (assess).

Alternative method: Side lying PKB (*d*), slump or PKB, bilateral PKB.

Normal response: Enough knee flexion to bring the heel to the buttocks, pulling in anterior thigh.

Positive response: Provokes or reproduces comparable signs or symptoms (pain, resistance, restriction of movement). Range of motion or symptom response is altered in one component when there is a release of another component.

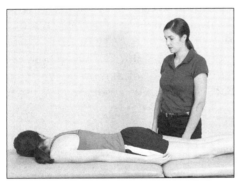

a

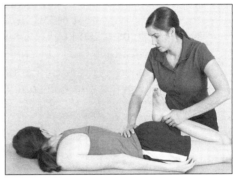

b

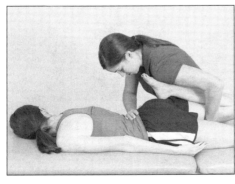

c

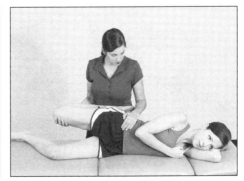

d

SLUMP

Patient position: Seated at the edge of the table with the knees at the edge and the hands behind the back (assess).

Clinician position: Standing to the side of the patient (*a*).

Method: Ask the patient to slump the trunk by flexion, keeping the cervical spine neutral and the sacrum vertical (assess) (*b*). Add neck flexion (assess) (no overpressure—support head in position (assess) (*c*), and add left knee extension (*d*) (asymptomatic side first, assess). If knee extension is full and painless, proceed and add ankle dorsiflexion (assess) (*e*). Add hip flexion (assess)—not pictured.

Sensitization: If knee extension is limited or reproduces pain (comparable to complaint), release neck flexion (assess). If symptoms are relieved or further knee extension is possible, a positive sign is present.

Alternative method: Alter the sequence, abduction of extended knee can reproduce groin symptoms of neurogenic origin (Butler), slump in long sitting.

Normal response: No symptoms or pulling at T8–T9 with trunk flexion or cervical flexion, pain behind knee and decreased knee extension with knee extension, increase in symptoms and decrease in range in DF with the added component of DF, decrease in symptoms and increase in range of knee extension and ankle DF with release of neck flexion.

Positive response: Provokes or reproduces comparable signs or symptoms (pain, resistance, restriction of movement). Range of motion or symptom response is altered in one component when there is a release of another component.

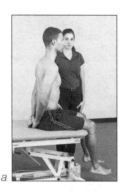 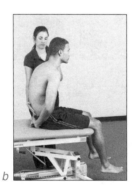 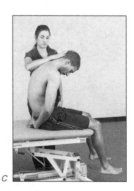

a   *b*   *c*

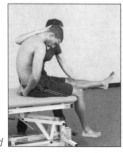 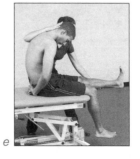

d   *e*

ULNT1

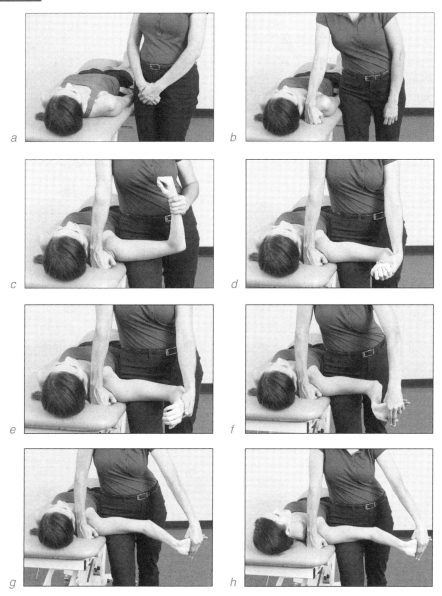

Patient position: Supine, no pillows, head in neutral position, shoulder near the edge of the table, and arm at the side (assess).

Clinician position: Standing to the side of the patient, facing the patient's head (*a*).

Method: Stabilize the shoulder girdle—fist into table (*b*) (assess), add glenohumeral abduction in slight extension to 90–110° (assess) (*c*), add glenohumeral lateral rotation to comfortable end range (assess) (*d*), add forearm supination (assess) (*e*), add wrist and finger extension (assess) (*f*), and add elbow extension (assess) (*g*).

Sensitization: Cervical lateral flexion away or toward (assess) (*h*). Lateral flexion away increases symptoms 70–90% of normal and lateral flexion toward decreases symptoms (70% of normal). Can also sensitize by putting opposite arm in the ULNT1 position and SLR.

Alternative method: Alter the sequence.

Normal response: Deep stretch or ache in cubital fossa, anterior forearm, and into the radial aspect of the hand; tingling in the thumb and first three fingers. Stretch across anterior shoulder (small percentage).

Positive response: Provokes or reproduces comparable signs or symptoms (pain, resistance, restriction of movement). Range of motion or symptom response is altered in one component when there is a release of another component.

ULNT2 (MB)—MEDIAN NERVE BIAS

Patient position: Supine, no pillows, head in neutral position, lying diagonally, scapula off the edge of the table, arm at the side (assess) (*a*).

Clinician position: Standing to the side of the patient facing the end of the bed, supporting the patient's arm at the elbow and wrist (assess) (*b*).

Method: Add shoulder girdle depression with the clinician's thigh on the superior aspect of the shoulder and the patient's arm in slight abduction (assess) (*b*). Add elbow extension (assess) (*c*), add glenohumeral lateral rotation—whole arm (assess) (*d*), add wrist or finger extension (assess) (*e*), and add glenohumeral abduction (*f*)—be careful (assess).

Sensitization: Sensitize with release of shoulder depression, release of wrist extension (assess).

Alternative method: Alter the sequence.

Normal response: Symptoms in the C5–7 dermatome and median nerve distribution.

Positive response: Provokes or reproduces comparable signs or symptoms (pain, resistance, restriction of movement). Range of motion or symptom response is altered in one component when there is a release of another component.

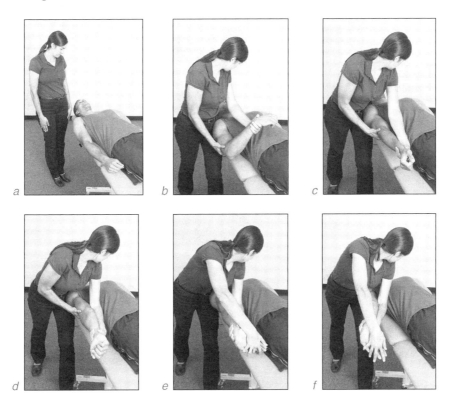

Patient position: Supine, no pillows, head in neutral position, lying diagonally, scapula off the edge of the table (assess) (*a*).

Clinician position: Standing to the side of the patient facing the end of the bed, cradling the patient's arm (assess).

Method: Add shoulder girdle depression with the clinician's thigh on the superior aspect of the shoulder and the patient's arm in slight abduction (assess) (*b*). Add elbow extension (assess) (*c*), add forearm pronation and shoulder internal rotation simultaneously (assess) (*d*), add wrist flexion (assess) (*e*), and add thumb flexion and ulnar deviation (assess) (*f*).

Sensitization: Sensitize with lateral flexion of the neck, shoulder abduction (40° available) (*g*), SLR (assess).

Alternative method: Alter sequence.

Normal response: Symptoms in the radial nerve distribution—stretch over lateral elbow or forearm, dorsum of the hand, lateral upper arm, and biceps brachii.

Positive response: Provokes or reproduces comparable signs or symptoms (pain, resistance, restriction of movement). Range of motion or symptom response is altered in one component when there is a release of another component.

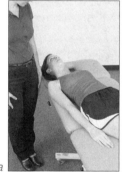

a

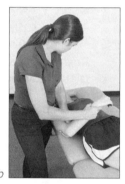

b

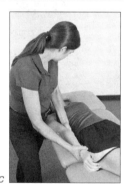

c

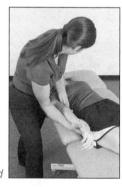

d

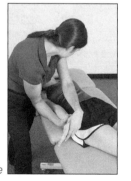

e

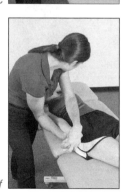

f

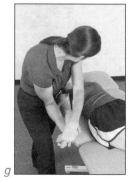

g

Patient position: Supine, no pillows, head in neutral position, shoulder near the edge of the table, arm at the side (assess).

Clinician position: Standing to the side of the patient facing the end of the bed (assess) (*a*).

Method: Stabilize the shoulder girdle by placing the fist into the table (assess) (*b*), add full elbow flexion (*c*), rest the elbow in the groin of the examiner (assess), add wrist extension (assess) (*d*), add forearm pronation (assess) (*e*), and add glenohumeral lateral rotation (assess) (*f*).

Sensitization: Sensitize with lateral flexion toward or away (*g*), scapular position, trunk side flexion, PKB, contralateral ULNT (assess).

Alternative method: Alter sequence.

Normal response: Symptoms in C8–T1 dermatome and ulnar nerve distribution.

Positive response: Provokes or reproduces comparable signs or symptoms (pain, resistance, restriction of movement). Range of motion or symptom response is altered in one component when there is a release of another component.

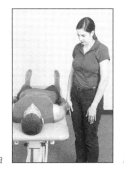

a

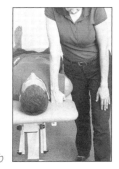

b

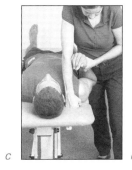

c

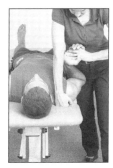

d

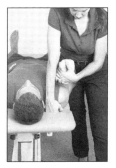

e

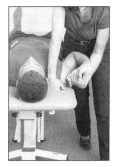

f

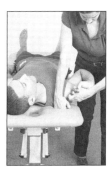

g

Intervention

The goal of intervention is to restore nervous system mobility and normalize the sensitivity of the system.

General   The clinician should refer to neurodynamic techniques as mobilization rather than stretching techniques. Severity and irritability should be established before treatment. In addition, the clinician can determine the origin of dysfunction (intraneural versus extraneural). The two conditions may coexist with one being predominant. The clinician can treat with through-range techniques (grade II, III) for extraneural pathologies and with end-range techniques (IV) for intraneural pathologies. Before initiating treatment the clinician needs to communicate to the patient what to expect with the treatment. For example, the clinician should communicate to a nonirritable patient potential exacerbation of symptoms that resolve in seconds (if the symptoms linger, the clinician may need to decrease the vigor of the technique or select another technique). The clinician should not cause the irritable patient to experience any exacerbation of symptoms. The clinician should treat joint signs and soft-tissue components first; if the treatment is not effective, treatment of the neurodynamic component can follow. Treatment to related soft tissue can be close to the site of injury (nonirritable) or farther from the site of injury (irritable). The clinician should reassess objective asterisks after treatment to monitor the effectiveness of treatment choice.

Nervous System Mobilization

Interventions for a Severe or Irritable Dysfunction

- Patient must be relaxed and comfortable.
- Do not start treatment using the neurodynamic test position.
- Initially, the mobilizing tension technique should be nonprovoking.
- Begin with a mobilizing tension technique removed from the symptomatic area (i.e., contralateral wrist extension)
- Oscillatory mobilizing techniques are used rather than sustained techniques.
- Suggested grades of movement: slow, rhythmic oscillations with maximal respect for symptoms.
- Bout: 15–60 seconds.
- Progression of intervention: gentle oscillations for 15–20 seconds, reassess, progress time; amplitude of technique can be increased; repeat technique with nervous system in more tension; technique could applied closer to the source of symptom area.

Intervention for a Nonsevere or Nonirritable Dysfunction

- The initial mobilizing neurodynamic technique will need to be into some resistance.
- Bout: 1–3 minutes.
- Progression of intervention: The starting technique can be performed longer (sustained no longer than 10 seconds and bout duration increased), the technique can be performed with other components in different positions, and the technique can be performed closer to symptoms.

Ahn, D.S. 2001. Hand elevation: a new test for carpal tunnel syndrome. *Annals of Plastic Surgery* 46:120–124.

Anderson, A.F., and A.B. Lipscomb. 1986. Clinical diagnosis of meniscal tears. Description of a new manipulative test. *American Journal of Sports Medicine* 14 (4):291–3.

Andrews, J.R., and J.A. Whiteside. 1993. Common elbow problems in the athlete. *Journal of Orthopaedic and Sports Physical Therapy* 17 (6):289–95.

Aprill, C., A. Dwyer, and N. Bogduk. 1990. Cervical zygapophyseal joint pain patterns. II: A clinical evaluation. *Spine* 15 (6):458–61.

Basmajian, J.V. 1979. *Muscles alive*. 4th ed. Baltimore: Williams and Wilkins.

Boeree, N.R., and C.E. Ackroyd. 1991. Assessment of the menisci and cruciate ligaments: An audit of clinical practice. *Injury* 22 (4):291–4.

Bogduk, N. 1994. Innervation and pain patterns of the cervical spine. Ed. R. Grant. 2nd ed., *Clinics in physical therapy: Physical therapy of the cervical and thoracic spine*. New York: Churchill Livingstone.

———. 1997. *Clinical anatomy of the lumbar spine and sacrum*. 3rd ed. New York: Churchill Livingstone.

Bowling, R.W., and P. Rockar. 1997. The elbow complex. Ed. T. Malone, T. McPoil, and A.J. Nitz. 3rd ed., *Orthopedic and sports physical therapy*. St. Louis: Mosby.

Boyling, J.D., and N. Palastanga. 1998. The vertebral column. 2nd ed. *Grieve's Modern Manual Therapy*. New York: Churchill Livingstone.

Braatz, J., and P. Gogia. 1987. The mechanics of pitching. *Journal of Orthopaedic and Sports Physical Therapy* 9:56.

Butler, D.B. 1991. *Mobilisation of the nervous system*. New York: Churchill Livingstone.

Cabaud, H.E., and D.B. Slocum. 1977. The diagnosis of chronic anterolateral rotary instability of the knee. *American Journal of Sports Medicine* 5 (3):99–105.

Caillet, R. 1966. *Shoulder pain*. Philadelphia: Davis.

Calis, M., K. Akgun, M. Birtane, I. Karacan, H. Calis, and F. Tuzun. 2000. Diagnostic values of clinical diagnostic tests in subacromial impingement syndrome. *Annals of the Rheumatic Diseases* 59 (1):44–7.

Carmichael, S.W., and D.L. Hart. 1985. Anatomy of the shoulder joint. *Journal of Orthopaedic and Sports Physical Therapy* 16:225–228.

Cavanagh, P.R., and M.A. Lafortune. 1980. Ground reaction forces in distance running. *Journal of Biomechanics* 13 (5):397–406.

Constant, C.R., and A.H.G. Murley. 1987. A clinical method of functional assessment of the shoulder. *Clinical Orthopedics Related Research* 214:160–164.

Conwell, E. 1970. Injuries to the wrist. *Clinical Symposia* 2:3–30.

Coplan, J.A. 1989. Rotational motion of the knee: A comparison of normal and pronating subjects. *Journal of Orthopaedic and Sports Physical Therapy* 10:366–369.

Craig, S.M. 1992. Anatomy of the joints of the fingers. *Hand Clinics* 8:693–700.

Crowninshield, R.D., R.C. Johnston, J.G. Andrews, and R.A. Brand. 1978. A biomechanical investigation of the human hip. *Journal of Biomechanics* 11 (1–2):75–85.

Cyriax, J. 1982. *Textbook of orthopaedic medicine: Diagnosis of soft tissue lesions*. Vol. 1. London: Bailliere Tindall.

Czerniecki, J.M. 1988. Foot and ankle biomechanics in walking and running. *American Journal of Physical Medicine and Rehabilitation* 67:246–252.

DiStefano, B. 1981. Anatomy and biomechanics of the ankle and foot. *Athletic Training* 16:43–47.

Donatelli, R. 1985. Normal biomechanics of the foot and ankle. *Journal of Orthopaedic and Sports Physical Therapy* 7 (91–95).

———. 1987. *Physical therapy of the shoulder*. New York: Churchill Livingstone.

Donatelli, R., and M. Wooden. 1989. *Orthopaedic physical therapy*. New York: Churchill Livingstone.

Dostal, W.F., and J.G. Andrews. 1981. A three-dimensional biomechanical model of hip musculature. *Journal of Biomechanics* 14 (11):803–12.

Dutton, M. 2002. *Manual therapy of the spine: An integrated approach*. New York: McGraw-Hill.

Dutton, Mark. 2004. *Orthopaedic examination, evaluation, and intervention*. New York: McGraw-Hill.

Dwyer, A., C. Aprill, and N. Bogduk. 1990. Cervical zygapophyseal joint pain patterns. I: A study in normal volunteers. *Spine* 15 (6):453–7.

Evans, P.J., G.D. Bell, and C. Frank. 1993. Prospective evaluation of the McMurray test. *American Journal of Sports Medicine* 21 (4):604–8.

Ferrari, D.A. 1990. Capsular ligaments of the shoulder. Anatomical and functional study of the anterior superior capsule. *American Journal of Sports Medicine* 18 (1):20–4.

Fisk, G.R. 1980. An overview of the injuries of the wrist. *Clinical Orthopaedics* 149:37–143.

Fleisig, G.S., C.J. Dillman, and J.R. Andrews. 1991. A biomechanical description of the shoulder joint during pitching. *American Journal of Sports Medicine* 18:20–24.

Fowler, P.J., and J.A. Lubliner. 1989. The predictive value of five clinical signs in the evaluation of meniscal pathology. *Arthroscopy* 5 (3):184–6.

Frankel, V.H., and A.H. Burstein. 1970. *Orthopedic biomechanics*. Philadelphia: Lea and Febiger.

Fukubayashi, T., and H. Kurosawa. 1980. The contact area and pressure distribution pattern of the knee. A study of normal and osteoarthrotic knee joints. *Acta Orthopaedica Scandinavica* 51 (6):871–9.

Goodfellow, J., D.S. Hungerford, and M. Sindel. 1976. Patellofemoral joint mechanics and pathology: Functional anatomy of the patellofemoral joint. *Journal of Bone and Joint Surgery (American Volume)* 58-B: 287–290.

Gowan, I.D., F.W. Jobe, J.E. Tibone, J. Perry, and D.R. Moynes. 1987. A comparative electromyographic analysis of the shoulder during pitching. Professional versus amateur pitchers. *American Journal of Sports Medicine* 15 (6):586–90.

Grimsby, O. 1995. *Fundamentals of manual therapy: A course workbook*. San Diego, CA: The Sorlandets Institute.

Guanche, C.A., and D.C. Jones. 2003. Clinical testing for tears of the glenoid labrum. *Arthroscopy* 19 (5):517–23.

Halbach, J.W, and R.T. Tank. 1997. The shoulder. Ed. T. Malone, T. McPoil, and A.J. Nitz. 3rd ed., *Orthopedic and sports physical therapy*. St. Louis: Mosby.

Hamilton, J.J., and K. Ziermer. 1981. Functional anatomy of the human ankle and foot. Ed. R. Kiene, *Proceedings of the AAOS symposium on the foot and ankle*. St. Louis: Mosby.

Harris, W.H. 1969. Traumatic arthritis of the hip after dislocation and acetabular fractures: treatment by mold arthroplasty. An end-result study using a new method of result evaluation. *Journal of Bone and Joint Surgery (American Volume)* 51 (4):737–55.

Hart, D.L., and S.W. Carmichael. 1985. Biomechanics of the shoulder. *Journal of Orthopaedic and Sports Physical Therapy* 16:229–278.

Hawkins, R.J., and J.C. Kennedy. 1980. Impingement syndrome in the absence of rotator cuff tear (stages 1 & 2). *Orthopedic Clinics of North America* 18:151.

Hoppenfeld, S. 1976. *Physical examination of the spine and extremities*. New York: Appleton-Century-Crofts.

Hoppenfeld, S., and V.L. Murthy. 2000. *Treatment and rehabilitation of fractures*. Philadelphia: Lippincott Williams and Wilkins.

Horn, C. 1997. Whiplash part I: Etiology and pathology. *Journal of Manual and Manipulative Therapy* 5 (2):114–120.

———. 1997. Whiplash part II: Clinical presentation, approaches to management and prevention. *Journal of Manual and Manipulative Therapy* 5 (3):121–128.

———. 1997. Whiplash part III: Subacute whiplash—a case study. *Journal of Manual and Manipulative Therapy* 5 (3):129–133.

Hughes, L.Y. 1985. Biomechanical analysis of the foot and ankle for predisposition to developing stress fractures. *Journal of Orthopaedic and Sports Physical Therapy* 7:96–101.

Hunt, G.C. 1997. Examination of lower extremity dysfunction. Ed. T. Malone, T. McPoil, and A.J. Nitz. 3rd ed. *Orthopedic and sports physical therapy*. St. Louis: Mosby.

Janda, V. 1983. On the concept of postural muscles and posture in man. *Australian Physiotherapy* 29:83–85.

Jobe, F.W., and J.P. Bradley. 1989. The diagnosis of no-operative treatment of shoulder injuries in athletes. *Office Practice of Sports Medicine* 8:419–433.

Jobe, F.W., D.R. Moynes, J.E. Tibone, and J. Perry. 1984. An EMG analysis of the shoulder in pitching. A second report. *American Journal of Sports Medicine* 12 (3):218–20.

Jobe, F.W., J.E. Tibone, J. Perry, and D. Moynes. 1983. An EMG analysis of the shoulder in throwing and pitching. A preliminary report. *American Journal of Sports Medicine* 11 (1):3–5.

Jones, L.A. 1989. The assessment of hand function: a critical review of techniques. *Journal of Hand Surgery (American Volume)* 14 (2 Pt 1):221–8.

Kaltenborn, F.M. 1980. *Mobilization of the extremity joints: Examination and basic treatment techniques*. Oslo: Olaf Norlis Bokhandel.

Kampner, S.L., and H.A. Wissinger. 1972. Anterior slipping of the capital femoral epiphysis. Report of a case. *Journal of Bone and Joint Surgery (American Volume)* 54 (7):1531–6.

Kapandji, I.A. 1983. *The physiology of the joints*. New York: Churchill Livingstone.

Kauer, J.M. 1980. Functional anatomy of the wrist. *Clinical Orthopaedics and Related Research* (149): 9–20.

Kendall, F.P., E.K. McCreary, and P.G. Provance. 1993. *Muscles: Testing and function*. Baltimore: Williams and Wilkins.

Kessler, R.M., and D. Hertling. 1983. *Management of common musculoskeletal disorders*. Philadelphia: Harper & Row.

Kisner, C., and L.A. Colby. 1996. *Therapeutic exercise: Foundations and techniques*. 3rd ed. Philadelphia: Davis.

Kulund, D. 1982. *The injured athlete*. Toronto: Lippincott.

Lafortune, M.A., P.R. Cavanagh, H.J. Sommer, 3rd, and A. Kalenak. 1992. Three-dimensional kinematics of the human knee during walking. *Journal of Biomechanics* 25 (4):347–57.

Lee, D. 2003. *Thorax: An integrated approach*. Delta, British Columbia, Canada: DOPC.

———. 2004. *The pelvic girdle*. 3rd ed. New York: Churchill Livingstone.

Lundborg, G. 2005. *Nerve injury and repair*. 2nd ed. Churchill Livingstone.

Lysholm, J., and Gillquist, J. 1982. Evaluation of the knee ligament surgery results with special emphasis on use of a scoring scale. *American Journal of Sports Medicine* 10:150–154.

MacConnaill, M.A., and J.V. Basmajian. 1977. *Muscles and movements: A basis for human kinesiology*. Baltimore: Williams and Wilkins.

MacDonald, P.B., P. Clark, and K. Sutherland. 2000. An analysis of the diagnostic accuracy of the Hawkins and Neer subacromial impingement signs. *Journal of Shoulder and Elbow Surgery* 9 (4):299–301.

MacKinnon, C.D., and D.A. Winter. 1993. Control of whole body balance in the frontal plane during human walking. *Journal of Biomechanics* 26 (6):633–44.

Maffulli, N. 1998. The clinical diagnosis of subcutaneous tear of the Achilles tendon. A prospective study in 174 patients. *American Journal of Sports Medicine* 26 (2):266–70.

Magee, David. 2002. *Orthopaedic physical assessment*. 4th ed. Philadelphia: Saunders.

Maitland, G.D. 1986. *Vertebral Manipulation*. 5th ed. Boston: Butterworth-Hienemann.

———. 1991. *Peripheral Manipulation*. 3rd ed. Boston: Butterworth-Heinemann.

———. 1994. *Peripheral Manipulation*. Boston: Butterworth.

McFadyen, B.J., and D.A. Winter. 1988. An integrated biomechanical analysis of normal stair ascent and descent. *Journal of Biomechanics* 21 (9):733–44.

McPoil, T., and R.S. Brocato. 1997. The foot and ankle: Biomechanical evaluation and treatment. Ed. T. Malone, T. McPoil, and A.J. Nitz. 3rd ed. *Orthopedic and sports physical therapy*. St. Louis: Mosby.

Meadows, J. 1999. *Orthopedic differential diagnosis in physical therapy*. New York: McGraw-Hill.

Morrey, B.F. 1985. *The elbow and its disorders*. Philadelphia: Saunders.

Morrey, B.F., L.J. Askew, and E.Y. Chao. 1981. A biomechanical study of normal functional elbow motion. *Journal of Bone and Joint Surgery (American Volume)* 63 (6):872–7.

Moynes, D.R., J. Perry, D.J. Antonelli, and F.W. Jobe. 1986. Electromyography and motion analysis of the upper extremity in sports. *Physical Therapy* 66 (12):1905–11.

Murray, M.P., A.B. Drought, and R.C. Kory. 1964. Walking patterns of normal men. *Journal of Bone and Joint Surgery (American Volume)* 46:335–60.

Neer, C.S., 2nd. 1983. Impingement lesions. *Clinical Orthopaedics and Related Research* (173):70–7.

Nirschl, R.P., and F.A. Pettrone. 1979. Tennis elbow. The surgical treatment of lateral epicondylitis. *Journal of Bone and Joint Surgery (American Volume)* 61 (6A):832–9.

Nissel, R. 1985. Mechanics of the knee. A study of joint and muscle load with clinical application. *Journal of Biomechanics* 13:375–381.

Nordin, M., and V.H. Frankel. 1989. *Basic biomechanics of the musculoskeletal system*. Philadelphia: Lea & Febiger.

Norkin, C., and P. Levangie. 1992. *Joint structure and function*. Philadelphia: Davis.

Novak, C.B., G.W. Lee, S.E. Mackinnon, and L. Lay. 1994. Provocative testing for cubital tunnel syndrome. *Journal of Hand Surgery (American Volume)* 19 (5):817–20.

Noyes, F.R., McGinniss, G.H., and Mooar, L.A. 1984. Functional disability in the anterior cruciate insufficient knee syndrome. *Sports Medicine* 1:287–288.

Nuber, G.W. 1988. Biomechanics of the foot and ankle during gait. *Clinical Sports Medicine* 7 (1):1–13.

O'Driscoll, S.W., R.L. Lawton, and A.M. Smith. 2005. The "moving valgus stress test" for medial collateral ligament tears of the elbow. *American Journal of Sports Medicine* 33 (2):231–9.

O'Sullivan, S.B., and T.J. Schmitz. 1998. *Physical rehabilitation assessment and treatment*. 3rd ed. Philadelphia: Davis.

Oldreive, W.L. 1995. A critical review of the literature on the tests of the sacroiliac joint. *Journal of Manual and Manipulaive Therapy* 3 (4):157–161.

Palmer, M.L., and M. Epler. 1990. *Clinical assessment procedures in physical therapy*. Philadelphia: Lippincott.

Paris, S. 1994. Course notes. St. Augustine, FL.

Paulos, L., F.R. Noyes, and M. Malek. 1980. A practical guide to the initial evaluation and treatment of knee ligament injuries. *Journal of Trauma* 20 (6):498–506.

Pearl, M.L., J. Perry, L. Torburn, and L.H. Gordon. 1992. An electromyographic analysis of the shoulder during cones and planes of arm motion. *Clinical Orthopaedics and Related Research* (284):116–27.

Peat, M. 1986. Functional anatomy of the shoulder complex. *Physical Therapy* 66 (12):1855–65.

Perry, J. 1978. Normal upper extremity kinesiology. *Physical Therapy* 58 (3):265–78.

———. 1992. *Gait analysis: Normal and pathological function*. Thorofare, NJ: Slack.

Poppen, N.K., and P.S. Walker. 1976. Normal and abnormal motion of the shoulder. *Journal of Bone and Joint Surgery (American Volume)* 58 (2):195–201.

Radin, E.L. 1980. Biomechanics of the human hip. *Clinical Orthopaedics and Related Research* (152):28–34.

Regan, W.D., S.L. Korinek, B.F. Morrey, and K.N. An. 1991. Biomechanical study of ligaments around the elbow joint. *Clinical orthopaedics and related research* (271):170–9.

Reid, D.C. 1992. *Sports injury: Assessment and rehabilitation*. New York: Churchill Livingstone.

Robinson, M.G. 1998. The McKenzie method of spinal pain management. Ed. Grieve, *Modern manual therapy: The vertebral column*. New York: Churchill Livingstone.

Romanes, G.J. 1981. *Cunningham's textbook of anatomy*. New York: Oxford Press.

Roy, S., and R. Irvin. 1983. *Sports medicine: Prevention, evaluation, management, and rehabilitation*. Englewood Cliffs, NJ: Prentice Hall.

Rubinstein, R.A., Jr., K.D. Shelbourne, J.R. McCarroll, C.D. VanMeter, and A.C. Rettig. 1994. The accuracy of the clinical examination in the setting of posterior cruciate ligament injuries. *American Journal of Sports Medicine* 22 (4):550–7.

Russek, L.N. 1999. Hypermobility syndrome. *Physical Therapy* 79 (6):591–9.

Sarrafian, S.K., J.L. Melamed, and G.M. Goshgarian. 1977. Study of wrist motion in flexion and extension. *Clinical orthopaedics and related research* (126):153–9.

Saudek, C.E. 1997. The hip. Ed. T. Malone, T. McPoil, and A.J. Nitz. 3rd ed. *Orthopedic and sports physical therapy*. St. Louis: Mosby.

Saunders, H.D. 1993. *Evaluation, treatment and prevention of musculoskeletal disorders*. 3rd ed. Bloomington: Educational Opportunities.

Schenkman, M., and V.R. DeCartava. 1987. Kinesiology of the shoulder complex. *Journal of Orthopaedic and Sports Physical Therapy* 8:438–450.

Sebastian, D. 2000. The anatomical and physiological variations in the sacroiliac joint of the male and female: Clinical implications. *Journal of Manual and Manipulaive Therapy* 8 (3):127–134.

Seligson, D., Sassman, J., and Pope, M. 1980. Ankle instability: Evaluation of lateral ligaments. *American Journal of Sports Medicine* 8:39.

Soderberg, G.L. 1986. *Kinesiology: Application to pathological motion*. Baltimore: Williams and Wilkins.

Stockwell, R.A. 1981. Cunningham's textbook of anatomy. Ed. G. Romanes, *Joints*. Oxford: Oxford University Press.

Stroyan, M., and K.E. Wilk. 1993. The functional anatomy of the elbow complex. *Journal of Orthopaedic and Sports Physical Therapy* 17 (6):279–88.

Tank, R., and J.W. Halbach. 1982. Physical therapy evaluation of the shoulder complex in athletes. *Journal of Orthopaedic and Sports Physical Therapy* 3:108–119.

Thein, L.S. 1989. Impingement syndrome and its conservative management. *Journal of Orthopaedic and Sports Physical Therapy* 11:183–191.

Timm, K.E. 1994. Knee. Ed. J. Richardson and Z. Iglarsh, *Clinical orthopaedic physical therapy*. Philadelphia: Saunders.

Upton, A.R., and A.J. McComas. 1973. The double crush in nerve entrapment syndromes. *Lancet* 2 (7825):359–62.

van Dijk, C.N., B.W. Mol, L.S. Lim, R.K. Marti, and P.M. Bossuyt. 1996. Diagnosis of ligament rupture of the ankle joint. Physical examination, arthrography, stress radiography and sonography compared in 160 patients after inversion trauma. *Acta Orthopaedica Scandinavica* 67 (6):566–70.

Van Wijmen, P.M. 1998. The use of repeated movements in the McKenzie method of spinal examination. Ed. Grieve. 2nd ed. *Modern manual therapy: The vertebral column*. New York: Churchill Livingstone.

Volz, R.G., M. Lieb, and J. Benjamin. 1980. Biomechanics of the wrist. *Clinical Orthopaedics and Related Research* (149):112–7.

Wadsworth, C.T. 1983. Clinical anatomy and mechanics of the wrist and hand. *Journal of Orthopaedic and Sports Physical Therapy* 4:206–216.

———. 1997. The wrist and hand. Ed. T. Malone, T. McPoil, and A.J. Nitz. 3rd ed. *Orthopedic and sports physical therapy*. St. Louis: Mosby.

Wallace, L.A., R.E. Mangine, and T.R. Malone. 1997. The knee. Ed. T. Malone, T. McPoil, and A.J. Nitz. 3rd ed. *Orthopedic and sports physical therapy*. St. Louis: Mosby.

Williams, P., and R. Warwick. 1980. *Gray's anatomy*. Philadelphia: Saunders.

Wright, D.G., S.M. Desai, and W.H. Henderson. 1964. Action of the subtalar and ankle-joint complex during the stance phase of walking. *Journal of Bone and Joint Surgery (American Volume)* 46:361–82.

Youm, Y., T.E. Gillespie, A.E. Flatt, and B.L. Sprague. 1978. Kinematic investigation of normal MCP joint. *Journal of Biomechanics* 11 (3):109–18.

Youm, Y., R.Y. McMurthy, A.E. Flatt, and T.E. Gillespie. 1978. Kinematics of the wrist. I. An experimental study of radial-ulnar deviation and flexion-extension. *Journal of Bone and Joint Surgery (American Volume)* 60 (4):423–31.

Young, S. 2000. Characteristics of a mechanical assessment for chronic lumbar facet joint pain. *Journal of Manual and Manipulaive Therapy* 8 (2):78–84.

Note: The italicized *f* and *t* following page numbers refer to figures and tables, respectively.